ORTHOPEDIC CLINICS OF NORTH AMERICA

www.orthopedic.theclinics.com

Evidence-Based Medicine

April 2018 • Volume 49 • Number 2

ELSEVIER

1600 John F. Kennedy Boulevard • Suite 1800 • Philadelphia, Pennsylvania, 19103-2899.

http://www.orthopedic.theclinics.com

ORTHOPEDIC CLINICS OF NORTH AMERICA Volume 49, Number 2
April 2018 ISSN 0030-5898, ISBN-13: 978-0-323-58312-1

Editor: Lauren Boyle
Developmental Editor: Kristen Helm

Orthopedic Clinics of North America (ISSN 0030-5898) is published quarterly by Elsevier Inc., 360 Park Avenue South, New York, NY 10010-1710. Months of issue are January, April, July, and October. Business and Editorial Offices: 1600 John F. Kennedy Blvd., Suite 1800, Philadelphia, PA 19103-2899. Customer Service Office: 3251 Riverport Lane, Maryland Heights, MO 63043. Periodicals postage paid at New York, NY and additional mailing offices. Subscription prices are $332.00 per year for (US individuals), $713.00 per year for (US institutions), $391.00 per year (Canadian individuals), $870.00 per year (Canadian institutions), $464.00 per year (international individuals), $870.00 per year (international institutions), $100.00 per year (US students), $220.00 per year (Canadian and international students). Foreign air speed delivery is included in all *Clinics* subscription prices. All prices are subject to change without notice. **POSTMASTER:** Send change of address to *Orthopedic Clinics of North America*, **Elsevier Health Sciences Division, Subscription Customer Service, 3251 Riverport Lane, Maryland Heights, MO 63043. Customer Service (orders, claims, online, change of address): Elsevier Health Sciences Division, Subscription Customer Service, 3251 Riverport Lane, Maryland Heights, MO 63043. Tel: 1-800-654-2452 (U.S. and Canada); 314-447-8871 (outside U.S. and Canada). Fax: 314-447-8029. E-mail:** journalscustomerservice-usa@elsevier.com **(for print support);** journalsonlinesupport-usa@elsevier.com **(for online support).**

Reprints. For copies of 100 or more, of articles in this publication, please contact the Commercial Reprints Department, Elsevier Inc., 360 Park Avenue South, New York, NY 10010-1710. Tel.: 212-633-3874; Fax: 212-633-3820; E-mail: reprints@elsevier.com.

Orthopedic Clinics of North America is covered in *MEDLINE/PubMed (Index Medicus)*, *Cinahl, Excerpta Medica*, and *Cumulative Index to Nursing and Allied Health Literature*.

ii

PROGRAM OBJECTIVE

Orthopedic Clinics of North America offers clinical review articles on the most cutting-edge technologies and techniques in the field, including knee and hip reconstruction, hand and wrist, pediatrics, trauma, shoulder and elbow, and foot and ankle.

TARGET AUDIENCE

Practicing orthopedic surgeons, orthopedic residents, and other healthcare professionals who specialize in orthopedic technologies and techniques for knee and hip reconstruction, hand and wrist, pediatrics, trauma, shoulder and elbow, and foot and ankle.

LEARNING OBJECTIVES

Upon completion of this activity, participants will be able to:
1. Review current evidence in bundle payment for musculoskeletal care
2. Discuss topics in prophylaxis and prevention of surgical site infections
3. Recognize current uses of evidence based medicine and treatment options for pediatric spine surgery and orthopaedic trauma

ACCREDITATION

The Elsevier Office of Continuing Medical Education (EOCME) is accredited by the Accreditation Council for Continuing Medical Education (ACCME) to provide continuing medical education for physicians.

The EOCME designates this enduring material for a maximum of 15 *AMA PRA Category 1 Credit*(s)™. Physicians should claim only the credit commensurate with the extent of their participation in the activity.

All other healthcare professionals requesting continuing education credit for this enduring material will be issued a certificate of participation.

DISCLOSURE OF CONFLICTS OF INTEREST

The EOCME assesses conflict of interest with its instructors, faculty, planners, and other individuals who are in a position to control the content of CME activities. All relevant conflicts of interest that are identified are thoroughly vetted by EOCME for fair balance, scientific objectivity, and patient care recommendations. EOCME is committed to providing its learners with CME activities that promote improvements or quality in healthcare and not a specific proprietary business or a commercial interest.

The planning committee, staff, authors and editors listed below have identified no financial relationships or relationships to products or devices they or their spouse/life partner have with commercial interest related to the content of this CME activity:

William R. Aibinder, MD; Afshin A. Anoushiravani, MD; Darryl A. Auston, MD, PhD; Frederick M. Azar, MD; Tim R. Beals, DO; Michael J. Beebe, MD; Clayton C. Bettin, MD, BS; Vamsy Bobba, MD; Yelena Bogdan, MD; K. Keely Boyle, MD; Lauren Boyle; James H. Calandruccio, MD; Kevin K. Chen, MA; Bonnie Y. Chien, MD; Christopher DiGiovanni, MD; Joshua S. Dines, MD; Tonya Dixon, MD, MPH; Thomas R. Duquin, MD; Ameer M. Elbuluk, BA; Todd Frush, MD; Benjamin J. Grear, MD; Daniel Guss, MD, MBA; Robert Harris, MD; David L. Helfet, MD; Pooya Hosseinzadeh, MD; Elizabeth W. Hubbard, MD; Aaron Huser, DO; Alison Kemp; Kelvin Y. Kim, BA; David Knesek, DO; Ryan Kozlowski, MD; Eric Lakey, MD; Kenneth M. Lin, MD; Benjamin M. Mauck, MD; William M. Mihalko, MD, PhD; Michelle Mo, MD, PhD; Matthew E. Oetgen, MD, MBA; Meghan A. Piccinin, MSc; Anthony I. Riccio, MD; Zain Sayeed, MSc, MHA; Jeyanthi Surendrakumar; Colin W. Swigler, MD; Norfleet B. Thompson, MD; Patrick C. Toy, MD; Dean Wang, MD.

The planning committee, staff, authors and editors listed below have identified financial relationships or relationships to products or devices they or their spouse/life partner have with commercial interest related to the content of this CME activity:

Kenneth J. Hunt, MD is a consultant/advisor for the Orthopaedic Foot & Ankle Outcomes Research Network
Richard Iorio, MD is a consultant/advisor for Zimmer Biomet, MCS ActiveCare, DJO, and Medtronic, owns stock in Zimmer Biomet, MCS ActiveCare
Joaquin Sanchez-Sotelo, MD, PhD receives royalties/holds patents with Stryker Corporation
Jeffrey R. Sawyer, MD is a speaker for NuVasive and Orthopaediatrics; receives royalties from Elsevier
Ran Schwarzkopf, MD, MSc is a consultant/advisor for Smith&Nephew and Intelijoint; has stock ownership in Intelijoint and Gauss Surgical; received a research grant from Smith&Nephew
Thomas (Quin) Throckmorton, MD is a speaker for Zimmer Biomet; is a consultant/advisor for Zimmer Biomet and Pacira; he owns stock in Gilead
John C. Weinlein, MD receives royalties/holds patents with Elsevier

UNAPPROVED/OFF-LABEL USE DISCLOSURE

The EOCME requires CME faculty to disclose to the participants:
1. When products or procedures being discussed are off-label, unlabelled, experimental, and/or investigational (not US Food and Drug Administration [FDA] approved); and
2. Any limitations on the information presented, such as data that are preliminary or that represent ongoing research, interim analyses, and/or unsupported opinions. Faculty may discuss information about pharmaceutical agents that is outside of FDA-approved labelling. This information is intended solely for CME and is not intended to promote off-label use of these medications. If you have any questions, contact the medical affairs department of the manufacturer for the most recent prescribing information.

TO ENROLL

To enroll in the *Orthopedic Clinics of North America* Continuing Medical Education program, call customer service at 1-800-654-2452 or sign up online at http://www.theclinics.com/home/cme. The CME program is available to subscribers for an additional annual fee of USD 215.

METHOD OF PARTICIPATION

In order to claim credit, participants must complete the following:

1. Complete enrolment as indicated above.
2. Read the activity.
3. Complete the CME Test and Evaluation. Participants must achieve a score of 70% on the test. All CME Tests and Evaluations must be completed online.

CME INQUIRIES/SPECIAL NEEDS

For all CME inquiries or special needs, please contact elsevierCME@elsevier.com.

EDITORIAL BOARD

CONTRIBUTORS

AUTHORS

WILLIAM R. AIBINDER, MD
Department of Orthopedic Surgery, Mayo
Clinic, Rochester, Minnesota

AFSHIN A. ANOUSHIRAVANI, MD
Adult Reconstruction Research Fellow,
Department of Orthopaedic Surgery, Hospital
for Joint Diseases, NYU Langone Medical
Center, New York, New York

DARRYL A. AUSTON, MD, PhD
Hughston Clinic – Trauma Division at Orange
Park, Orange Park, Florida

TIM R. BEALS, DO
Department of Orthopedic Surgery, Jack
Hughston Memorial Hospital, Phenix City,
Alabama

VAMSY BOBBA, MD
Department of Orthopaedics, Musculoskeletal
Institute of Surgical Excellence, Detroit
Medical Center, Detroit, Michigan

YELENA BOGDAN, MD
Department of Orthopaedic Trauma,
Geisinger Holy Spirit, Camp Hill,
Pennsylvania

K. KEELY BOYLE, MD
Department of Orthopaedics, University at
Buffalo, The State University of New York,
Erie County Medical Center, Buffalo,
New York

JAMES H. CALANDRUCCIO, MD
Associate Professor, Department of
Orthopaedic Surgery and Biomedical
Engineering, Campbell Clinic, The University
of Tennessee, Memphis, Tennessee

KEVIN K. CHEN, MA
Adult Reconstruction Research Fellow,
Department of Orthopaedic Surgery, Hospital
for Joint Diseases, NYU Langone Medical
Center, New York, New York

BONNIE Y. CHIEN, MD
Resident, Harvard Combined Orthopaedic
Residency Program, Boston, Massachusetts

CHRISTOPHER DIGIOVANNI, MD
Associate Professor in Orthopaedic Surgery,
Chief of the Foot and Ankle Service, Foot and
Ankle Center, Massachusetts General Hospital
Orthopaedics, Boston, Massachusetts;
Newton-Wellesley Hospital, Newton,
Massachusetts

JOSHUA S. DINES, MD
Associate Professor, Sports Medicine and
Shoulder Service, Hospital for Special Surgery,
New York, New York

TONYA DIXON, MD, MPH
Foot and Ankle Fellow, Foot and Ankle
Center, Massachusetts General Hospital
Orthopaedics, Boston, Massachusetts

THOMAS R. DUQUIN, MD
Clinical Assistant Professor of Orthopaedics,
Director of Medical Student Education
Department of Orthopaedics, University at
Buffalo, The State University of New York, Erie
County Medical Center, Buffalo, New York

AMEER M. ELBULUK, BA
Adult Reconstruction Research Fellow,
Department of Orthopaedic Surgery, Hospital
for Joint Diseases, NYU Langone Medical
Center, New York, New York

TODD FRUSH, MD
Department of Orthopaedics, Musculoskeletal
Institute of Surgical Excellence, Detroit
Medical Center, Detroit, Michigan

DANIEL GUSS, MD, MBA
Assistant Professor in Orthopaedic Surgery,
Foot and Ankle Center, Massachusetts
General Hospital Orthopaedics, Boston,
Massachusetts; Newton-Wellesley Hospital,
Newton, Massachusetts

ROBERT HARRIS, MD
Department of Orthopedic Surgery,
Hughston Clinic –Trauma Division at
Midtown, Orthopedic Program Director, Jack
Hughston Memorial Hospital, Phenix City,
Alabama

DAVID L. HELFET, MD
Department of Orthopaedic Trauma,
Hospital for Special Surgery, New York,
New York

POOYA HOSSEINZADEH, MD
Assistant Professor, Department of
Orthopaedic Surgery, Washington
University School of Medicine in St. Louis,
St. Louis Children's Hospital, St Louis,
Missouri

ELIZABETH W. HUBBARD, MD
Assistant Professor, Department of
Orthopaedic Surgery, University of Kentucky
College of Medicine, Shriners Hospitals for
Children, Lexington, Kentucky

KENNETH J. HUNT, MD
Associate Professor and Chief, Foot and Ankle
Surgery, Department of Orthopaedic Surgery,
University of Colorado School of Medicine,
Aurora, Colorado

AARON HUSER, DO
Pediatric Orthopaedic Fellow, Department
of Orthopaedic Surgery, Washington
University School of Medicine in St. Louis,
St. Louis Children's Hospital, St Louis,
Missouri

RICHARD IORIO, MD
Chief of Division of Adult Reconstruction,
William and Susan Jaffe Professor of
Orthopaedic Surgery, Department of
Orthopaedic Surgery, Hospital for Joint
Diseases, NYU Langone Medical Center,
New York, New York

KELVIN Y. KIM, BA
Adult Reconstruction Research Fellow,
Department of Orthopaedic Surgery, Hospital
for Joint Diseases, NYU Langone Medical
Center, New York, New York

DAVID KNESEK, DO
Department of Orthopaedics, Musculoskeletal
Institute of Surgical Excellence, Detroit
Medical Center, Detroit, Michigan

RYAN KOZLOWSKI, MD
Department of Orthopaedics, Musculoskeletal
Institute of Surgical Excellence, Detroit
Medical Center, Detroit, Michigan

ERIC LAKEY, BS
Department of Orthopaedic Surgery,
University of Colorado School of Medicine,
Aurora, Colorado

KENNETH M. LIN, MD
Sports Medicine and Shoulder Service,
Hospital for Special Surgery, New York,
New York

BENJAMIN M. MAUCK, MD
Hand and Upper Extremity Surgeon, Staff,
Department of Orthopaedic Surgery,
Campbell Clinic Orthopaedics, Memphis,
Tennessee

MICHELLE MO, MD, PhD
Resident Physician, Department of
Orthopaedic Surgery, Washington University
School of Medicine in St. Louis, St. Louis
Children's Hospital, St Louis, Missouri

MATTHEW E. OETGEN, MD, MBA
Chief, Division of Orthopaedic Surgery and
Sports Medicine, Children's National Health
System, Associate Professor of Orthopaedic
Surgery, George Washington University
School of Medicine & Health Sciences,
Washington, DC

MEGHAN A. PICCININ, MSc
College of Osteopathic Medicine, Michigan
State University, Detroit Medical Center,
Detroit, Michigan

ANTHONY I. RICCIO, MD
Associate Professor, Department of
Orthopaedic Surgery, The University of Texas
Southwestern Medical Center, Texas Scottish
Rite Hospital for Children, Dallas, Texas;
Adjunct Associate Professor of Surgery,
Uniformed Services University of the Health
Sciences, Bethesda, Maryland

JOAQUIN SANCHEZ-SOTELO, MD, PhD
Consultant and Professor, Department of
Orthopedic Surgery, Mayo Clinic, Rochester,
Minnesota

ZAIN SAYEED, MD, MHA
Department of Orthopaedics, Institute of
Innovations and Clinical Excellence, Detroit
Medical Center, Detroit, Michigan

RAN SCHWARZKOPF, MD, MSc
Adult Reconstruction Assistant Professor,
Department of Orthopaedic Surgery, Hospital
for Joint Diseases, NYU Langone Medical
Center, New York, New York

COLIN W. SWIGLER, MD
Resident, PGY4, Orthopaedic Surgery
Residency, Campbell Clinic, The University of
Tennessee, Memphis, Tennessee

NORFLEET B. THOMPSON, MD
Instructor, Department of Orthopaedic
Surgery and Biomedical Engineering,
Campbell Clinic, The University of Tennessee,
Memphis, Tennessee

DEAN WANG, MD
Sports Medicine and Shoulder Service,
Hospital for Special Surgery, New York,
New York

CONTENTS

Knee and Hip Reconstruction
Patrick C. Toy and William M. Mihalko

> The objective of this study was to evaluate the efficacy of respiratory synchronized compression devices (RSCDs) versus nonsynchronized intermittent pneumatic compression devices (NSIPCDs) in preventing venous thromboembolism (VTE) after total joint arthroplasty. A systematic literature review was conducted. Data regarding surgical procedure, deep vein thrombosis, pulmonary embolism, mortality, and adverse events were abstracted. Compared with control groups, the risk ratio of deep vein thrombosis development was 0.51 with NSIPCDs and 0.47 with RSCDs. This article demonstrates that RSCDs may be marginally more effective at preventing VTE events than NSIPCDs. Furthermore, the addition of mechanical prophylaxis to any chemoprophylactic regimen increases VTE prevention.

> In the face of escalating costs and variations in quality of care, bundled payment models for total joint arthroplasty procedures are becoming increasingly common, both through the Centers for Medicare & Medicaid Services and private payer organizations. The effective implementation of these payment models requires cooperation between multiple service providers to ensure economic viability without deterioration in care quality. This article introduces a stepwise model for the financial analysis of bundled contracts for use in negotiations between hospitals and private payer organizations.

> In an effort to rein in expenditures and improve quality of care, the Centers for Medicare & Medicaid Services (CMS) has initiated bundled reimbursement programs for total joint arthroplasty (TJA) procedures. The success of CMS's bundled payment models has prompted some private insurers to collaborate with provider organizations to institute similar bundled contracts for TJA. The authors review the experiences of orthopedic groups in the implementation of bundled payments for primary and revision TJA through both public and private payers. The authors also discuss the potential benefits, risks, and barriers groups may encounter under this novel payment model.

Trauma
John C. Weinlein and Michael J. Beebe

Although tourniquets are commonly used in patients with limb trauma, both in the acute and elective settings, no set protocols exist for their indications, contraindications, or proper use. This article addresses the current literature on optimal pressure, timing, cuff design, and complications of tourniquets in patients with trauma. General issues are discussed, followed by those specific to upper and lower extremities. Lastly, serious complications, such as pulmonary embolism, are described.

Intraarticular fractures carry a significant risk for posttraumatic osteoarthritis, and this risk varies across different joint surfaces of the lower extremity. These differences are likely due to the anatomic and biomechanical specifics of each joint surface. High-quality human studies are lacking to delineate the threshold articular incongruity that significantly increases risk for posttraumatic osteoarthritis and diminished clinical outcomes for many joint surfaces. Even with anatomic reduction of the articular surface, close attention must be paid to mechanical axis and joint stability to optimize outcomes.

Pediatrics
Jeffrey R. Sawyer

The hip is the second most common involved joint in cerebral palsy. Hip displacement occurs in more than 33% of children with cerebral palsy, with a higher prevalence in nonambulatory children. Hip displacement in this population is typically progressive. Hip dislocation can result in pain and difficulty with sitting and perineal care. Because early stage of hip displacement can be silent, hip surveillance programs are recommended. Most programs use the degree of hip dysplasia and Growth Motor Function Classification System level for screening recommendations. Treatment depends on the degree of dysplasia, functional status of the patient, and patient's age.

Evidence-based medicine (EBM) is a process of decision making aimed at making the best clinical decisions as they relate to patients' health. The current use of EBM in pediatric spine surgery is varied, based mainly on the availability of high-quality data. The use of EBM is limited in idiopathic scoliosis, whereas EBM has been used to investigate the treatment of pediatric spondylolysis. Studies on early-onset scoliosis are of low quality, making EBM difficult in this condition. Future focus and commitment to study quality in pediatric spinal surgery will likely increase the role of EBM in these conditions.

The management of pediatric fractures has evolved over the past several decades, and many injuries that were previously being managed nonoperatively are now being treated surgically. The American Academy of Orthopaedic Surgeons has developed clinical guidelines to help guide decision making and streamline patient care for certain injuries, but many topics remain controversial. This article analyzes the evidence regarding management of 5 of the most common and controversial injuries in pediatric orthopedics today.

Hand and Wrist
Benjamin M. Mauck and James H. Calandruccio

Distal radius fractures are one of the most commonly treated fractures in the United States. The highest rates are seen among the elderly, second only to hip fractures. With the increasing aging population these numbers are projected to continue to increase. Distal radius fractures include a spectrum of injury patterns encountered by general practitioners and orthopedists alike. This evidence-based review of distal radius fractures incorporates the current and available literature on the diagnosis, management, and treatment of fractures of the distal radius.

Carpal tunnel syndrome (CTS) is one of the most common musculoskeletal disorders of the upper extremity. Comorbidities associated with the development of CTS include diabetes and obesity. Although a high rate of repetitive hand/wrist motions is a risk factor, there is insufficient evidence to implicate computer use in the development of CTS. Initial treatment generally is nonoperative, with the strongest evidence supporting bracing/splinting. Strong evidence supports operative treatment, regardless of technique, as superior to nonoperative treatment. Complications are infrequent and most are minor and transient.

Shoulder and Elbow
Thomas (Quin) Throckmorton

Rotator cuff disease affects a large proportion of the overall population and encompasses a wide spectrum of pathologies, including subacromial impingement, rotator cuff tendinopathy or tear, and calcific tendinitis. Various injection therapies have been used for the treatment of rotator cuff disease, including corticosteroid, prolotherapy, platelet-rich plasma, stem cells, and ultrasound-guided barbotage for calcific tendinitis. However, the existing evidence for these therapies remains controversial or sparse. Ultimately, improved understanding of the underlying structural and compositional deficiencies of the injured rotator cuff tissue is needed to identify the biological needs that can potentially be targeted with injection therapies.

Infection after orthopedic procedures is a devastating and serious complication associated with significant clinical and financial challenges to the health care system and unfortunate patient. The time- and resource-intensive nature of treating infection after orthopedic procedures has turned attention toward enhancing prevention and establishing quality improvement measures. Prevention strategies throughout the perioperative period include host optimization, risk mitigation, reducing bacterial burden, and proper wound management. Understanding the most common offending organisms of the shoulder, *Propionibacterium acnes* and coagulase-negative *Staphylococcus* species, and their hypothesized mechanism of infection is crucial to selecting appropriate preventative measures.

The incidence of venous thromboembolic events (VTEs) complicating shoulder surgery is difficult to estimate. Case reports, retrospective studies, prospective studies, and systematic reviews vary in terms of separating symptomatic versus asymptomatic VTEs, those occurring in the upper versus lower extremities, and those leading to pulmonary embolism. Reported rates vary between 0.02% and 13%. Arthroplasty is associated with a higher incidence than arthroscopy. Surgery for fracture presents increased risk. Mechanical prophylaxis using compression devices could be considered given its favorable risk-benefit profile. Chemical prophylaxis should be considered for high-risk patients. Evidence-based criteria cannot be obtained from the current literature on VTEs after shoulder surgery.

Foot and Ankle
Clayton C. Bettin and Benjamin J. Grear

There are limited data to guide the use of venous thromboembolism disease (VTED) prophylaxis after foot and ankle surgery. Although there is general consensus that the overall risk is lower than after hip or knee replacement, subpopulations of patients may be at relatively heightened risk. Furthermore, existing data are often conflicting regarding the efficacy of prophylaxis, with little acknowledgment of the trade-offs between VTED prophylaxis and potential complications associated with the use of such medications. This article provides an overview of currently available evidence to guide decision making regarding VTED prophylaxis in patients who undergo foot and ankle surgery.

Patient-reported outcomes (PROs) are a measure of health care quality that empowers patients to share their health care perceptions with their providers. In orthopedic foot and ankle surgery, these measures can range from global assessments of pain or satisfaction to complex questionnaires designed to assess the function of specific anatomic regions or the recovery from specific procedures. This article seeks to characterize the use of PROs in foot and ankle surgery, describe some of the most commonly used measures, discuss implementation in everyday clinical practice, and explore the future of PROs in foot and ankle orthopedics.

EVIDENCE-BASED MEDICINE

PREFACE

Evidence-Based Medicine

In the current health care environment, physicians are under increasing pressure to provide quality care in the most cost-effective way possible. This dual focus—morbidity and money—is driving an emphasis on evidence-based clinical decision-making. Simply stated, evidence-based medicine combines the best research evidence with clinical expertise and patient values and preferences. The articles in this issue provide information to assist orthopedic surgeons in developing evidence-based guidelines for their particular practice situations.

Despite developments in anticoagulation therapies, thromboembolic complications remain a concern after total joint arthroplasty. Elbuluk and colleagues analyzed the available literature and determined that respiratory-synchronized compression devices may be marginally more effective at preventing thromboembolic events than standard intermittent pneumatic compression devices, but the addition of any mechanical prophylaxis increases prevention over chemoprophylaxis alone. In an effort to reduce expenditures and improve quality of care, the Centers for Medicare and Medicaid Services has initiated bundled reimbursement programs for total joint arthroplasty procedures. The two-part discussion by Piccinin and colleagues explains benefits and risks of bundled payment plans and provides a model for the financial analysis of bundled contracts for use in negotiations between hospitals and private payer organizations.

Because of the variety of injury and patient characteristics, as well as the multiple treatment options, development of evidence-based guidelines for trauma is difficult. Bogdan and Helfet provide an in-depth discussion of indications, contraindications, and complications of the use of tourniquets in limb trauma, and Beals and colleagues point out the importance of considering the mechanical axis and joint stability in addition to anatomic reduction to optimize outcomes of intraarticular fractures.

Children with cerebral palsy commonly have hip displacement, typically progressing to dislocation, which can result in pain and sitting difficulty. Huser and colleagues provide information about hip surveillance programs and surgical treatment of hip dysplasia. As Oetgen points out, the development of evidence-based guidelines for pediatric spine surgery is limited by the small number of quality articles on adolescent idiopathic scoliosis, early-onset scoliosis, and spondylolysis. Hubbard and Riccio discuss the American Academy of Orthopaedic Surgeons clinical guidelines for the treatment of a number of pediatric fractures, noting five areas that remain controversial.

Distal radial fractures and carpal tunnel syndrome are two of the most common musculoskeletal problems in the hand and wrist. Choosing between operative and nonoperative treatment for distal radial fractures and selecting the appropriate fixation device can be difficult. Mauck and Swigler provide information on the diagnosis and treatment of these common injuries. Calandruccio and Thompson provide evidence on the treatment of carpal tunnel syndrome, noting that strong evidence supports operative treatment.

Shoulder and elbow injuries encompass a wide variety of musculoskeletal pathologies, one of the most common being rotator cuff disorders. Lin and colleagues discuss the various injection therapies developed to avoid operative treatment; however, existing evidence for these is sparse or controversial. When operative treatment is indicated for shoulder or elbow disorders, preventing complications is paramount. Boyle and Duquin describe measures to prevent surgical site infections, and Aibinder and Sanchez-Sotelo provide information about venous thromboembolism (VTE) prophylaxis.

VTE prophylaxis also is a concern with foot and ankle surgery, and Chien and colleagues provide an overview of currently available evidence for decision-making regarding prophylaxis in patients who have foot and ankle surgery. As part of the evidence-based trio (evidence + experience + patient perceptions), patient-reported outcomes are

Orthop Clin N Am 49 (2018) xvii–xviii
https://doi.org/10.1016/j.ocl.2017.12.002
0030-5898/18/© 2017 Published by Elsevier Inc.

important measures of health care quality. Hunt and Lakey describe some of the most commonly used measures and discuss their implementation into everyday clinical practice.

Overall, the authors in this issue have provided a wealth of information on evidence-based medicine in a variety of subspecialty situations, and we hope this will help clinicians develop evidence-based guidelines for their patients.

Frederick M. Azar, MD
Campbell Clinic, Inc
University of Tennessee–Campbell Clinic
Department of Orthopaedic Surgery &
Biomedical Engineering
1211 Union Avenue, Suite 510
Memphis, TN 38104, USA

E-mail address:
fazar@campbellclinic.com

Knee and Hip Reconstruction

Respiratory Synchronized Versus Intermittent Pneumatic Compression in Prevention of Venous Thromboembolism After Total Joint Arthroplasty

A Systematic Review and Meta-Analysis

Ameer M. Elbuluk, BA, Kelvin Y. Kim, BA,
Kevin K. Chen, MA, Afshin A. Anoushiravani, MD,
Ran Schwarzkopf, MD, MSc, Richard Iorio, MD*

KEYWORDS

- Total joint arthroplasty • Venous thromboembolism • Deep venous thrombi • Pulmonary emboli
- Thromboprophylaxis • Respiratory synchronized compression
- Intermittent pneumatic compression devices

KEY POINTS

- Mechanical compression devices serve as an alternative and conjunctive therapy to chemoprophylaxis in prevention of thromboembolic events after total joint arthroplasty. There is still uncertainty, however, regarding the safest and most effective thromboprophylactic strategy.
- Nonsynchronized intermittent pneumatic compression devices (NSIPCDs) function by providing pressure at a constant cycle, whereas continuous enhanced circulation therapy devices function in a synchronized manner with a patient's own respiratory cycle (respiratory synchronized compression devices [RSCDs]).
- RSCDs may be marginally more effective at preventing venous thromboembolism events (VTEs) than NSIPCDs. The addition of mechanical prophylaxis to any chemoprophylactic regimen further increases VTE prevention.
- Although the sole use of compression devices has been shown to decrease the risk of bleeding and other associated complications, there is not enough evidence to support mechanical compression as a sole means of VTE prophylaxis.

Source of Funding: No external funds were received in support of this study.

Investigation performed at the New York University (NYU) Langone Medical Center, Hospital for Joint Diseases, New York, NY.

Department of Orthopaedic Surgery, Hospital for Joint Diseases, NYU Langone Medical Center, 301 East 17th Street, New York, NY 10003, USA

* Corresponding author. Department of Orthopaedic Surgery, NYU Langone Medical Center, Hospital for Joint Diseases, 301 East 17th Street, Suite 1402, New York, NY 10003.

E-mail address: richard.iorio@nyumc.org

Orthop Clin N Am 49 (2018) 123–133
https://doi.org/10.1016/j.ocl.2017.11.001
0030-5898/18/© 2017 Elsevier Inc. All rights reserved.

INTRODUCTION

Venous thromboembolism (VTE), including deep vein thrombosis (DVT) and pulmonary embolism (PE), is a serious and potentially life-threatening complication after total joint arthroplasty (TJA).[1–10] Hip and knee replacements are at particularly high risk for VTE, largely due to obstructed venous blood flow during surgery and reduced patient mobility during recovery.[11] In current practice, nearly every patient undergoing TJA is prophylactically treated to prevent thromboembolic events with the use of anticoagulants and, in some cases, with or without mechanical prophylaxis, such as sequential or intermittent pneumatic compression devices.[12] There is still uncertainty, however, regarding the safest and most effective thromboprophylactic strategy after TJA.

Several studies have shown that the morbidity rate of chemoprophylaxis treatment may be equal or worse than the complications associated with perioperative thromboembolic events.[13–18] Pharmacologic prophylaxis (ie, low-molecular-weight heparin [LMWH], aspirin, or warfarin) is not a benign intervention and is often associated with an increased risk for major bleeding, wound drainage, and periprosthetic joint infection.[19] Many of these complications result in hospital readmission and additional surgical interventions for patients, resulting in a greater economic burden on the health care system.[20] As a result, the American Academy of Orthopaedic Surgeons has recently published conservative thromboprophylaxis guidelines supporting less aggressive chemoprophylactic regimens after TJA.[21,22] Mechanical compression devices serve as an alternative and conjunctive therapy to chemoprophylaxis. They function primarily by compressing blood vessels in the lower extremities, which decreases venous stasis and enhances fibrinolysis.

Different types of nonsynchronized intermittent pneumatic compression devices (NSIPCDs) have been used for thromboprophylaxis after TJA. These devices generally function by providing a pressure gradient that facilitates venous blood flow based on automatic or constant time lengths. In contrast, respiratory synchronized compression devices (RSCDs) function synchronously with a patient's respiratory phase.[23,24] The devices are capable of monitoring respiratory-related venous flow and do not pump during inspiration when levels of right heart filling are low but rather pump during the expiratory phase when levels of right heart filling are greater. Despite the widely accepted use of these modalities of mechanical prophylaxis, the effectiveness of these thromboprophylactic devices after TJA remains unclear. The aim of this systematic review was to comparatively evaluate the efficacy of RSCDs to NSIPCDs in prevention of thromboembolic events after TJA.

MATERIALS AND METHODS

Search Strategy

A systematic literature search was performed in accordance with the Preferred Reporting Items for Systematic Reviews and Meta-Analyses guidelines (Fig. 1). Two reviewers independently searched 3 online databases (PubMed, Cochrane, and Embase) to identify all relevant articles published between January 2000 and August 2016. Reference lists of included studies were examined for additional articles that could have been missed. The search terms and inclusion/exclusion criteria were established a priori (Box 1, Table 1). Eligible studies were included based on the following criteria:

1. Levels I, II, and III evidence
2. Studies published in English
3. Human studies
4. Primary and revision TJA
5. Studies reporting DVT or PE
6. Full-text availability

Exclusion criteria were as follows:

1. Studies on any hip or knee arthroplasty secondary to trauma
2. Studies not reporting any VTE events
3. Potential overlap of patient populations when study was by same investigators or institutions
4. Nonhuman studies
5. Non–English language studies

Data Extraction

Two of the authors (A.M.E. and K.Y.K) reviewed all titles and abstracts independently to determine eligibility and extract relevant data, including number of patients and DVT/PE rate. In addition, any information on complications (eg, major bleeding) or adverse events was documented. Disagreements were resolved by discussion between the 2 authors, and, if a consensus could not be reached, a more senior reviewer (A.A.A. or R.I.) helped resolve the discrepancy. The final decision on inclusion was made based on the full-text article.

Qualitative Analysis

The quality of studies was assessed with the use of the Methodological Index for Non-Randomized Studies (MINORS) criteria.

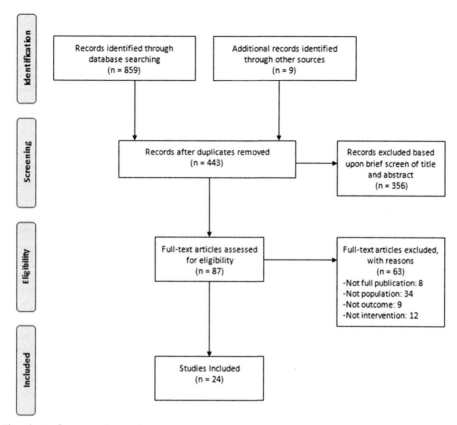

Fig. 1. Flowchart of systematic search strategy.

MINORS is a validated scoring tool to assess internal and external validity for nonrandomized studies.[25] Studies are assigned 0, 1, or 2 with a maximum of 24 for comparative studies and 16 for noncomparative studies. Studies

Box 1 Search criteria
1. WizAir AND arthroplasty
2. ActiveCare AND arthroplasty
3. Mobile intermittent pneumatic compression
4. Portable intermittent pneumatic compression
5. Pneumatic compression AND arthroplasty
6. Sequential compression AND arthroplasty
7. External compression AND arthroplasty
8. Pumps AND arthroplasty
9. Venous thromboembolism AND arthroplasty
10. Deep venous thrombosis AND arthroplasty
11. Pulmonary embolism AND arthroplasty
Search engines: Pubmed, Cochrane, and Embase.

were not excluded, however, from the systematic review on the basis of their quality.

Quantitative Analysis

All statistical analysis, including assessment of heterogeneity, was performed using Review Manager 5.3 (Cochrane, London, United Kingdom). The I^2 statistic was used to evaluate heterogeneity, and a fixed-effect model was used based on the I^2 value. Analysis of relative risk (RR) was performed by evaluation of studies that compared NSIPCDs with any control chemoprophylaxis regimen or RSCDs with any control chemoprophylaxis regimen. The authors used risk ratio to express the effectiveness of RSCDs to NSIPCDs in preventing DVT or PE. The results of the analyses were expressed as forest plots, illustrating the relative risk for thromboembolic events after TJA with a 95% CI for each study, and a cumulative weighted mean effect for all the studies in the analyses. Inter-reviewer agreement for article screening was evaluated with use of the kappa value: $\kappa > 0.60$ indicated substantial agreement; $0.21 \leq \kappa \leq 0.60$ was moderate agreement; and $\kappa < 0.21$ indicated slight agreement.

Table 1
Inclusion and exclusion criteria

Study Characteristic	Inclusion Criteria	Exclusion Criteria
Population	Primary or revision TJA	No fracture surgery
Intervention	NSIPCD or RSCD used for ≥24 h, with or without pharmacologic prophylaxis	GCS, foot pumps
Comparator	Pharmacologic prophylaxis or NSIPCD or RSCD (or both)	
Outcome	Primary: VTE events (DVT and/or PE) Secondary: mortality and adverse events (major or minor bleeding)	No VTE event recorded
Design	RCTs or cohort studies	Case studies
Other	Publication years 2000–present English-language publication	Cadaver or nonhuman study

RESULTS

Studies Included

The initial search protocol identified 868 studies, of which 425 were duplicates. The titles and abstracts of the remaining 443 studies were reviewed and resulted in the exclusion of 357 studies that were not relevant to the study. The full-text articles of the remaining 87 studies were critically appraised in their entirety for eligibility, resulting in the exclusion of an additional 63 studies. No other studies were extracted from the reference lists of these studies. The reasons for exclusion were that a study did not report a VTE outcome (14%), was not the desired patient population (54%), reported wrong intervention (19%), and did not have full-text publication (13%). The 24 included articles identified by the 2 independent reviewers were then evaluated by a third reviewer to ensure that the strict eligibility criteria had been met. There was excellent agreement among reviewers involving the title (κ = 0.91; 95% CI, 0.89–0.93), abstract (κ = 0.85; 95% CI, 0.81–0.89), and full text (κ = 0.97; 95% CI, 0.95–0.99). There was no disagreement between the reviewers regarding the definitive inclusion of final studies.

Study Quality

Of the 24 studies that were used, 13 studies represented level I evidence and 11 studies represented level III evidence. There was significant agreement among the quality assessment scores based on the MINORS criteria (κ = 0.94; 95% CI, 0.91–0.96). The included studies had a mean MINORS score (and SD) of 12.8 ± 3.6, which indicates average quality of evidence.

Study Characteristics

Six different compression devices and manufacturers were represented in this study.

RSCDs included ActiveCare (Medical Compression Systems, Or Akiva, Israel); and NSIPCDs included WizAir (Medical Compression Systems, Or Akiva, Israel), Deep Vein Thrombosis Kendall SCD (Kendall, Mansfield, Massachusetts), VenaFlow (Aircast, Summit, New Jersey), Flowtron (Huntleigh Healthcare, Luton, United Kingdom), and DVT (Daesung Maref, Gunpo, Korea). Three studies did not specify which brands of devices were used. Aspirin or LMWH was used in conjunction with compression devices in 11 studies evaluating the efficacy of RSCDs or NSIPCDs. Of the studies that evaluated RSCDs, 3 compared results to LMWH, 2 studies had no control group, 1 study to Flowtron plus LMWH, 1 study to warfarin, and 1 study to either warfarin or LMWH. Of the studies that investigated NSIPCDs, 8 studies compared results to other NSIPCDs, 5 studies had no control group, 2 studies compared with LMWH, 1 study compared with graduated compression stockings (GCS), 1 study compared with GCS plus LMWH, and 1 study compared with an NSIPCD plus LMWH and rivaroxaban. There was a notable difference in length of treatment with compression devices between the 2 groups. RSCDs were used for a minimum of 10 days with only 1 study cohort using them for 28 days (Odeh and colleagues).[26] All studies using NSIPCDs were used for the length of hospitalization, which was 4.6 days on average.

Deep Vein Thrombosis Events

When RSCDs and NSIPCDs alone were compared with control chemoprophylactic groups, the RR of DVT development was 0.47 (95% CI, 0.27–0.80;

$I^2 = 0\%$) for RSCDs and 0.51 (95% CI, 0.39–0.67; $I^2 = 69\%$) for NSIPCDs. When aspirin plus RSCDs or NSIPCDs were compared with control chemoprophylaxis groups, the RSCDs group showed a higher RR of 0.72 (95% CI, 0.31–1.64; $I^2 = 0\%$) compared with 0.41 (95% CI, 0.26–0.63; $I^2 = 38\%$) for the NSIPCDs group. Further analysis of these data indicated that when RSCDs and NSIPCDs were used in conjunction with a more aggressive chemoprophylaxis agent (ie, LMWH, warfarin, or heparin), RSCDs showed a lower RR of 0.36 (95% CI, 0.18–0.75; $I^2 = 0\%$) compared with an RR of 0.44 (95% CI, 0.27–0.70; $I^2 = 78\%$) observed in the NSIPCD group. The main form of aggressive chemoprophylaxis used in this group of RSCDs studies was LMWH whereas a combination of either LMWH, warfarin, or heparin was used in the NSIPCDs studies. Forest plots were designed to illustrate the data analysis comparing DVT events in RSCDs or NSIPCDs with a chemoprophylaxis group (Fig. 2).

Pulmonary Embolism Events

The RR for developing a PE in the RSCDs cohort, regardless of the type of chemoprophylaxis used in conjunction with the compression device, was 0.62 (95% CI, 0.29–1.32; $I^2 = 0\%$) whereas the risk in the NSIPCDs group was 0.24 (95% CI, 0.04–1.47; $I^2 = 0\%$). PE data regarding RSCDs-alone and NSIPCDs-alone could not be calculated given the limited number of studies that fit these criteria. When aspirin was used with RSCDs, the RR for a PE event was 0.65 (95% CI, 0.29–1.45; $I^2 = 0\%$) compared with a risk of 0.34 (95% CI, 0.03–3.28; $I^2 = 0\%$) when aspirin was used with NSIPCDs. When the risk of PEs was assessed in regard to the use of more aggressive chemoprophylaxis agents, an RR of 0.50 (95% CI, 0.07–3.56; $I^2 = 0\%$) was found when RSCDs were used with LMWH. The risk of PE events in the NSIPCDs plus aggressive chemoprophylaxis group could not be evaluated given the lack of studies that made this particular comparison.

When stratifying each study by the use or nonuse of spiral CT imaging to detect PE events, RSCDs were found to have an RR of 0.66 (95% CI, 0.29–1.47; $I^2 = 0\%$) when PE detection was done with spiral CT. The risk for PEs in the NSIPCDs group could not be evaluated due to the limited number of studies that used spiral CTs for PE detection. Finally, when all imaging

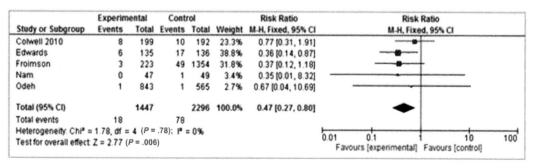

A

Study or Subgroup	Experimental Events	Total	Control Events	Total	Weight	Risk Ratio M-H, Fixed, 95% CI
Ben Galim	0	25	0	25		Not estimable
Chin	9	110	6	110	4.4%	1.50 [0.55, 4.07]
Eisele	3	266	10	170	8.9%	0.19 [0.05, 0.69]
Froimson	3	323	49	1081	16.4%	0.20 [0.06, 0.65]
Gelfer	4	61	17	61	12.4%	0.24 [0.08, 0.66]
Jiang	10	60	11	60	8.0%	0.91 [0.42, 1.98]
Koo	1	24	4	11	4.0%	0.11 [0.01, 0.91]
Lachiewicz 2004	16	206	36	217	25.6%	0.47 [0.27, 0.82]
Ryan	4	54	11	50	8.3%	0.34 [0.11, 0.99]
Silbersack	18	48	18	57	12.0%	1.19 [0.70, 2.01]
Total (95% CI)		1177		1842	100.0%	0.51 [0.39, 0.67]
Total events	68		162			

Heterogeneity: Chi² = 25.79, df = 8 (P = .001); I² = 69%
Test for overall effect: Z = 4.81 (P<.00001)

0.01 0.1 1 10 100
Favours [experimental] Favours [control]

B

Study or Subgroup	Experimental Events	Total	Control Events	Total	Weight	Risk Ratio M-H, Fixed, 95% CI
Colwell 2010	8	199	10	192	23.3%	0.77 [0.31, 1.91]
Edwards	6	135	17	136	38.8%	0.36 [0.14, 0.87]
Froimson	3	223	49	1354	31.8%	0.37 [0.12, 1.18]
Nam	0	47	1	49	3.4%	0.35 [0.01, 8.32]
Odeh	1	843	1	565	2.7%	0.67 [0.04, 10.69]
Total (95% CI)		1447		2296	100.0%	0.47 [0.27, 0.80]
Total events	18		78			

Heterogeneity: Chi² = 1.78, df = 4 (P = .78); I² = 0%
Test for overall effect: Z = 2.77 (P = .006)

0.01 0.1 1 10 100
Favours [experimental] Favours [control]

Fig. 2. (A) NSIPCDs versus chemoprophylaxis and (B) RSCDs versus chemoprophylaxis in prevention of DVT.

modalities other than spiral CT were used to detect PEs, there was a 0.50 (95% CI, 0.07–3.56; $I^2 = 0\%$) risk in the RSCDs group compared with a slightly lower risk of 0.34 (95% CI, 0.04–3.26; $I^2 = 0\%$) in the NSIPCDs cohort. Forest plots were designed to demonstrate the risk of PE events between RSCDs or NSIPCDs and chemoprophylaxis cohorts (Fig. 3).

Complications

In the 4 of 7 studies that evaluated the complication rates of RSCDs, there was a 0% (0 of 722 patients) rate of any major bleeding events, and 10.2% (74 of 722 patients) rate of minor bleeding. Of the 8 of 14 studies that evaluated complications in NSIPCDs, there was also a 0% (0 of 3063 patients) rate of major bleeding events, whereas 33 of 3063 (1.1%) patients were reported to have minor bleeds. A meta-analysis of the studies that reported minor bleeds suggests that there is a higher risk with RSCDs versus NSIPCDs (RR 9.51; 95% CI, 6.36–14.22). It should be noted, however, that there were no consistent criteria used to define major or minor bleeding throughout the studies and that chemoprophylaxis regimens varied in each study.

Mortality

There were 2 reported deaths in the RSCDs group; however, none of them was due to PE.

The NSIPCDs group reported 3 total deaths with 1 that was caused by a PE.

DISCUSSION

As the number of elective TJA continues to increase, the importance of VTE rises as well. DVT resulting in PE remains the most common cause of readmission and death after TJA.[27–29] Several clinical trials have shown that even asymptomatic DVT after major joint surgery can be significantly reduced with VTE prophylaxis to approximately 20% to 40%.[30] Although many orthopedic surgeons recognize the importance of prophylaxis for VTE, controversy remains regarding the most effective method. Chemoprophylaxis reduces the incidence of DVT after TJA but also increases the risk for major postoperative bleeding. As an alternative, many orthopedic surgeons have used NSIPCDs in conjunction with chemoprophylaxis. Pneumatic compression pumps are seen as advantageous because they are less invasive and are associated with a lower complication profile than pharmacologic agents.

The purpose of this study was to compare the effectiveness of 2 methods of mechanical prophylaxis in preventing VTE events: RSCDs versus NSIPCDs. There were 4 major findings in the study. First, when compared with the control

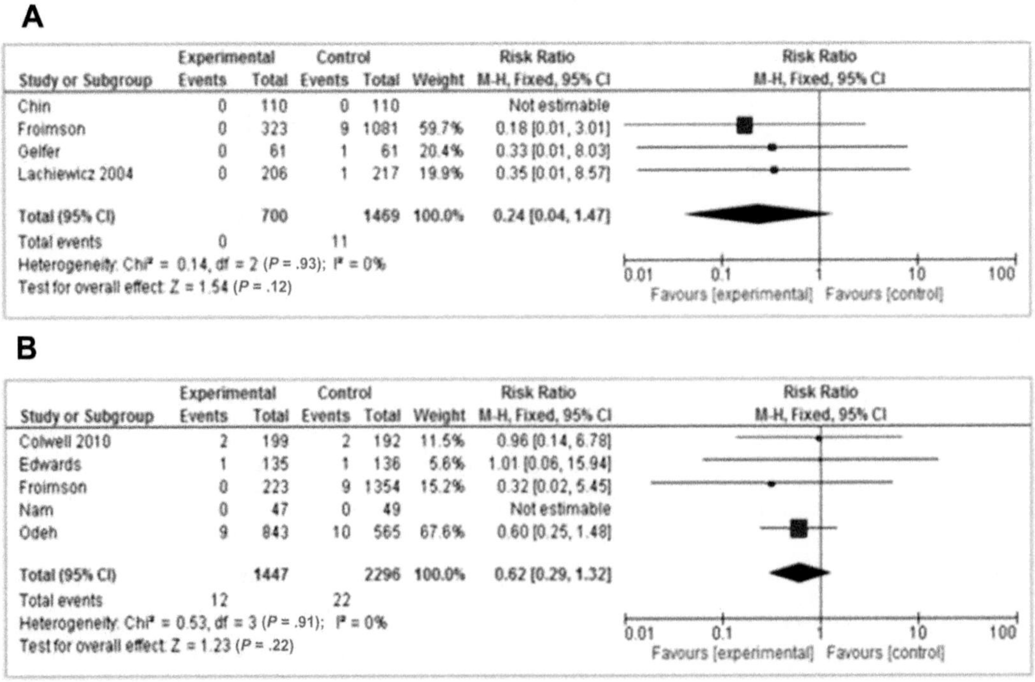

A

B

Fig. 3. (A) NSIPCDs versus chemoprophylaxis and (B) RSCDs versus chemoprophylaxis in prevention of PE.

Table 2
Results of studies reporting venous thromboemolic events

Device/Investigators	Control	No. of Cases	Type of Study	Type of Arthroplasty	Chemoprophylaxis	Deep Vein Thrombosis Rate (%)	Pulmonary Embolism Rate (%)
Respiratory synchronized devices							
ActiveCare + SFT							
Colwell et al, 2014	N/A	3060	Retrospective	THA/TKA	ASA	0.75	0.16
Colwell et al, 2010	LMWH	199	RCT	THA	ASA	5	1
Edwards et al, 2008	LMWH	135	RCT	THA/TKA	LMWH	4.3	0.71
Froimson et al	Flowtron + LMWH	223	Retrospective	THA/TKA	LMWH	1.3	0
Hardwick et al	LMWH	198	RCT	THA	ASA	4.1	1
Levy et al	N/A	287	Retrospective	TKA	—	3.1	3.6
Nam et al	Warfarin	47	Retrospective	TKA	ASA	0	0
Odeh et al	Warfarin/LMWH	843	Retrospective	THA/TKA	ASA	0.12	0
	Enoxaparin	—	—	—	—	—	—
Nonsynchronized devices							
WizAir							
Ben-Galim et al	Kendall	25	RCT	THA/TKA	Heparin	0	0
Gelfer et al	Enoxaparin	61	RCT	THA/TKA	ASA	6.5	0

(continued on next page)

Device/Investigators	Control	No. of Cases	Type of Study	Type of Arthroplasty	Chemoprophylaxis	Deep Vein Thrombosis Rate (%)	Pulmonary Embolism Rate (%)
Kendall							
Choi et al	DVT	27	RCT	TKA	—	55.6	—
Koo et al	DVT	13	RCT	TKA	—	7.7	—
Lachiewicz 2007	N/A	599	Retrospective	TKA	ASA	9.3	0.5
Lachiewicz 2006	N/A	936	Retrospective	THA	ASA	3.9	0.7
Lachiewicz 2004	VenaFlow	217	RCT	TKA	—	15	0.47
VenaFlow							
Eisele et al	LMWH	266	RCT	THA/TKA	LMWH	1.1	—
Lachiewicz 2004	Kendall	206	RCT	TKA	—	6.9	0
Ryan et al	Stockings	50	RCT	THA	ASA	8	—
Silbersack et al	GCS + LMWH	68	RCT	THA/TKA	LMWH	0	0
Flowtron							
Froimson et al	ActiveCare	1081	Retrospective	THA/TKA	LMWH	3.6	0.66
Morris	N/A	120	Retrospective	TKA	ASA	4.2	0.83
DVT							
Choi et al	Kendall	27	RCT	TKA	—	51.9	—
Kim et al	N/A	459	Retrospective	THA	—	4.8	0.7
Others							
Chin et al	Enoxaparin	110	RCT	TKA	—	8	0
Jiang et al	LMWH + rivaroxaban	60	RCT	TKA	ASA	16.7	—
Keeney et al	N/A	705	Retrospective	THA	Warfarin	3.5	0

Abbreviations: ASA, aspirin; GCS, graduated compression stockings; THA, Total Hip Arthroplasty; TKA, Total Knee Arthroplasty.

Table 3
Evidence profile of studies in systematic review

Characteristics	Respiratory Synchronized Compression Devices	Nonsynchronized Intermittent Pneumatic Compression Devices
No. of studies	3 RCTs; 5 retrospective	10 RCTs; 6 retrospective
No. of patients	4104	5030
Average length of follow-up (d)	86.5	92.6
Duration of use (d)	10.1	4.6

chemoprophylactic groups, the RR of DVT development was 0.51 (95% CI, 0.39–0.67) with NSIPCDs and 0.47 (95% CI, 0.27–0.80) with RSCDs. Second, the RRs for development of PE in these groups respectively were 0.24 (95% CI, 0.04–1.47) versus 0.62 (95% CI, 0.29–1.32).The authors hypothesized, however, that this slight increase in PE rate could be due to the rise in spiral CT usage in detection of PE.[31] Thus, studies were analyzed separately based on whether spiral CT was used. Results showed that for both RSCDs and NSIPCDs, studies that use spiral CT for PE detection demonstrated higher PE rates. Although this finding supports the authors' theory regarding spiral CTs, results still suggest that NSIPCDs may be slightly more effective at preventing PE events than RSCDs. Only 1 study met inclusion criteria for NSIPCDs with spiral CT, which does not represent a fair analysis in comparison to RSCDs, which had 4 studies using spiral CTs. Third, compared with chemoprophylaxis alone, compression devices seem to reduce the incidence of all VTEs after TJA, although statistical significance was only observed with DVT prevention. Lastly, the addition of pumps to any chemoprophylaxis agent (ie, aspirin, LMWH, or warfarin) decreased the overall rate of VTE events.

The 2012 American College of Chest Physicians evidence-based clinical practice guidelines for antithrombotic therapy and prevention of thrombosis highlight the clinical challenge of providing effective VTE prophylaxis without excessive bleeding.[32] These guidelines also recommend the use of NSIPCDs instead of no prophylaxis for the prevention of VTE after TJA. The authors' study, however, specifically aimed to assess whether there was a significant difference in VTE events with RSCDs, which are sequenced to the respiratory cycle, in comparison to other NSIPCDs, which are sequenced by constant time cycles. Studies have already shown that RSCDs are

significantly safer than LMWH with regard to major bleeding (P<.05).[20] The authors' findings support previously reported data which proved the effectiveness of both methods alone or in combination with a pharmacologic prophylaxis. The authors' study also showed a slightly higher rate of PE in patients using respiratory synchronized technology. RSCDs, however, are relatively new, which concurrently aligns with an increase in PE detection via spiral CT scanners that were not readily available for many previous studies examining PE events with NSIPCDs. Lastly, studies have emphasized the high compliance of RSCDs, a mobile compression device that can be used after hospitalization, to be greater than NSIPCDs, which are used only in-hospital settings and cannot be worn out of bed during ambulation.[24] The authors' analysis showed, however, that although RSCDs were used for nearly twice the duration of NSIPCDs (10 days vs 5 days on average), each device reported similar rates of DVT prevention. As length of stay for TJA continues to decrease, the compliance of in-hospital NSIPCD use comes into greater focus, because these devices are not mobile compared with RSCDs. Nonetheless, regardless of type of SCD, the underlying issue remains that methods must be found to identify which low-risk patients would benefit from sole use of mechanical prophylaxis.

Limitations

There are several limitations in the authors' study. First, not all studies included in the analysis were randomized controlled trials (RCTs). For a more comprehensive analysis, retrospective studies were included to increase the number of patients in each cohort. In doing so, the quality of evidence provided by the conclusions was reduced. As a result, definitive conclusions regarding the various interventions are not possible. Larger and higher-quality RCTs would be needed to confirm the findings. Second, there was high heterogeneity (>50%) among the NSIPCDs cohort, which makes it difficult to compare the different studies and their outcomes. This marked heterogeneity could be due to the lack of a standardized protocol in VTE prophylaxis after TJA. Third, although studies were combined for analysis, the sample size of the authors' study might not be enough to distinguish the true difference of DVT and PE incidence between patients and controls. By increasing the sample size through a systematic review, however, the authors' combined results allow for more accurate results. Furthermore, the original studies do not represent all patient populations because the landscape of patients undergoing TJA continues to change. Lastly, each hospital follows its own VTE protocol and although most protocols follow evidence-based clinical guidelines, this variability could change the effect on outcomes.

SUMMARY

Regardless of compression methodology, the authors' study supports previous literature on the adjunctive use of compression devices to pharmacologic agents in reducing VTE events (Table 2).[24] Although the sole use of compression devices has been shown to decrease the risk of bleeding and other associated complications, there is not enough evidence to support mechanical compression as a sole means of VTE prophylaxis.[24] In conclusion, this systematic review of patients undergoing TJA demonstrated similar rates of DVT in patients who used RSCDs compared with those who used NSIPCDs (Table 3). In conclusion, this systematic review of patients undergoing TJA demonstrated similar rates of DVT in patients who used RSCDs compared to those who used NSIPCDs.

REFERENCES

1. Charnley J. Low friction arthroplasty of the hip: theory and practice. Berlin: Springer; 1979. p. 308.
2. Coventry MB, Beckenbaugh RD, Nolan DR, et al. 2,012 total hip arthroplasties. A study of postoperative course and early complications. J Bone Joint Surg Am 1974;56(2):273–84.
3. Coventry MB, Nolan DR, Beckenbaugh RD. "Delayed" prophylactic anticoagulation: a study of results and complications in 2,012 total hip arthroplasties. J Bone Joint Surg Am 1973;55(7):1487–92.
4. Insall JN. Surgery of the knee. New York: Churchill Livingstone; 1984. p. 646–7.
5. Johnson R, Green JR, Charnley J. Pulmonary embolism and its prophylaxis following the Charnley total hip replacement. Clin Orthop Relat Res 1977;127:123–32.
6. Murray DW, Carr AJ, Bulstrode CJ. Pharmacological thromboprophylaxis and total hip replacement. J Bone Joint Surg Br 1995;77(1):3–5.
7. Pellegrini VD Jr, Donaldson CT, Farber DC, et al. The John Charnley Award: prevention of readmission for venous thromboembolic disease after total hip arthroplasty. Clin Orthop Relat Res 2005;441(441):56–62.
8. Pellegrini VD Jr, Donaldson CT, Farber DC, et al. The Mark Coventry Award: prevention of readmission for venous thromboembolism after total knee arthroplasty. Clin Orthop Relat Res 2006;452(452):21–7.
9. Stulberg BN, Insall JN, Williams GW, et al. Deep-vein thrombosis following total knee replacement. An analysis of six hundred and thirty-eight arthroplasties. J Bone Joint Surg Am 1984;66(2):194–201.
10. Turpie AG, Lassen MR, Davidson BL, et al, Fisher WDRECORD4 Investigators. Rivaroxaban versus enoxaparin for thromboprophylaxis after total knee arthroplasty (RECORD4): a randomised trial. Lancet 2009;373(9676):1673–80.
11. Warwick D, Martin AG, Glew D, et al. Measurement of femoral vein blood flow during total hip replacement. Duplex ultrasound imaging with and without the use of a foot pump. J Bone Joint Surg Br 1994;76(6):918–21.
12. Budhiparama NC, Abdel MP, Ifran NN, et al. Venous thromboembolism (VTE) prophylaxis for hip and knee arthroplasty: changing trends. Curr Rev Musculoskelet Med 2014;7(2):108–16.
13. Callaghan JJ, Dorr LD, Engh GA, et al. Prophylaxis for thromboembolic disease: recommendations from the American College of Chest Physicians—are they appropriate for orthopaedic surgery? J Arthroplasty 2005;20:273.
14. Parvizi J, Azzam K, Rothman RH. Deep venous thrombosis prophylaxis for total joint arthroplasty: American Academy of Orthopaedic Surgeons guidelines. J Arthroplasty 2008;23(7 Suppl):2.
15. Burnett RS, Clohisy JC, Wright RW, et al. Failure of the American College of Chest Physicians-1A protocol for lovenox in clinical outcomes for thromboembolic prophylaxis. J Arthroplasty 2007;22:317.
16. Sharrock NE, Gonzalez Della Valle A, Go G, et al. Potent anticoagulants are associated with a higher all-cause mortality rate after hip and knee arthroplasty. Clin Orthop Relat Res 2008;466:714.
17. Walsh M, Preston C, Bong M, et al. Relative risk factors for requirement of blood transfusion after total hip arthroplasty. J Arthroplasty 2007;22:1162.
18. Freedman KB, Brookenthal KR, Fitzgerald RH Jr, et al. A metaanalysis of thromboembolic prophylaxis

following elective total hip arthroplasty. J Bone Joint Surg Am 2000;82-A:929.

19. Mortazavi SM, Hansen P, Zmistowski B, et al. Hematoma following primary total hip arthroplasty: a grave complication. J Arthroplasty 2013;28(3):498–503.

20. Schairer WW, Vail TP, Bozic KJ. What are the rates and causes of hospital readmission after total knee arthroplasty? Clin Orthop Relat Res 2014;472(1):181–7.

21. American Academy of Orthopaedic Surgeons. Preventing venous thromboembolic disease in patients undergoing elective hip and knee arthroplasty: evidence-based guideline and evidence report. 2011. Available at: http://www.aaos.org.ezproxy.med.nyu.edu/research/gui. Accessed September 16, 2016.

22. Pitto RP, Hamer H, Heiss-Dunlop W, et al. Mechanical prophylaxis of deep-vein thrombosis after total hip replacement a randomised clinical trial. J Bone Joint Surg Br 2004;86:639–42.

23. Edwards JZ, Pulido PA, Ezzet KA, et al. Portable compression device and lowmolecular-weight heparin compared with low-molecular-weight heparin for thromboprophylaxis after total joint arthroplasty. J Arthroplasty 2008;23:1122.

24. Colwell CW Jr, Froimson MI, Anseth SD, et al. A mobile compression device for thrombosis prevention in hip and knee arthroplasty. J Bone Joint Surg Am 2014;96:177.

25. Slim K, Nini E, Forestier D, et al. Methodological index for non-randomized studies (minors): development and validation of a new instrument. ANZ J Surg 2003;73(9):712–6.

26. Odeh K, Doran J, Yu S, et al. Risk-Stratified Venous Thromboembolism Prophylaxis After Total Joint Arthroplasty: Aspirin and Sequential Pneumatic Compression Devices vs Aggressive Chemoprophylaxis. J Arthroplasty 2016.

27. Geerts WH, Pineo GF, Heit JA, et al. Prevention of venous thromboembolism: the Seventh ACCP Conference on Antithrombotic and Thrombolytic Therapy. Chest 2004;126:338s.

28. Kahn SR, Hirsch A, Shrier I. Effect of postthrombotic syndrome on health-related quality of life after deep venous thrombosis. Arch Intern Med 2002;162:1144.

29. Pengo V, Lensing AW, Prins MH, et al. Incidence of chronic thromboembolic pulmonary hypertension after pulmonary embolism. N Engl J Med 2004;350:2257.

30. Geerts WH, Heit JA, Clagett GP, et al. Prevention of venous thromboembolism. Chest 2001;119(Suppl 1):132S–75S.

31. Schoepf UJ, Goldhaber SZ, Costello P. Spiral computed tomography for acute pulmonary embolism. Circulation 2004;109(18):2160–7.

32. Geerts WH, Bergqvist D, Pineo GF, et al, American College of Chest Physicians. Prevention of venous thromboembolism: American College of Chest Physicians evidence-based clinical practice guidelines (8th edition). Chest 2008;133(6 Suppl):381S–453S.

Bundle Payment for Musculoskeletal Care
Current Evidence (Part 1)

Meghan A. Piccinin, MSc[a], Zain Sayeed, MD, MHA[b,*],
Ryan Kozlowski, MD[c], Vamsy Bobba, MD[c],
David Knesek, DO[c], Todd Frush, MD[c]

KEYWORDS

- Total joint arthroplasty • Total knee arthroplasty • Bundle payments • Bundled contracts • BPCI
- Value-based care • Financial analysis

KEY POINTS

- The implementation of the Bundled Payments for Care Improvement (BPCI) program by the Centers for Medicare & Medicaid Services demonstrated significant cost savings and improvements in quality of care.
- A thorough financial analysis of bundled contracts incorporates the evaluation of settings of care, episode period, patient population, revenue and quality terms, and distribution of payments to ensure the economic viability of the payment model.
- Preoperative risk factor modification, enhanced coordination of care, standardization of implant costs, and optimized postacute care utilization may allow orthopedic groups to maximize the advantages of bundled payment models on both costs and care quality.

INTRODUCTION

In the United States, total knee arthroplasty and total hip arthroplasty are 2 commonly occurring surgeries expected to undergo significant growth through 2021.[1–3] Although the Centers for Medicare & Medicaid Services (CMS) remain the largest payer for these procedures, private insurance providers comprise a majority of financers for lower-extremity total joint arthroplasty (TJA) patients under 65 year old.[4,5]

Traditionally, TJAs have been reimbursed through fee-for-service (FFS) models, incentivizing the quantity of services rendered rather than quality of care or cost control, which has been a primary contributor to high health care costs in the United States.[6] In the face of the anticipated future surge in TJA procedures, CMS has begun to transition from FFS reimbursement to alternate payment models (APMs).[7] One of the most widely instituted of these APMs is bundled reimbursement models, including the Bundled Payments for Care Improvement (BCPI) and Comprehensive Care for Joint Replacement (CJR) initiatives. Many institutions have experimented with the implementation of bundled payment models, with a majority realizing cost savings and quality improvements.[8–12]

Funding Sources: No additional funding sources were used for this article.
Conflicts of Interest: No conflicts of interest are evident for authors of this article.
[a] Department of Orthopaedic Surgery, College of Osteopathic Medicine, Michigan State University, Detroit Medical Center, 4707 St Antoine Street, Detroit, MI 48201, USA; [b] Department of Orthopaedics, Institute of Innovations and Clinical Excellence, Detroit Medical Center, 4201 St Antoine Street, Detroit, MI 48201, USA; [c] Department of Orthopaedics, Musculoskeletal Institute of Surgical Excellence, Detroit Medical Center, 4201 St Antoine Street, Detroit, MI 48201, USA
* Corresponding author.
E-mail address: zainsayeed@gmail.com

Orthop Clin N Am 49 (2018) 135–146
https://doi.org/10.1016/j.ocl.2017.11.002

Because Medicare is the largest payer of health care costs in the United States, changes to the CMS reimbursement systems are able to drive provider and hospital financial decisions.[13] With the implementation and preliminary successes of BPCI and CJR, hospitals, providers, and patients seem to be embracing the notion of bundled payment models due to the improved quality, decreased costs, enhanced coordination of care, and simplicity.[14] Many orthopedic surgeons believe that bundled payments are the most successful payment model in decreasing costs and enhancing quality.[15] With 83% of hospitals interested or already participating in bundles, the opportunity is presented for private payers to similarly take advantage of the cost savings anticipated to be provided by these models.[14] Although CMS' implementation of bundled payments involved primarily unilateral determination of target pricing, for private payers to make use of this model, they must collaborate with hospitals and provider groups to negotiate mutually beneficial reimbursement schedules. This article presents a stepwise model (Box 1) for the financial analysis of bundled contracts for use in the negotiations between hospitals and private payer organizations.

FINANCIAL ANALYSIS OF BUNDLED CONTRACTS
Define the Bundle Clinically
Of premiere importance in negotiating bundled payments is the precise determination of what procedures the contract is to cover. In orthopedic surgery, the primary episodes considered for bundles are Medicare Severity Diagnosis Related Groups (MS-DRG) 469 and 470 (major joint replacement or reattachment of the lower extremity with and without major complications and comorbidities, respectively), which have several unique qualities that allow for feasible implementation of bundles, as described previously. Some other orthopedic surgeries, such as spinal surgery episodes, were available for implementation under BPCI but failed to produce cost savings or quality improvement and actually led to a significant increase in Medicare claims.[8] Selection of the episode of care to be included in the bundle must ensure that there is adequate potential for cost savings to be realized to ensure economic viability of the contract for all involved stakeholders.

Additionally, it is crucial to establish accountability and to outline the responsibilities of each stakeholder involved in care delivery. All of those involved need to share the common goal

Box 1
Outline of financial analysis of bundled contracts with private payer organizations

1. Define the bundle clinically

   Identify primary episodes of care

   Outline stakeholder responsibilities

   Define inclusions and exclusions of the care agreement

2. Determine the different settings of care

   Determine inclusion or exclusion of inpatient stay, outpatient care, and PAC settings

3. Identify the episode period to be included

   Determine episode start date

   Determine episode end date

   Incorporate rate and cost of readmissions

4. Refine the patient population for analysis

   Stratify patients based on risk factors

   Optimize modifiable risk factors

5. Incorporate bundled payment revenue and quality terms

   Evaluate impact of more streamlined care pathways on episode volume

   Integrate provisions for financial outlier cases

   Evaluate costs of administrative and procedural changes

6. Perform the financial analysis

   Calculate episode payment required for desired margin of profitability

   Identify areas of potential cost reductions or quality improvements

7. Determine how to distribute payments

   Involve surgeons, administrators, and other stakeholders in development of reimbursement models

   Develop guidelines to evaluate provider performance

of quality improvement and cost reduction and collaboration in the provision of care. Determinations need to be made regarding specific inclusions and exclusions of the care agreement, conditions of any warranties, definitions of cost parameters, and best clinical protocols/standard of care.[16]

Determine the Different Settings of Care
Medicare's BPCI and CJR programs offer the option of several different models, consisting

of acute inpatient hospital stay, postacute care (PAC), or both. These settings include claims for hospital inpatient, hospital outpatient, physician services (inpatient, outpatient, and office), rehabilitation services, and external claims. The specific duties, inclusions, and exclusions of each participant in the provision of the bundled episode must be clearly delineated to ensure compliance with the aims of the program.

Selection of the settings of care to be covered by the bundle depends on the duration of coverage dictated by the terms of the bundle and the hospital's evaluation of where cost reductions remain to be found. More than 70% of patients undergoing TJA are discharged to PAC, with 54% of this cohort using home health agencies and 37% discharged to skilled nursing facilities (SNFs).[17] PAC costs were the most rapidly growing proportion of Medicare spending between 1994 and 2009 and account for the largest variation in spending between episodes, indicating the opportunity for optimization in the postdischarge setting.[18-21] Medicare payments for MS-DRG 470 averaged between $14,372 for episodes with discharge to the community and $43,772 for episodes with discharge to a long-term care facility.[20] Despite the frequent utilization and high costs of inpatient rehabilitation and SNFs, discharge to these facilities has not demonstrated improved health outcomes, suggesting that a shift toward lower-cost discharge settings may allow for cost savings without sacrificing quality of care.[22,23]

Identify the Episode Period to be Included

Currently, there are a variety of defined episodes of care used in CMS-provided and private bundled contracts. Contract start dates tend to begin 30 days or 3 days prior to anchor admission, at the time of the anchor admission, or after discharge from the anchor admission as under BPCI Model 3. Postdischarge coverage periods are similarly variable, including options for 0 days as under BPCI Model 1, 30 days, 60 days, or 90 days after discharge.

The selection of postdischarge coverage period should seek to maximize the likelihood that readmissions are resultant from the original episode of care rather than patients' preexisting medical conditions.[24] As such, it may be necessary to use a longer window for essentially healthy patients and a shorter duration for those with recurring comorbidities. Shorter coverage periods reduce hospitals' potential exposure to postoperative complications included in the bundle, resulting in a lower financial risk but at the expense of the greater profit margins

realized in 60-day or 90-day postdischarge coverage models. A majority of readmissions and PAC costs were accrued within 30 days of discharge, with low payments from days 31 to 90.[25-27] Longer episodes of care capture more costs and readmissions but add a smaller degree of financial risk, potentially making longer postdischarge care windows a more profitable model for hospitals and providers.[25] To minimize the risk of financial losses, programs should attempt to design interventions that target the specific causes of readmission or high PAC costs at their institution. Successful implementation of such measures may allow institutions to elect bundles with a higher risk, which can result in a greater potential profit.

Readmissions are a common and expensive consequence of TJAs and their costs must be incorporated into the price of the bundle in order for the contract to be economically sustainable.[28-30] The readmission rate for a specific episode of care within the selected postdischarge period and the average cost of these readmissions must be determined to calculate the amount required to supplement the base payment to cover the cost of readmissions.[24] Additionally, readmissions unrelated to the original episode of care should be excluded from the bundle.

Refine the Patient Population for Analysis

Although there is a trend of demographic shift with younger patients undergoing TJA, the typical TJA candidates tend to be old, obese, and sick, with a significant number of comorbid conditions.[31,32] Due to the nature of the procedures and patient factors, TJAs are somewhat commonly plagued by suboptimal postoperative outcomes, including surgical sequelae, such as surgical site infection, arthrofibrosis, cellulitis, and dislocation, as well as medical complications, such as pulmonary embolism, pneumonia, urinary tract infection, and *Clostridium difficile* colitis.[29,30,33-37]

The viability of bundled contracts depends on the reduction in the quantity and severity of poor outcomes of TJAs. Understanding the many risk factors that predispose to complications is critical in preventing sequelae. Higher costs, prolonged length of stay, and discharge to inpatient rehabilitation have been associated with older age, female gender, nonwhite race, low socioeconomic status, and American Society of Anesthesiologists class 3 or greater.[33,38-41] Additionally, health habits (such as smoking, alcohol misuse, chronic opioid use, and suboptimal nutritional status) and comorbidities (such as diabetes, cardiac, and cerebrovascular and pulmonary diseases) also contribute to poor postoperative outcomes in patients undergoing TJA.[42–47]

The known associations between certain risk factors and poor outcomes has prompted some to hypothesize that providers will preferentially avoid more complex cases that may pose a greater financial risk to the provider and the hospital.[15,48] A 2016 study by Ellimoottil and colleagues[49] demonstrated an inverse relationship between patient complexity and reconciliation payments, stressing the importance of appropriate risk stratification procedures in determining reimbursement. To circumvent potential limitations in care for complex cases, it may be beneficial for patients to undergo preoperative risk stratification to identify instances in which deviations from the standard approach may be required to optimize care. Such variations from the usual standard of care based on patient severity may be reflected in the reimbursement schedule. Cases in which risk factor modification is inappropriate or ineffectual may necessitate exclusion of such episodes from the bundle agreement.[50,51] Furthermore, risk stratification is necessary to accurately compare surgeons and monitor postoperative outcome measures. Utilization of risk stratification tools may assist orthopedic surgeons in evaluating comorbidities and physical status to better predict patient outcomes. Such tools include the Charnley classification, American Society of Anesthesiologists physical status classification system, Charlson Comorbidity Index, and Outpatient Arthroplasty Risk Assessment Score.[52,53] Additionally, the readmission risk assessment tool and LACE index may provide accurate evaluations of the potential for postdischarge rehospitalization in TJA patients.[54,55]

Based on the outcomes of the risk stratification, it is beneficial that patients undergo preoperative medical status optimization to improve their candidacy for TJA. Orthopedic providers may find benefit in collaborating with other specialists to optimize medication and functional status in patients with comorbidities that may have an adverse impact on TJA outcomes. Delaying elective TJA until successful control of risk factors may be a worthwhile endeavor that may reduce complications, readmissions, and expenditures. Additionally, involvement of the patient in their health care management through enhancing patient activation and risk factor reduction can contribute to improved outcomes and lowered costs.[56–58]

A retrospective pilot study found that 59% of patients with obesity, smoking, or poorly controlled diabetes mellitus were able to beneficially modify these risk factors prior to TJA, demonstrating the willingness of a significant proportion of patients to actively work toward improving their surgical outcomes.[59] An open trial of energy-protein supplements given to elderly patients undergoing surgery for hip fracture observed that greater protein intake was associated with decreased postoperative complications.[60] A randomized controlled trial investigating 4-week preoperative smoking cessation demonstrated a 49% risk reduction in postoperative complications after general or orthopedic surgeries.[61] Both preoperative physical therapy and smoking cessation programs have demonstrated cost reductions in TJA episodes, primarily driven by decreases in PAC utilization.[62,63] Risk stratification protocols have also been instituted to identify and prophylactically manage TJA patients at an increased risk of venous thromboembolism, successfully reducing the incidence of thromboembolism and the need for aggressive anticoagulation therapy.[64]

An increasingly prevalent risk factor necessitating stratification for TJA bundles is opiate dependence. Habitual preoperative use of opiate medications has been associated with greater risks of postoperative complications and revisions, prolonged recoveries, and continued postoperative opiate use after TJA.[65–69] Additionally, preoperative opiate users reported less pain relief after TJA than nonusers.[70,71] TJA patients on methadone maintenance also demonstrate greater postoperative opiate requirements and more pain management referrals relative to control patients.[72] Successful weaning of opiates preoperatively has been shown to significantly improve pain and activity indices in TJA patients.[73]

Obesity, in particular morbid obesity and superobesity, is another important modifiable risk factor influencing outcomes of TJA. Obesity has been associated with increased operating room time as well as a greater risk of complications and inferior postoperative function.[74,75] Increases in body mass index beyond 30 results in significant increases in direct medical costs relating to TJAs.[76,77] In addition to the direct implications of obesity on the results of TJAs, obese patients also have a greater number of comorbidities, further complicating TJA procedures and outcomes.[78] Although obesity is an critical determinant of postoperative outcomes, weight loss should be encouraged through dietary and lifestyle changes rather than through bariatric surgical approaches, which have a greater risk of complications, infections, and need for revisions in TJAs relative to both obese and nonobese patients.[79–81] This discrepancy is believed to be the result of gastrointestinal malabsorption leading to a state of malnutrition, which impairs immune system function.[79,81]

Incorporate Bundled Payment Revenue and Quality Terms

When entering into bundled contracts with Medicare, there is rarely an allowance for hospital input into the determination of the target price. The CMS sets the relative weight of an MS-DRG based on the national costs of patient care within each MS-DRG category. The CMS accounts for regional variations, which is then adjusted based on budget goals.[24] As of 2014, the average Medicare payments for 30-day TJAs were $37,575 for MS-DRG 469 and $25,568 for MS-DRG 470.[48] Because hospitals' cost margins for Medicare-reimbursed TJAs are low, any reduction in these margins through high complication or readmission rates may result in economic unsustainability of the procedures.[28,82] Due to the lack of negotiation power of the hospitals, providers may benefit from investigating whether they are able to provide the outlined services at the target price or be subjected to financial disincentives.

In establishing contracts with private payers, however, hospitals have significant negotiating power in setting their reimbursement structure. Hospitals must assess the impact of bundled contract implementation on the volume of new episodes being performed. Reductions in cost, streamlined care pathways, and improvement in patient outcome measures should result in ability to increase volume of performed procedures, hence adding to the positive financial contribution margins.[16]

Also to be incorporated into the contract are provisions for financial outlier cases, with costs significantly exceeding the median expenditure for a specified service. Among total knee arthroplasties performed for Medicare patients, 2% had payments in excess of $50,000, 0.2% had payments greater than $100,000, and 0.01% had payments greater than $200,000.[83] Although infrequent, particularly expensive episodes can have disastrous financial consequences on low-volume or underprepared hospitals and providers. For this reason, many bundled contracts include policies for outlier payments for cases falling in excess of a specified threshold, typically episode payments greater than 2 SDs from the average regional episode payment. This provision limits the financial risks to providers if an episode of care falls significantly above the targeted price.

There are also important expenditures to recognize unrelated to direct patient care. The institution of novel payment models is associated with administrative costs and structural and procedural changes that may undermine potential profitability, particularly in the early stages of model implementation.[84,85] Under CMS' CJR model, a stop-loss limit was included to moderate hospital's repayment responsibility over the initial years of the program. The stop-loss limit allows for minimization of annual variability in episode severity that can skew procedural cost distributions.

Once hospitals assess the financial aspects of the bundle, a detailed understanding of risk factors that drive high costs, and a plan to address these, serves beneficial for an organization. Factors associated with increased episode expenditures include comorbidities, readmissions, infections, and discharge to long-term care or an SNF.[20,28,36,86–88] Taking direct steps to reduce the incidence of these contributors through the implementation of stringent quality-control measures can result in improved profitability and patient outcomes. Such quality outcome measures include the Patient Safety for Selected Indicators (PSI 90), compliance with Surgical Care Improvement Project measures, Hospital Consumer Assessment of Healthcare Providers and Systems scores, and the BPCI Continuity Assessment Record and Evaluation (B-CARE) Item Set. B-CARE provides streamlined standardization of the acute and postacute evaluation of patients' functional, medical, cognitive, and social support status, specifically for use in CMS' BPCI models.[89] Additionally, adverse event rates, readmission rates, and patient satisfaction markers should also be incorporated to assess program performance. These measures of quality of care and patient outcomes could also be incorporated into bundled contract negotiations to adjust for provider performance and as an annual target measure that delineates gainsharing among participating physicians.

Perform the Financial Analysis

Stakeholders may improve value in a care episode by conducting a thorough financial analysis of the bundle terms to establish an episode payment that will prove financially sustainable. Hospitals must calculate what the payment must be to achieve their desired margin of profitability, which in itself is dependent on several contributors. Elimination of variability in costs is a key to maximizing profitability and financial predictability. Analyses by Ejaz and colleagues[90] identified significant variability in reimbursements for TJA, with large variation specifically in the surgeon and hospital payments. Standardization of fair market value reimbursement from these procedures and gainsharing incentives could effectively offer substantial cost savings for bundled contracts.[16]

Understanding the direct costs associated with each care setting is critical to localizing areas that could be subject to cost reduction measures. One of the primary drivers of hospital inpatient costs is the price of joint implants.[91,92] Implants are costly, comprising up to 47% of total 30-day episode cost yet also highly variable in price due to hospital and physician preferences rather than patient factors.[16,93] Additionally, the cost of implants is increasing at a pace greater than the growth in Medicare payments for TJAs.[94] More expensive, premium implants have not been shown to improve rates of revision or survival compared with standard implants.[95] Efforts to decrease the average cost of implants include standardizing implant options within a hospital, establishing a price cap, and including physicians in the negotiation of discounts for implants from vendors. Additionally, gainsharing in bundled contracts make surgeons financially responsible for their expenditures, which can motivate them to elect for more cost-effective alternatives.

Unplanned readmissions due to operative complications and medical decompensation are an integral source of expenses in the post-acute management of TJA.[20] Episodes with readmissions resulted in a $1324 lower profit margin.[96] The readmission rate and event costs are widely variable among orthopedic groups and emulating best practices in the preoperative, perioperative, and postoperative care of patients may decrease the associated expenditures.[29,86,97] Preoperative risk management and perioperative considerations to reduce the incidence of infections and complications can assist in the reduction of readmissions as well.[98] Collaborative involvement of multidisciplinary teams is critical in effectively managing patient comorbidities presurgery and postsurgery to minimize the incidence of complications.[99] Implementation of rapid recovery protocols also significantly reduced likelihood of readmission.[100,101] Patient education regarding postsurgical expectations prior to surgery and scheduled follow-up appointments with the surgeon and the patient's primary care provider are other avenues by which readmissions can successfully be diminished.[102]

PAC costs account for a large and variable proportion of the total costs of TJA.[26] Discharge to inpatient rehabilitation units or SNFs is associated with significantly greater costs than discharge to home but has a minimal effect on outcomes.[19–21] Some studies have found decreased readmission rates in those patients discharged to home care rather than those discharged to subacute inpatient facilities.[103,104] Strategies that guide discharges toward less intensive alternatives have been an effective mechanism by which orthopedic groups successfully mitigate waste in the PAC setting. Tessier and colleagues[105] reported that implementation of well-defined PAC pathways resulted in a per-episode decrease of $3189 and $2466 for total hip and knee arthroplasties, respectively. Additionally, Snow and colleagues[62] noted that preoperative physical therapy was associated with a 29% reduction in PAC utilization, resulting in a per-episode cost reduction of $871. Other investigators have found that by extending the acute hospital stay by up to 5 days, patients could be discharged to home rather than inpatient facility, which still managed to yield lower overall costs.[106] Through the exploratory implementation of the various strategies that have successfully reduced PAC utilization and costs in other programs, stakeholders can optimize their institution's clinical pathway to maximize cost savings and profitability.

As hospitals institute more streamlined care pathways at a lower cost, realization of a competitive advantage in the health care marketplace ensues.[27] A larger episode volume is desirable under a bundled model because it enables fixed costs to be distributed among a greater number of cases, reducing the per-episode burden of overhead costs while simultaneously mitigating the interyear variability in the number and severity of cases.[26] Additionally, high-volume centers have been shown most cost effective and have better outcomes than low-volume institutions.[107–109]

Determine How to Distribute Payments

Fundamental to the notion of bundled payments is collaboration between multidisciplinary teams to achieve ideal outcomes. Gainsharing incentivizes surgeons and other providers to actively recognize and institute cost reductions by sharing the financial responsibility and risks. Under the FFS payment model, physicians face no incentive to assist in the containment of hospital costs. Although reductions in costs are a leading priority, they must not result from a deterioration in quality of care. As such, and in alignment with the aim of improving quality and decreasing cost of care, reimbursement models must incorporate outcome metrics into providers' performance assessment.

In a survey of the American Association of Hip and Knee Surgeons members, Kamath and colleagues[15] noted that 79% of respondents reported uncertainty regarding revenue sharing as a barrier to the implementation of APMs. One of the challenges in the implementation of bundled contracts is the nature of single-reimbursement distribution for each case among all stakeholders involved in the episode of care. Typical physician compensation structure based on the quantity and complexity of services rendered is antithetical to bundled care models as they continue to reward volume over value.[110] Potential reimbursement strategies may focus on quantity of patients under a physician's care, retention of patients, quality of care, and patient satisfaction with a bonus or deduction based on overall performance.

It is critical for orthopedic surgeons to work in conjunction with hospital administrators and other stakeholders to develop a set of predetermined guidelines to evaluate the performance of providers in various settings of care. A common apprehension of surgeons in regarding bundled payments is the erosion of their autonomy; the involvement of surgeons in the development of performance and reimbursement metrics is prudent to ensure transparency, objectivity, and impartiality.[111] The development of preset evaluation standards served as the foundation for the Joint Utilization Management Program (JUMP) coordinated by the orthopedics group at the Detroit Medical Center.[10] Within BPCI Model 2, JUMP involved the development of scorecards for PAC centers and surgeons to follow the postoperative progression of patients, including PAC utilization and length of stay.[10] Attainment of annual targets and provider performance served as the basis for gainsharing among the physicians.[10]

"WHAT IF" ANALYSIS

The implementation of any number of procedural or organizational changes can drastically affect the cost and quality of care delivery. Preoperative identification and optimization of risk factors for infections and common postsurgical complications have been shown to improve the outcomes of arthroplasties.[64,112,113] One study found that more than 50% of all Medicare readmissions within 30 days of discharge had no contact with a physician between their discharge and readmission, suggesting that poor communication and coordination of care may be partially responsible for rehospitalizations.[114]

Considering the wide range in physician payments and outcome measures, there is opportunity for improvement through the emulation of evidence-based best practices. Much of the choice regarding implant is based on physician preferences and hospital factors rather than patient characteristics.[93] Through a sole source agreement with a vendor, the Reno Orthopaedic Clinic was able to obtain a 30% discount on implants, allowing 100% attainment of the surgical cost-saving target.[11] Another group at the New York University Hospital for Joint Diseases implemented implant price standardization, reducing intersurgeon variation in implant costs.[115] Average implant cost decreased by $876 for total hip arthroplasties and $1042 for total knee arthroplasties, resulting in more than $2 million in savings in the initial year of the program.[115] The orthopedic group at Lahey Hospital & Medical Center in Massachusetts took advantage of the spirit of bundled contracts to parlay that into bundled negotiations with its implant vendors to supply all of the instruments, implants, and disposable tools required for an orthopedic surgery at a preset price.[116] Through this program, implant costs were decreased by 32% and 23% for total hip arthroplasties and total knee arthroplasties, respectively.[116]

Many of the facilities participating in bundled payment models obtained a large proportion of their cost savings due to shifting of discharge disposition from expensive inpatient rehabilitation and SNFs to home health care services and home self-care.[9,11,27,117–122] PAC costs can also be reduced through improved patient education regarding options of discharge facilities, earlier follow-up with the surgeon, and daily, rather than weekly, evaluation of readiness for discharge.[11] Establishing well-defined clinical PAC pathways after TJAs are also integral in efforts to reduce episode cost and PAC resource utilization.[105]

SUMMARY

With the rapidly inflating costs and projected increase in demand for health care services, identifying novel payment strategies that reward value rather than volume are critical. TJAs are ideal services for early implementation of APMs due to their variation in payments and quality, capability for standardization and reproducibility, and large case volume. Migrating from an FFS payment system to bundled contracts is estimated to result in a 10% decrease in health care spending and a 5% to 15% reduction in the utilization of services.[123]

In the first 21 months of the BPCI initiative, participating hospitals reduced their payments to Medicare compared with nonparticipating hospitals, with no significant differences in quality measures.[118] Many provider organizations have implemented bundled payment systems, with a majority successfully reducing costs, primarily through decreases in PAC expenditures.

The early success of CMS' bundled payment models provides an opportunity for private payers to collaborate with hospitals to negotiate their own bundled contracts that can mutually advantageous. Implementation of bundles without thorough financial analysis of the incorporated terms can be detrimental to the potential for profitability and feasibility of the system, yet successful integration can promote improved economic and quality outcomes, while fostering a culture of collaboration and accountability among providers.

REFERENCES

1. Williams SN, Wolford ML, Bercovitz A. Hospitalization for total knee replacement among inpatients aged 45 and over: United States, 2000–2010. Hyattsville (MD): National Center for Health Statistics; 2015.

2. Wolford ML, Paslo K, Bercovitz A. Hospitalization for total hip replacement among inpatients aged 45 and over: United States, 2000–2010. Hyattsville (MD): National Center for Health Statistics; 2015.

3. Odum S, Van Doren B, Curtin B, et al. Projections for total joint arthroplasty demand for the next generation. Value Health 2016;19(3):A86.

4. Centers for Medicare and Medicaid Services. Comprehensive care for joint replacement model. 2017. Available at: https://innovation.cms.gov/initiatives/cjr. Accessed February 6, 2017.

5. Matlock D, Earnest M, Epstein A. Utilization of elective hip and knee arthroplasty by age and payer. Clin Orthop Relat Res 2008;466(4):914–9.

6. Laugesen MJ, Glied SA. Higher fees paid to US physicians drive higher spending for physician services compared to other countries. Health Aff 2011;30(9):1647–56.

7. Shatto JD. Center for medicare and medicaid innovation's methodology and calculations for the 2016 estimate of fee-for-service payments to

alternative payment models [press release]. Baltimore (MD): Centers for Medicare and Medicaid Services; 2016.

8. The Lewin Group. CMS bundled payments for care improvement intiative models 2-4: year 2 evaluation & monitoring annual report. Baltimore (MD): Centers for Medicare and Medicaid Services; 2016.

9. Iorio R, Bosco J, Slover J, et al. Single institution early experience with the bundled payments for care improvement initiative. J Bone Joint Surg Am 2017;99(1):e2.

10. El-Othmani MM, Sayeed Z, Ramsey J, et al. Medicare's bundle payment for care improvement initiative model 2: the Joint Utilization Management Program (JUMP) Experience. J Arthroplasty. [E-pub ahead of Print].

11. Althausen PL, Mead L. Bundled payments for care improvement: lessons learned in the first year. J Orthop Trauma 2016;30:S50–3.

12. Navathe AS, Troxel AB, Liao JM, et al. Cost of joint replacement using bundled payment models. JAMA Intern Med 2017;177(2):214–22.

13. Das D. Impact of changes in Medicare payments on the financial condition of nonprofit hospitals. J Health Care Finance 2013;40(1):11–39.

14. PricewaterhouseCoopers. Strategy& annual bundles survey - 2015/2016 results: hospitals, employers, and consumers. New York: PwC; 2016.

15. Kamath AF, Courtney PM, Bozic KJ, et al. Bundled payment in total joint care: survey of AAHKS membership attitudes and experience with alternative payment models. J Arthroplasty 2015; 30(12):2045–56.

16. Froimson MI, Rana A, White RE, et al. Bundled payments for care improvement initiative: the next evolution of payment formulations: AAHKS Bundled Payment Task Force. J Arthroplasty 2013;28(8):157–65.

17. Tian W. An all-payer view of hospital discharge to postacute care, 2013. In: HCUP statistical brief 205. Rockville (MD): Agency for Healthcare Research and Quality; 2016. Available at: http://www.hcup-us.ahrq.gov/reports/statbriefs/sb205-Hospital-Discharge-Postacute-Care.pdf.

18. Chandra A, Dalton MA, Holmes J. Large increases in spending on postacute care in medicare point to the potential for cost savings in these settings. Health Aff 2013;32(5):864–72.

19. IMPAQ International LLC, Urdapilleta O, Weinberg D, et al. Evaluation of the medicare acute care episode (ACE) demonstration - Final evaluation report. Baltimore (MD): Centers for Medicare and Medicaid Services; 2013.

20. Dobson A, DaVanzo JE, Heath S, et al. Medicare payment bundling: insights from claims data and

policy implications. Vienna (VA): Dobson DaVanzo & Associates, LLC; 2012.

21. Lavernia CJ, D'Apuzzo MR, Hernandez VH, et al. Postdischarge costs in arthroplasty surgery. J Arthroplasty 2006;21(6):144–50.

22. Bini SA, Fithian DC, Paxton LW, et al. Does discharge disposition after primary total joint arthroplasty affect readmission rates? J Arthroplasty 2010;25(1): 114–7.

23. Buntin MB, Deb P, Escarce J, et al. Comparison of medicare spending and outcomes for beneficiaries with lower extremity joint replacements. Arlington (VA): RAND Health; 2005.

24. Luft HS. Economic incentives to promote innovation in healthcare delivery. Clin Orthop Relat Res 2009;467(10):2497–505.

25. Sood N, Huckfeldt PJ, Escarce JJ, et al. Medicare's bundled payment pilot for acute and post-acute care: analysis and recommendations on where to begin. Health Aff 2011;30(9):1708–17.

26. Kivlahan C, Orlowski JM, Pearce J, et al. Taking risk: early results from teaching hospitals' participation in the Center for Medicare and Medicaid Innovation Bundled Payments for Care Improvement Initiative. Acad Med 2016;91(7):936–42.

27. Doran JP, Zabinski SJ. Bundled payment initiatives for Medicare and non-Medicare total joint arthroplasty patients at a community hospital: bundles in the real world. J Arthroplasty 2015; 30(3):353–5.

28. Bosco JA, Karkenny AJ, Hutzler LH, et al. Cost burden of 30-day readmissions following Medicare total hip and knee arthroplasty. J Arthroplasty 2014;29(5):903–5.

29. Schairer WW, Sing DC, Vail TP, et al. Causes and frequency of unplanned hospital readmission after total hip arthroplasty. Clin Orthop Relat Res 2014; 472(2):464–70.

30. Schairer WW, Vail TP, Bozic KJ. What are the rates and causes of hospital readmission after total knee arthroplasty? Clin Orthop Relat Res 2014; 472(1):181–7.

31. Cram P, Lu X, Kaboli PJ, et al. Clinical characteristics and outcomes of Medicare patients undergoing total hip arthroplasty, 1991-2008. JAMA 2011; 305(15):1560–7.

32. Fehring TK, Odum SM, Griffin WL, et al. The obesity epidemic: its effect on total joint arthroplasty. J Arthroplasty 2007;22(6):71–6.

33. Belmont PJ, Goodman GP, Waterman BR, et al. Thirty-day postoperative complications and mortality following total knee arthroplasty. J Bone Joint Surg Am 2014;96(1):20–6.

34. Cholewinski P, Putman S, Vasseur L, et al. Long-term outcomes of primary constrained condylar knee arthroplasty. Orthop Traumatol Surg Res 2015;101(4):449–54.

35. Bozic KJ, Grosso LM, Lin Z, et al. Variation in hospital-level risk-standardized complication rates following elective primary total hip and knee arthroplasty. J Bone Joint Surg 2014;96(8):640–7.

36. Plate JF, Brown ML, Wohler AD, et al. Patient factors and cost associated with 90-day readmission following total hip arthroplasty. J Arthroplasty 2016;31(1):49–52.

37. Pulido L, Parvizi J, Macgibeny M, et al. In hospital complications after total joint arthroplasty. J Arthroplasty 2008;23(6):139–45.

38. Courtney PM, Huddleston JI, Iorio R, et al. Socioeconomic risk adjustment models for reimbursement are necessary in primary total joint arthroplasty. J Arthroplasty 2017;32(1):1–5.

39. Bradley BM, Griffiths SN, Stewart KJ, et al. The effect of obesity and increasing age on operative time and length of stay in primary hip and knee arthroplasty. J Arthroplasty 2014;29(10):1906–10.

40. Tayne S, Merrill CA, Smith EL, et al. Predictive risk factors for 30-day readmissions following primary total joint arthroplasty and modification of patient management. J Arthroplasty 2014;29(10):1938–42.

41. SooHoo NF, Li Z, Chan V, et al. The importance of risk adjustment in reporting total joint arthroplasty outcomes. J Arthroplasty 2016;31(3):590–5.

42. Everhart JS, Altneu E, Calhoun JH. Medical comorbidities are independent preoperative risk factors for surgical infection after total joint arthroplasty. Clin Orthop Relat Res 2013; 471(10):3112–9.

43. Kremers HM, Kremers WK, Berry DJ, et al. Social and behavioral factors in total knee and hip arthroplasty. J Arthroplasty 2015;30(10):1852–4.

44. Alfargieny R, Bodalal Z, Bendardaf R, et al. Nutritional status as a predictive marker for surgical site infection in total joint arthroplasty. Avicenna J Med 2015;5(4):117.

45. Hansen CA, Inacio MC, Pratt NL, et al. Chronic use of opioids before and after total knee arthroplasty: a retrospective cohort study. J Arthroplasty 2017; 32(3):811–7.e1.

46. Best MJ, Buller LT, Gosthe RG, et al. Alcohol misuse is an independent risk factor for poorer postoperative outcomes following primary total hip and total knee arthroplasty. J Arthroplasty 2015;30(8):1293–8.

47. Rosas S, Sabeh KG, Buller LT, et al. Medical comorbidities impact the episode-of-care reimbursements of total hip arthroplasty. J Arthroplasty 2017;32(7):2082–7.

48. Bozic KJ, Ward L, Vail TP, et al. Bundled payments in total joint arthroplasty: targeting opportunities for quality improvement and cost reduction. Clin Orthop Relat Res 2014;472(1):188–93.

49. Ellimoottil C, Ryan AM, Hou H, et al. Medicare's new bundled payment for joint replacement may

penalize hospitals that treat medically complex patients. Health Aff (Millwood) 2016;35(9):1651–7.

50. Painter MW, Burns ME, Bailit MH. Bundled payment across the US today: status of implementations and operational findings. Newtown (CT): Health Care Incentives Improvement Institute; 2012.

51. Rozell JC, Courtney PM, Dattilo JR, et al. Should all patients be included in alternative payment models for primary total hip arthroplasty and total knee arthroplasty? J Arthroplasty 2016;31(9):45–9.

52. Bjorgul K, Novicoff WM, Saleh KJ. Evaluating comorbidities in total hip and knee arthroplasty: available instruments. J Orthop Traumatol 2010; 11(4):203–9.

53. Meneghini RM, Ziemba-Davis M, Ishmael MK, et al. Safe selection of outpatient joint arthroplasty patients with medical risk stratification: the "outpatient arthroplasty risk assessment score". J Arthroplasty 2017;32(8):2325–31.

54. Iorio R, Boraiah S, Inneh I, et al. A readmission risk assessment tool to manage modifiable risk factors prior to primary hip and knee arthroplasty. Bone Joint J 2016;98(Supp 9):44.

55. van Walraven C, Dhalla IA, Bell C, et al. Derivation and validation of an index to predict early death or unplanned readmission after discharge from hospital to the community. Can Med Assoc J 2010;182(6):551–7.

56. Tzeng A, Tzeng TH, Vasdev S, et al. The role of patient activation in achieving better outcomes and cost-effectiveness in patient care. JBJS Rev 2015;3(1):e4.

57. Greene J, Hibbard JH. Why does patient activation matter? An examination of the relationships between patient activation and health-related outcomes. J Gen Intern Med 2012;27(5):520–6.

58. Hibbard JH, Greene J, Overton V. Patients with lower activation associated with higher costs; delivery systems should know their patients''scores'. Health Aff 2013;32(2):216–22.

59. DeFroda S, Rubin L, Jenkins D. Modifiable risk factors in total joint arthroplasty: a pilot study. R I Med J (2013) 2015;99(5):28–31.

60. Botella-Carretero JI, Iglesias B, Balsa JA, et al. Perioperative oral nutritional supplements in normally or mildly undernourished geriatric patients submitted to surgery for hip fracture: a randomized clinical trial. Clin Nutr 2010;29(5): 574–9.

61. Lindström D, Azodi OS, Wladis A, et al. Effects of a perioperative smoking cessation intervention on postoperative complications: a randomized trial. Ann Surg 2008;248(5):739–45.

62. Snow R, Granata J, Ruhil AV, et al. Associations between preoperative physical therapy and post-acute care utilization patterns and cost in

total joint replacement. J Bone Joint Surg Am 2014;96(19):e165.

63. Hejblum G, Atsou K, Dautzenberg B, et al. Cost-benefit analysis of a simulated institution-based preoperative smoking cessation intervention in patients undergoing total hip and knee arthroplasties in France. Chest 2009;135(2):477–83.

64. Nam D, Nunley RM, Johnson SR, et al. The effectiveness of a risk stratification protocol for thromboembolism prophylaxis after hip and knee arthroplasty. J Arthroplasty 2016;31(6):1299–306.

65. Zywiel MG, Stroh DA, Lee SY, et al. Chronic opioid use prior to total knee arthroplasty. J Bone Joint Surg Am 2011;93(21):1988–93.

66. Sing DC, Barry JJ, Cheah JW, et al. Long-acting opioid use independently predicts perioperative complication in total joint arthroplasty. J Arthroplasty 2016;31(9):170–4.e1.

67. Zarling BJ, Yokhana SS, Herzog DT, et al. Preoperative and postoperative opiate use by the arthroplasty patient. J Arthroplasty 2016;31(10):2081–4.

68. Bedard NA, Pugely AJ, Westermann RW, et al. Opioid use after total knee arthroplasty: trends and risk factors for prolonged use. J Arthroplasty 2017;32(8):2390–4.

69. Rozell JC, Courtney PM, Dattilo JR, et al. Preoperative opiate use independently predicts narcotic consumption and complications after total joint arthroplasty. J Arthroplasty 2017;32(9):2658–62.

70. Smith SR, Bido J, Collins JE, et al. Impact of preoperative opioid use on total knee arthroplasty outcomes. J Bone Joint Surg Am 2017;99(10): 803–8.

71. Aasvang EK, Lunn TH, Hansen T, et al. Chronic pre-operative opioid use and acute pain after fast-track total knee arthroplasty. Acta Anaesthesiol Scand 2016;60(4):529–36.

72. Chan FJ, Schwartz AM, Wong J, et al. Use of chronic methadone before total knee arthroplasty. J Arthroplasty 2017;32(7):2105–7.

73. Nguyen LCL, Sing DC, Bozic KJ. Preoperative reduction of opioid use before total joint arthroplasty. J Arthroplasty 2016;31(9):282–7.

74. Liu W, Wahafu T, Cheng M, et al. The influence of obesity on primary total hip arthroplasty outcomes: a meta-analysis of prospective cohort studies. Orthop Traumatol Surg Res 2015;101(3): 289–96.

75. Springer BD, Parvizi J, Austin M, et al. Obesity and total joint arthroplasty a literature based review. J Arthroplasty 2013;28(5):714–21.

76. Kremers HM, Visscher SL, Kremers WK, et al. Obesity increases length of stay and direct medical costs in total hip arthroplasty. Clin Orthop Relat Res 2014;472(4):1232–9.

77. Kremers HM, Visscher SL, Kremers WK, et al. The effect of obesity on direct medical costs in total

knee arthroplasty. J Bone Joint Surg Am 2014; 96(9):718–24.

78. Odum SM, Springer BD, Dennos AC, et al. National obesity trends in total knee arthroplasty. J Arthroplasty 2013;28(8):148–51.

79. Nickel BT, Klement MR, Penrose CT, et al. Lingering risk: bariatric surgery before total knee arthroplasty. J Arthroplasty 2016;31(9):207–11.

80. Inacio MC, Paxton EW, Fisher D, et al. Bariatric surgery prior to total joint arthroplasty may not provide dramatic improvements in post-arthroplasty surgical outcomes. J Arthroplasty 2014;29(7):1359–64.

81. Martin J, Watts C, Taunton M. Bariatric surgery does not improve outcomes in patients undergoing primary total knee arthroplasty. Bone Joint J 2015;97(11):1501–5.

82. Healy WL, Rana AJ, Iorio R. Hospital economics of primary total knee arthroplasty at a teaching hospital. Clin Orthop Relat Res 2011;469(1): 87–94.

83. Cram P, Lu X, Li Y. Bundled payments for elective primary total knee arthroplasty an analysis of medicare administrative data. Geriatr Orthop Surg Rehabil 2015;6(1):3–10.

84. Cromwell J, Dayhoff DA, McCall NT, et al. Medicare Participating Heart Bypass Center Demonstration. Baltimore (MD): Centers for Medicare and Medicaid Services; 1998.

85. Ridgely MS, De Vries D, Bozic KJ, et al. Bundled payment fails to gain a foothold in California: the experience of the IHA bundled payment demonstration. Health Aff 2014;33(8):1345–52.

86. Clair AJ, Evangelista PJ, Lajam CM, et al. Cost analysis of total joint arthroplasty readmissions in a bundled payment care improvement initiative. J Arthroplasty 2016;31(9):1862–5.

87. González-Vélez A, Romero-Martín M, Villanueva-Orbalz R, et al. The cost of infection in hip arthroplasty: a matched case–control study. Rev Esp Cir Ortop Traumatol 2016;60(4):227–33.

88. Hustedt JW, Goltzer O, Bohl DD, et al. Calculating the cost and risk of comorbidities in total joint arthroplasty in the United States. J Arthroplasty 2017;32(2):355–61.e1.

89. Centers for Medicare and Medicaid Services. CARE item set and B-CARE. 2015. Available at: https://www.cms.gov/Medicare/Quality-Initiatives-Patient-Assessment-Instruments/Post-Acute-Care-Quality-Initiatives/CARE-Item-Set-and-B-CARE.html. Accessed February 6, 2017.

90. Ejaz A, Gani F, Kim Y, et al. Variation in inpatient hospital and physician payments among patients undergoing general versus orthopedic operations. Surgery 2016;160(6):1657–65.

91. Kremers HM, Visscher SL, Moriarty JP, et al. Determinants of direct medical costs in primary and revision total knee arthroplasty. Clin Orthop Relat Res 2013;471(1):206–14.

92. Meyers SJ, Reuben JD, Cox DD, et al. Inpatient cost of primary total joint arthroplasty. J Arthroplasty 1996;11(3):281–5.

93. Robinson JC, Pozen A, Tseng S, et al. Variability in costs associated with total hip and knee replacement implants. J Bone Joint Surg Am 2012; 94(18):1693–8.

94. Belatti DA, Pugely AJ, Phisitkul P, et al. Total joint arthroplasty: trends in Medicare reimbursement and implant prices. J Arthroplasty 2014;29(8): 1539–44.

95. Gioe TJ, Sharma A, Tatman P, et al. Do "premium" joint implants add value?: analysis of high cost joint implants in a community registry. Clin Orthop Relat Res 2011;469(1):48–54.

96. Clement RC, Derman PB, Graham DS, et al. Risk factors, causes, and the economic implications of unplanned readmissions following total hip arthroplasty. J Arthroplasty 2013;28(8):7–10.

97. Lavernia CJ, Villa JM. Readmission rates in total hip arthroplasty: a granular analysis? J Arthroplasty 2015;30(7):1127–31.

98. Hatz D, Anoushiravani AA, Chambers MC, et al. Approach to decrease infection following total joint arthroplasty. Orthop Clin North Am 2016; 47(4):661–71.

99. Huddleston JM, Long KH, Naessens JM, et al. Medical and surgical comanagement after elective hip and knee arthroplasty a randomized, controlled trial. Ann Intern Med 2004;141(1): 28–38.

100. Klingenstein G, Jain R, Schoifet S, et al. Rapid recovery protocol for primary total knee arthroplasty reduces length of stay and decreases hospital readmissions in a community setting. Bone Joint J 2016;98(Supp 8):109.

101. Stambough JB, Nunley RM, Curry MC, et al. Rapid recovery protocols for primary total hip arthroplasty can safely reduce length of stay without increasing readmissions. J Arthroplasty 2015; 30(4):521–6.

102. Flickinger M, Kates L, Shawna G. Project RED: a transformation approach to post-discharge care. Population Health Matters (Formerly Health Policy Newsletter) 2011;24(1):2.

103. Welsh RL, Graham JE, Karmarkar AM, et al. Effects of postacute settings on readmission rates and reasons for readmission following total knee arthroplasty. J Am Med Dir Assoc 2017;18(4):367.e1–10.

104. Ramos NL, Karia RJ, Hutzler LH, et al. The effect of discharge disposition on 30-day readmission rates after total joint arthroplasty. J Arthroplasty 2014; 29(4):674–7.

105. Tessier JE, Rupp G, Gera JT, et al. Physicians with defined clear care pathways have better discharge

disposition and lower cost. J Arthroplasty 2016; 31(9):54–8.

106. Slover JD, Mullaly KA, Payne A, et al. What is the Best strategy to minimize after-care costs for total joint arthroplasty in a bundled payment environment? J Arthroplasty 2016;31(12):2710–3.

107. Losina E, Walensky RP, Kessler CL, et al. Cost-effectiveness of total knee arthroplasty in the United States: patient risk and hospital volume. Arch Intern Med 2009;169(12):1113.

108. Katz JN, Losina E, Barrett J, et al. Association between hospital and surgeon procedure volume and outcomes of total hip replacement in the United States Medicare population. J Bone Joint Surg Am 2001;83(11):1622–9.

109. Katz JN, Barrett J, Mahomed NN, et al. Association between hospital and surgeon procedure volume and the outcomes of total knee replacement. J Bone Joint Surg Am 2004;86(9):1909–16.

110. Robinow A. The potential of global payment: insights from the field. New York: Commonwealth Fund; 2010.

111. Elbuluk AM, O'Neill OR. Private bundles: the nuances of contracting and managing total joint arthroplasty episodes. J Arthroplasty 2017;32(6): 1720–2.

112. van Kasteren ME, Mannien J, Ott A, et al. Antibiotic prophylaxis and the risk of surgical site infections following total hip arthroplasty: timely administration is the most important factor. Clin Infect Dis 2007;44(7):921–7.

113. Radcliff KE, Orozco FR, Quinones D, et al. Preoperative risk stratification reduces the incidence of perioperative complications after total knee arthroplasty. J Arthroplasty 2012;27(8):77–80.e1-8.

114. Jencks SF, Williams MV, Coleman EA. Rehospitalizations among patients in the Medicare fee-for-service program. N Engl J Med 2009;360(14): 1418–28.

115. Bosco JA, Alvarado CM, Slover JD, et al. Decreasing total joint implant costs and physician specific cost variation through negotiation. J Arthroplasty 2014;29(4):678–80.

116. Healy WL, Iorio R, Lemos MJ, et al. Single price/case price purchasing in orthopaedic surgery: experience at the Lahey Clinic. J Bone Joint Surg 2000;82(5):607–12.

117. Bolz NJ, Iorio R. Bundled payments: our experience at an Academic Medical Center. J Arthroplasty 2016;31(5):932–5.

118. Dummit LA, Kahvecioglu D, Marrufo G, et al. Association between hospital participation in a Medicare bundled payment initiative and payments and quality outcomes for lower extremity joint replacement episodes. JAMA 2016;316(12): 1267–78.

119. Dundon JM, Bosco J, Slover J, et al. Improvement in total joint replacement quality metrics. J Bone Joint Surg Am 2016;98(23):1949–53.

120. Froemke CC, Wang L, DeHart ML, et al. Standardizing care and improving quality under a bundled payment initiative for total joint arthroplasty. J Arthroplasty 2015;30(10):1676–82.

121. Iorio R. Strategies and tactics for successful implementation of bundled payments: bundled payment for care improvement at a large, urban, Academic Medical Center. J Arthroplasty 2015; 30(3):349–50.

122. Iorio R, Clair AJ, Inneh IA, et al. Early results of Medicare's bundled payment initiative for a 90-day total joint arthroplasty episode of care. J Arthroplasty 2016;31(2):343–50.

123. Hussey P, Mulcahy A, Schnyer C, et al. Closing the Quality Gap: Revisiting the State of the Science (Vol. 1: Bundled Payment: Effects on Health Care Spending and Quality). Rockville (MD): Agency for Healthcare Research and Quality; 2012.

Bundle Payment for Musculoskeletal Care
Current Evidence (Part 2)

Meghan A. Piccinin, MSc[a], Zain Sayeed, MD, MHA[b,*],
Ryan Kozlowski, MD[c], Vamsy Bobba, MD[c],
David Knesek, DO[c], Todd Frush, MD[c]

KEYWORDS

- Total joint arthroplasty • Total knee arthroplasty • Bundle payments • Bundled contracts • BPCI
- Comprehensive care for joint replacement • Private payers

KEY POINTS

- In general, orthopedic groups that elected to implement Model 2 of the Centers for Medicare and Medicaid Services' (CMS) Bundled Payments for Care Improvement (BPCI) program realized significant reductions in medical costs without deterioration in the quality of care.
- Bundled contracts between orthopedic groups and private payer organizations have demonstrated initial successes in reducing expenditures and improving outcome measures.
- The advantages realized through both the CMS's and private payers' experimentation with bundled payments are likely to be succeeded by further implementation of bundled reimbursement models.
- Before entering into a bundled contract, it is important to weigh the potential benefits of such an arrangement against the possible risks and barriers to implementation in order to determine if bundled reimbursement is a viable model for a specific institution.

INTRODUCTION

Total hip arthroplasty (THA) and total knee arthroplasty (TKA) are among the most commonly performed surgical procedures in the United States, with approximately 300,000 THA and 700,000 TKA procedures performed annually and a high patient satisfaction rate.[1–3] Although the annual number of the procedures has undergone significant growth since 1990, the number of lower extremity total joint arthroplasty (TJA) procedures performed is anticipated to increase exponentially through 2021 and beyond.[4–6] Most TJAs are reimbursed by the Centers for Medicare and Medicaid Services (CMS), with these procedures comprising the largest proportion of inpatient surgical procedures for Medicare beneficiaries.[5,7]

Despite its ubiquity, TJA is plagued by wide variations in cost and quality.[8–16] With such a vast volume of cases being performed annually, even a small global reduction in individual episode costs could yield a substantial financial impact on national health care resource consumption. The traditional fee-for-service (FFS) model used by various payers incentivizes the quantity of services provided, with less focus on the quality or cost of care, which may lead

---

Funding Sources: No additional funding sources were used for this article.
Conflicts of Interest: No conflicts of interest are evident for the authors of this article.
[a] College of Osteopathic Medicine, Michigan State University, Detroit Medical Center, 4707 St Antoine Street, Detroit, MI 48201, USA; [b] Department of Orthopaedics, Institute of Innovations and Clinical Excellence, Detroit Medical Center, 4201 St Antoine Street, Detroit, MI 48201, USA; [c] Department of Orthopaedics, Musculoskeletal Institute of Surgical Excellence, Detroit Medical Center, 4201 St Antoine Street, Detroit, MI 48201, USA
* Corresponding author.
E-mail address: zainsayeed@gmail.com

Orthop Clin N Am 49 (2018) 147–156
https://doi.org/10.1016/j.ocl.2017.11.003

to fragmented care with poor coordination and collaboration between stakeholders involved in care delivery.[17] With the anticipated forthcoming surge in demand for TJA, it has become imperative to overhaul Medicare's FFS payment system in favor of novel models that promote higher quality with simultaneous cost saving by hospitals and individual providers.

The CMS has already successfully transitioned more than 30% of payments from FFS to an alternative payment model (APM), with the goal of increasing this to 50% by 2018.[18,19] Of particular interest as an APM is bundled payment reimbursement models, which provide all necessary care required by patients during a defined episode of care over a specified duration for a predetermine price, rather than billing for discrete procedures and visits.[20] Optimistic estimates suggest that implementation of bundled payment systems could result in a 5.4% reduction in national health care spending.[21]

TJA represents the ideal procedure for bundling because of the significant variation in price and quality, potential for standardization and reproducibility, and high volume. The inconsistency in the CMS' disbursements and quality measures for TJA demonstrates that there is great potential for cost reductions through the emulation of best practices and care coordination.[22] The clear, evidence-based guidelines for TJA allow for accurate assessment of outcomes, which can provide guidance for distributing payments. Additionally, the large volume of procedures performed annually allows for the potential of a substantial savings margin, making the administrative costs of implementing an innovative payment model worthwhile. In this review, the authors assess the current economic and quality outcomes of various bundle payment programs for TJA and outline a financial analysis strategy for use in the negotiation of bundled contracts.

CENTERS FOR MEDICARE AND MEDICAID SERVICES' IMPLEMENTATION OF BUNDLED CONTRACTS

In 2011, the CMS instituted the Bundled Payments for Care Improvement (BPCI) initiative for several Medicare Severity-Diagnosis Related Groups (MS-DRGs) to test novel care delivery models aiming at reducing Medicare expenses while maintaining or improving the quality of care.[23] The episodes of care that BPCI participants were able to choose from included both MS-DRG 469 (major joint replacement or

reattachment of lower extremity with major complication or comorbidity) and MS-DRG 470 (major joint replacement or reattachment of lower extremity without major complication or comorbidity).[17] Providers voluntarily elected to participate in the initiative, selecting from 3 retrospective models and one prospective model outlined in Table 1.[17] Any cost savings realized less than the target price were to be shared among the providers, whereas expenditures in excess of the target price required repayment to Medicare. Ongoing outcome measures are monitored under BPCI, although there is no defined threshold for quality of care.[24]

Based on the preliminary results of the BPCI initiative, in April 2016, the CMS further implemented the Comprehensive Care for Joint Replacement Model (CJR) for TJA at 800 hospitals in 75 metropolitan statistical areas (MSA), excluding BPCI-participating hospitals.[25] The aim of this initiative was to support more efficient, high-quality care in TJA for Medicare beneficiaries while shifting from historical pricing to MSA-specific geographic pricing.[25,26] Although similar to the BPCI initiative, there are several important distinguishing features (Table 2).[24,25] Under the CJR, an episode of care begins with the admission of a Medicare beneficiary for an MS-DRG 469 or 470 to a

Table 1	
Medicare reimbursement schedules under the voluntary Bundled Payments for Care Improvement initiative	
Models	**Coverage**
Model 1	Retrospective payment covering acute inpatient hospital admission only
Model 2	Retrospective payment covering acute inpatient hospital stay & certain postdischarge care
Model 3	Retrospective payment covering 30 d of postdischarge care, excluding the acute inpatient hospital admission
Model 4	Prospective payment covering acute inpatient hospital admission only

BPCI-participating hospitals selected from one of 4 retrospective or prospective payment models. Most hospitals participating in the orthopedic surgery bundled payments elected to implement Model 2.[23]

Data from Centers for Medicare and Medicaid Services (CMS). Bundled payments for care improvement (BPCI) initiative: general information. Available at: https://innovation.cms.gov/initiatives/bundled-payments/ . Accessed January 30, 2017.

Table 2
Comparison of the bundled payments instituted under Centers for Medicare and Medicaid Services' Bundled Payments for Care Improvement and Comprehensive Care for Joint Replacement Model initiatives

	BPCI	CJR
Location	National	75 metropolitan statistical areas
Duration	3 y	5 y
Participation	Voluntary	Involuntary
Episodes	48 unique episode types	THA & TKA
Episode duration	30, 60, or 90 d	90 d
CMS discount	2% for 90-d bundles 3% for 30- or 60-d bundles	3% initially, increased or decreased based on quality score
Regional price variation	No	Yes
Risk adjustment	Based on MS-DRG	Based on MS-DRG & hip fracture status
Stop-gain limits	20%	0% (y 1), 5% (y 2), 10% (y 3), 20% (y 4–5)
Stop-loss limits	20%	0% (y 1), 5% (y 2), 10% (y 3), 20% (y 4–5)
Reconciliation	Quarterly	Annually
Quality measures	Monitored	Required for reconciliation payments

CJR is a mandatory program implemented in metropolitan hospitals for TJA only. Bundle payments vary with MS-DRG, hip fracture status, and geographic location and are reconciled annually. In order to be eligible for reconciliation payments, hospitals must meet a standard minimum quality threshold. There are also progressive stop-loss and stop-gain limits in place in the early years of the program.

Used with permission of American Hospital Association. Mechanic R. Medicare's Bundled Payment Initiatives: Considerations for Providers. © 2016 American Hospital Association. Available at: http://www.aha.org/content/16/issbrief-bundledpmt.pdf.

participating hospital and covers all related Medicare Part A and B expenses through 90 days after discharge.[25] Medicare determines target episode prices, including allowances for geographic variation and risk stratification within each diagnostic category.[25] Providers are compensated under the traditional FFS system for services rendered throughout the model year, which are then reconciled against the preset episode price for each hospital.[25] As with the BPCI model, any discrepancies between expected and actual expenditures are either rendered to the hospital or required to be repaid to the CMS.[25] As a condition of participation in this program, a minimum quality standard must be obtained in order to qualify for reconciliatory CMS payments.[24] Through a 5-year testing period, the CJR is expected to result in $343 million in savings to Medicare expenditures.[25]

BUNDLED PAYMENTS IN PRACTICE

Following their experiences with the BPCI and CJR initiatives, several orthopedic groups published the outcome of the implementation of bundled payments in their practices. In the following section, the authors discuss the early results various hospital groups have achieved under bundled reimbursement schemes.

Large-Scale Evaluation of Bundled Payments for Care Improvement at Multiple Hospitals

An overarching evaluation of the CMS's BPCI program through its second year in practice was prepared by The Lewin Group.[23] In this detailed report, the results of the various models for each broad MS-DRG category were assessed and analyzed. Because most of the hospitals participating in orthopedic bundles elected to implement Model 2, the results of that system are the focus of this discussion. At the national level, 82 hospitals participated in orthopedic surgery episodes under Model 2 for a total of 18,936 procedures, with 90% of these falling under MS-DRG 469 and 470. BPCI-participating hospitals were able to realize a 3% greater reduction in total Medicare expenditures through 90 days after discharge in comparison with nonparticipating facilities. These savings were achieved through changes in post–acute care (PAC) utilization, with shorter average stays in skilled nursing facilities (SNFs) and decreased discharge to institutional PAC settings. Importantly, these changes were not accompanied by any deviation in quality metrics, including

30- and 90-day readmissions, or emergency department visits, or 30-day mortality.

Dummit and colleagues[27] evaluated CMS payments using Medicare claims data and assessed utilization and quality from initial hospitalization up to 90 days after discharge in 31,700 BPCI episodes with MS-DRG 469 or 470 from October 2013 to June 2015 in comparison with pre-BPCI episodes and nonparticipating institutions. Although payments to both BPCI-participating and nonparticipating hospitals declined over the study period, payments to participating hospitals were on average $1166 lower than those to nonparticipating programs. Corroborating the results of The Lewin Group, most of the reduction in payments stemmed from the decreased utilization of institutional PAC in the postdischarge period, with no differences in 30- and 90-day quality measures.

Kivlahan and colleagues[28] reported the experiences of 19 academic institutions in the implementation of the 90-day BPCI Model 2 for major joint replacements, including hip fractures. The utilization of TJA bundles at the 19 hospitals in the study resulted in more than $4.5 million in savings for CMS ($4200 per episode). These savings were accomplished primarily through redirection of inpatient rehabilitation discharges to less costly alternatives, such as SNFs and home health agencies. Interestingly, bundles for other procedural groupings, such as percutaneous coronary intervention, stroke, and spinal fusion, incurred losses for Medicare.

Individual Institution Experiences with Centers for Medicare and Medicaid Services Bundles

Through several published reports, the experience of the specialized Hospital for Joint Diseases at the New York University Langone Medical Center with bundled payments has been well-documented. The Langone Medical Center elected to participate in the 90-day BPCI Model 2 for MS-DRG 469 and 470.[26,29–31] To ensure successful implementation, the group focused on several strategies to improve both quality and financial metrics. These improvements included preoperative risk factor management, patient education, standardization of clinical pathways, enhanced coordination of care, risk stratification and preventative protocols for major postoperative complications (such as venous thromboembolism and infection), emphasis on home discharge, and quality-dependent gainsharing among surgeons.[26,30,32] With 721 patients included in the first year of implementation, the institution

realized 8.1% cost savings for MS-DRG 469% and 17% for MS-DRG 470, with a concomitant 1.23-day decrease in hospital length of stay (LOS) and 41% reduction in discharge to inpatient rehabilitation facilities.[29,31] These improvements continued through to the third year of the program, generating a 20% decrease in 90-day episode costs relative to the first year of BPCI implementation, along with a decrease in 30-, 60-, and 90-day readmission rates.[30]

Currently under review, a report by El-Othmani and colleagues summarizes the experiences of the orthopedics group at the Detroit Medical Center (DMC) in their implementation of BPCI Model 2, covering care from the day of admission to 30 days after discharge for MS-DRG 469 and 470. (El-Othmani MM, Sayeed Z, Ramsey JnA, et al. Medicare's bundle payment for care improvement initiative model 2: the Joint Utilization Management Program (JUMP) Experience. J Arthroplasty. Submitted for publication.) With a primary focus on improving accountability and efficiency in postoperative care, the DMC's Joint Utilization Management Program (JUMP) was developed and instituted to optimize PAC utilization. JUMP established clear guidelines for determining the form of discharge and expectations for LOS in postacute rehabilitation facilities. PAC risk stratification was also used to predict the severity at discharge in order to establish a baseline for rehabilitation and optimize the transition between inpatient and postdischarge care and, hence, align providers in the in-hospital and PAC settings. The group also developed surgeon and PAC scorecards with annual target goals to follow patients' postoperative course, holding providers accountable for long-term outcomes. Over 2 years, 638 episodes of care were initiated under JUMP. This program was able to decrease the inpatient LOS by 1.21 days, decrease inpatient rehabilitation facility readmissions and LOS, increase home health care service utilization, and decrease 30-day readmission rates.

The Baptist Health System in San Antonio, Texas implemented BPCI Model 2 for 30-day episodes of care for MS-DRG 469 and 470. The 2017 study by Navathe and colleagues[33] discussed how bundled contracts instituted under BPCI and CMS's earlier Acute Care Episodes project (a voluntary bundled payment demonstration restricted to applicant hospitals in Texas, Oklahoma, New Mexico, and Colorado) affected quality, costs, and PAC spending over 3942 patient episodes. The group was successfully able to reduce Medicare expenditures by

13.8% for MS-DRG 469% and 20.8% for MS-DRG 470 episodes of care. Somewhat uniquely, most cost reductions came internally through decreases in implant costs, whereas 48.8% of the savings were achieved through lower spending on PAC. Quality measures were also improved, with a reduction in emergency department visits, readmissions, and proportion of episodes necessitating a prolonged LOS.

Althausen and Mead[34] published a report on the implementation of 90-day BPCI Model 2 at 5 hospitals under the Reno Orthopedic Clinic for 470 MS-DRG 469 and 470 as well as 176 MS-DRG 480, 481, and 482 (hip and femur procedures without major joint replacement). Despite sustaining $220,000 in implementation costs, the 5 hospitals were able to realize nearly $2,000,000 in savings over the 15-month intervention period, with an average of $1969 in savings for each TJA procedure. A gainsharing agreement allowed for a maximum disbursement of $492,442 based on these savings, although only $355,906 was available for gainsharing because of failure to achieve all quality targets. The source of these savings was primarily due to a decrease in implant costs and changes to PAC utilization, including a ranking system of SNFs, daily assessment of readiness for discharge, and earlier postoperative follow-up. Additional cost savings were realized through non-BPCI episodes of care due to the BPCI-implementation of algorithms, cost controls, and case management that positively benefited all patients.

A 2017 report by Edwards, Mears, and Barnes[35] chronicled the results of the orthopedic group at the University of Arkansas Medical Sciences following their implementation of 90-day BPCI Model 2 for 461 cases of MS-DRG 469 and 470.[35,36] During the 12-month program, the group realized a 14% decrease in costs per episode of care, primarily from reductions in PAC utilization, decreased LOS, and reduced readmission rates. Through these improvements, this group received a net CMS reconciliation payment of $1,012,962 for distribution among the participating physicians and facility. The investigators attributed their success under BPCI to the implementation of a standardized clinical pathway, price caps for implants, increased discharge to home, and mandatory preoperative education classes.

The experiences of BPCI implementation by North Carolina's OrthoCarolina group are discussed in a report by Curtin, Russell, and Odum.[37] Over the course of the 1-year program, 4757 Medicare patients underwent one of more than 20 orthopedic MS-DRG procedures bundled under BPCI Model 2. Relative to non-BPCI patients, the median expenditure per episode decreased from $22,193 to $19,472. Reductions in the readmission rate and PAC utilization largely contributed to these savings, with PAC costs declining by more than 21%.

Single-Institution Implementation of Private Bundled Contracts

Providence Health & Services in Portland, Oregon experimented with the implementation of a private payer bundled payment model for care of 317 instances of MS-DRG 469 or 470 from 30 days before surgery to 90 days postoperatively.[38] To optimize outcomes, the group implemented a standardized pathway that homogenizes patient care from the preoperative planning process to discharge and restricts direct costs by limiting the use of specific supplies and implants. A gainsharing agreement was also instituted, in which postreconciliatory savings are distributed based on obtaining Surgical Care Improvement Project and discharge disposition targets. These changes successfully reduced claims by 6%, decreased LOS by 18%, and shifted discharges from SNFs and home health care to home self-care. These targets were met while maintaining high patient satisfaction and a low mortality rate.

The experiences of a community hospital in bundle implementation have been presented by Doran and Zabinski[39] regarding the institution of a private payer bundled contract between Shore Orthopaedic University Associates and Horizon Healthcare Services of New Jersey. The group performs approximately 550 TJA annually, of which 55% are covered by Medicare. The episode period included in the coverage plan extended from 30 days before surgery to 90 days following discharge. Implementation of the bundled contract led to an increase in the number of TJA performed annually, alongside a $2262 reduction in the average cost per episode. The total cost savings over the 2-year program exceeded $524,000, with $262,445 in savings-based payments to the provider group. These savings were attributed to a decrease in inpatient LOS, a reduction in the use of nursing and inpatient rehabilitation facilities, lowered implant costs, and an improved readmission rate.

Whitcomb and colleagues[40] reported on the implementation of a private bundled contract in 2011 at Baystate Health in Springfield, Massachusetts for 45 episodes of elective THA procedures. The agreed on bundle was unique in that an episode was initiated at the time when a surgeon identified the need for a THA and covered services in support of that episode through the third postoperative visit, typically 10 to 14 weeks postoperatively, rather than a defined time frame. The plan also excluded coverage of postoperative complications. Efforts were made to begin postoperative physical therapy on postoperative day 0, reduce LOS to 2 days when appropriate, and discharge patients to home. Because of the pilot nature of this study, the hospitals and surgeons were protected from financial risk if costs exceeded the bundle price, although gainsharing of savings was permitted. Although median adjusted payments did not differ from the baseline, the project was successful in increasing the discharge to home, decreasing PAC expenditures, and improving adherence to care guidelines.

Blue Cross and Blue Shield of North Carolina (BCBSNC) partnered with Triangle Orthopaedic Associates (TOA) to implement bundled payment contracts for TKA in 2012 and THA in 2013, covering care from the inpatient period through 90 days postoperatively.[41] In the first year of the program, 100 bundled TKAs were performed, with fewer complications, lower medical costs, and a 97% patient satisfaction rate.[41] Given the success of this initial partnership, BCBSNC has since expanded their bundled payment program to encompass orthopedic procedures through OrthoCarolina and Novant in addition to TOA.[42]

Implementation of Bundled Payments for Care Improvement for Revision Total Joint Arthroplasty

The University of Pennsylvania implemented BPCI for revision TJA (MS-DRG 466, 467, or 468), which tends to be costlier and have less favorable outcomes than primary TJA.[43,44] The bundle included care from the time of index admission to 90 days after discharge for 50 revision TKAs and 41 revision THAs. The strategies used to facilitate cost and quality improvements included preoperative risk stratification programs, standardization of implant costs, provider education regarding the program, patient education regarding discharge expectations, increased emphasis on reducing LOS, and improved communication. Although this program successfully decreased LOS, they were unable to achieve a significant difference in total cost per episode of care. These findings intimate that bundles may be better left to procedures, such as primary TJA, that have larger episode volumes, more predictable outcomes, and an improved capacity for standardization and reproducibility.

CONSIDERATIONS IN IMPLEMENTATION OF BUNDLED PAYMENTS
Potential Benefits

The traditional FFS reimbursement model has contributed to high health care costs in the United States, rewarding volume over value, with no incentive to providers to moderate their expenditures.[45] The implementation of gainsharing agreements in bundled payments aligns the objectives of payers and providers. Gainsharing serves as motivation for stakeholders to pursue cost-saving measures and take definitive actions to reduce postoperative complications and readmissions. Furthermore, gainsharing can be tied to outcome measures, ensuring that high-quality care continues to be provided to patients.

Success under bundle agreements requires providers in multiple settings to improve communication and collaboration, which leads to superior patient outcomes.[46] Optimization of care coordination for patients covered by bundled payment systems also contributes to enhanced quality of care and reduced costs for patients under existing FFS models or other reimbursement systems. Under the CMS' current bundled models, requirements have been instituted to monitor outcome measures to ensure that cost savings do not result from inappropriate reductions to care quality.[47]

Potential Risks and Barriers

Despite the potential for significant cost savings under bundled payment models, there is also the possibility of a significant financial risk from several distinct sources. Losses may be incurred because of poor implementation or mismanagement of care episodes or monetary and time investments in redesigning care pathways and billing processes. Although physicians tend to be shielded from this risk by hospitals at present, this model may prove to be unsustainable in the long-term. Additionally, hospitals may attempt to recoup losses sustained under a bundle model by transitioning these costs to patients still using FFS payment systems.[48]

Occasional high-cost episodes also serve as an additional source of economic risk under bundled payments, in which providers would not be reimbursed for expenses in excess of the bundle price. This possibility may be mitigated through such strategies as outlier payments, reinsurance, and stop-loss limits to reduce hospitals' financial responsibility.[49]

Outlier payments are triggered after costs of care surpass a given threshold, wherein the payer covers a specified percentage of costs greater than the threshold.[50] Under reinsurance, the reinsurer is responsible for payment of patient care costs in excess of a specified limit.[51] Stop-loss provisions are activated once the costs of an episode exceed a specified threshold, then reverting back to an FFS payment, sheltering providers from extreme financial risk.

Although many institutions have demonstrated cost and quality improvements under BPCI, CJR, and private bundled contracts, not all institutions may be able to replicate these results. There is a wide disparity in TJA costs and quality across the United States, varying with geography, supply costs and hospital factors.[9,10] Particularly, low-volume hospitals have been reported to have higher complication rates and poorer outcomes, potentially offsetting the benefit that may be derived from bundled reimbursement models.[52–55] A larger quantity of TJA procedures performed allows for moderation of the costs of outlier cases, reducing volatility and increasing the predictability of economic forecasting.[28] It is recommended that providers should have a minimum of 100 cases per year to participate in bundled payment models in order to mitigate the effects of cost and outcome variability.[56]

In addition to financial risk, there is concern that flat-fee bundles may discourage providers from taking on complex cases that have a greater probability of exceeding the negotiated bundle price.[57] This cohort with more comorbidities and postoperative complications tends to disproportionately be of lower socioeconomic status, potentially eroding this population's access to health care services.[58] The incorporation of risk modification and stratification strategies to adjust bundle price based on anticipated resource utilization can be of use in eliminating this potential pitfall.[59]

Physician providers have also expressed concerns regarding the implementation of bundled payments.[60] Successful implementation of bundles is contingent on effective cooperation between patients, surgeons, anesthetists, hospitals, and other health care providers. Resistance of providers to sufficiently collaborate can prevent the realization of cost savings and negatively impact patient care. Some providers may be hesitant over the increasingly cooperative patient care necessitated by bundled payments, fearing an erosion of physician autonomy.[47] This concern is unfounded, however, because of the integral leadership role physicians play

in the management and redesign of care pathways and increased accountability demanded by bundled payment outcome measures.[61] Additionally, some physicians also report apprehension regarding the potential for malpractice liability through experimentation with novel health care delivery methods; thus, the implementation of bundled contracts should be met with reformation of medical jurisprudence.[62]

Despite these concerns, the implementation of bundled reimbursement has the potential to yield such significant cost savings that the benefits of bundle programs outweigh the drawbacks for many institutions. Many of the apprehensions regarding bundled contracts can be mitigated through sound financial risk management strategies and shifting physicians' perceptions to heighten their sense of accountability for the costs of the care that they provide.

SUMMARY

The preliminary results of BPCI and private bundled contract implementation demonstrate the advantages that may be realized by improved care coordination and collaboration between providers in the setting of TJA. Each institution applied a unique approach to the modification of care to realize these benefits, such as optimization of care pathways, reduction of implant costs, and alterations in PAC utilization. Overall, bundled reimbursement schemes resulted in benefits to patients through improved functional outcome measures and diminished complication and readmission rates, payers through reduced costs, and surgeons through gainsharing agreements.

Although participation in BCPI was voluntary, the implementation of mandatory bundled payment initiatives, such as CJR, emphasizes the importance of hospitals and providers that remain under FFS models to earnestly consider the appropriateness of bundles in their practices. All involved stakeholders must understand and endorse the fundamental changes necessary to render successful implementation of the bundle program. The preemptive evaluation of cost-saving measures, development of a culture of interdepartmental collaboration, optimization of care coordination, and establishment of the required administrative infrastructure can proactively enhance the successfulness of bundled models when they are introduced.

Following on the cost savings attained by CMS's bundled payment models, nongovernmental health care insurers are also eager to develop and implement their own mutually beneficial bundled contracts with hospital organizations. Within these private negotiations, hospitals and providers have greater power than they do with the CMS to set the parameters of the bundle, including price, duration, exclusions, risk mitigation strategies, and gainsharing agreements. As bundled payment models have demonstrated a benefit on patient outcomes, prospective the analysis of bundle components and early implementation of private and commercial bundled payment models serves as an opportunity for hospitals and providers to realize a financial benefit while concurrently improving patient care.

REFERENCES

1. Williams SN, Wolford ML, Bercovitz A. Hospitalization for total knee replacement among inpatients aged 45 and over: United States, 2000–2010. Hyattsville (MD): National Center for Health Statistics; 2015.

2. Wolford ML, Paslo K, Bercovitz A. Hospitalization for total hip replacement among inpatients aged 45 and over: United States, 2000–2010. Hyattsville (MD): National Center for Health Statistics; 2015.

3. Noble PC, Conditt MA, Cook KF, et al. The John Insall Award: patient expectations affect satisfaction with total knee arthroplasty. Clin Orthop Relat Res 2006;452:35–43.

4. Cram P, Lu X, Kates SL, et al. Total knee arthroplasty volume, utilization, and outcomes among Medicare beneficiaries, 1991-2010. JAMA 2012; 308(12):1227–36.

5. Kurtz SM, Ong KL, Lau E, et al. Impact of the economic downturn on total joint replacement demand in the United States. J Bone Joint Surg Am 2014;96(8):624–30.

6. Odum S, Van Doren B, Curtin B, et al. Projections for total joint arthroplasty demand for the next generation. Value Health 2016;19(3):A86.

7. Centers for Medicare and Medicaid Services. Comprehensive care for joint replacement model. 2017. Available at: https://innovation.cms.gov/initiatives/cjr. Accessed February 6, 2017.

8. Cram P, Lu X, Li Y. Bundled payments for elective primary total knee arthroplasty an analysis of Medicare administrative data. Geriatr Orthop Surg Rehabil 2015;6(1):3–10.

9. Haas DA, Kaplan RS. Variation in the cost of care for primary total knee arthroplasties. Arthroplasty Today 2016.

10. Li Y, Lu X, Wolf BR, et al. Variation of Medicare payments for total knee arthroplasty. J Arthroplasty 2013;28(9):1513–20.

11. Stryker LS, Odum SM, Fehring TK. Variations in hospital billing for total joint arthroplasty. J Arthroplasty 2014;29(9):155–9.

12. Thakore RV, Greenberg SE, Bulka CM, et al. Geographic variations in hospital charges and Medicare payments for major joint arthroplasty. J Arthroplasty 2015;30(5):728–32.

13. Miller DC, Gust C, Dimick JB, et al. Large variations in Medicare payments for surgery highlight savings potential from bundled payment programs. Health Aff (Millwood) 2011;30(11):2107–15.

14. Bozic KJ, Grosso LM, Lin Z, et al. Variation in hospital-level risk-standardized complication rates following elective primary total hip and knee arthroplasty. J Bone Joint Surg Am 2014;96(8): 640–7.

15. Tsai TC, Joynt KE, Orav EJ, et al. Variation in surgical-readmission rates and quality of hospital care. N Engl J Med 2013;369(12):1134–42.

16. Lurie JD, Bell JE, Weinstein J. What rate of utilization is appropriate in musculoskeletal care? Clin Orthop Relat Res 2009;467(10):2506–11.

17. Centers for Medicare and Medicaid Services. Bundled payments for care improvement (BPCI) initiative: general information. 2017. Available at: https://innovation.cms.gov/initiatives/bundled-payments/. Accessed January 30, 2017.

18. Centers for Medicare and Medicaid Services. Health care payment learning and action network. 2016. Available at: https://innovation.cms.gov/initiatives/Health-Care-Payment-Learning-and-Action-Network/. Accessed February 6, 2017.

19. Shatto JD. Center for Medicare and Medicaid innovation's methodology and calculations for the 2016 estimate of fee-for-service payments to alternative payment models [press release]. Baltimore (MD): Centers for Medicare and Medicaid Services; 2016.

20. de Brantes F, Rosenthal MB, Painter M. Building a bridge from fragmentation to accountability—the Prometheus payment model. N Engl J Med 2009; 361(11):1033–6.

21. Hussey PS, Eibner C, Ridgely MS, et al. Controlling US health care spending—separating promising from unpromising approaches. N Engl J Med 2009;361(22):2109–11.

22. Sood N, Huckfeldt PJ, Escarce JJ, et al. Medicare's bundled payment pilot for acute and postacute care: analysis and recommendations on where to begin. Health Aff (Millwood) 2011;30(9):1708–17.

23. The Lewin Group. CMS bundled payments for care improvement initiative models 2-4: year 2 evaluation & monitoring annual report. Baltimore (MD): Centers for Medicare and Medicaid Services; 2016.

24. Mechanic R. Medicare's bundled payment initiatives: considerations for providers. Washington, DC: American Hospital Association; 2016.

25. Centers for Medicare & Medicaid Services (CMS), HHS. Medicare program: comprehensive care for joint replacement payment model for acute care hospitals furnishing lower extremity joint

replacement services. Final rule. Fed Regist 2015; 80(226):73273.

26. Iorio R, Bosco J, Slover J, et al. Single institution early experience with the bundled payments for care improvement initiative. J Bone Joint Surg Am 2017;99(1):e2.

27. Dummit LA, Kahvecioglu D, Marrufo G, et al. Association between hospital participation in a Medicare bundled payment initiative and payments and quality outcomes for lower extremity joint replacement episodes. JAMA 2016;316(12): 1267–78.

28. Kivlahan C, Orlowski JM, Pearce J, et al. Taking risk: early results from teaching hospitals' participation in the Center for Medicare and Medicaid innovation bundled payments for care improvement initiative. Acad Med 2016;91(7):936–42.

29. Bolz NJ, Iorio R. Bundled payments: our experience at an academic medical center. J Arthroplasty 2016; 31(5):932–5.

30. Dundon JM, Bosco J, Slover J, et al. Improvement in total joint replacement quality metrics. J Bone Joint Surg Am 2016;98(23):1949–53.

31. Iorio R, Clair AJ, Inneh IA, et al. Early results of Medicare's bundled payment initiative for a 90-day total joint arthroplasty episode of care. J Arthroplasty 2016;31(2):343–50.

32. Kim K, Iorio R. The 5 clinical pillars of value for total joint arthroplasty in a bundled payment paradigm. J Arthroplasty 2017;32(6):1712–6.

33. Navathe AS, Troxel AB, Liao JM, et al. Cost of joint replacement using bundled payment models. JAMA Intern Med 2017;177(2):214–22.

34. Althausen PL, Mead L. Bundled payments for care improvement: lessons learned in the first year. J Orthop Trauma 2016;30:S50–3.

35. Edwards PK, Mears SC, Barnes CL. BPCI: everyone wins, including the patient. J Arthroplasty 2017; 32(6):1728–31.

36. Kee JR, Edwards PK, Barnes CL. Effect of risk acceptance for bundled care payments on clinical outcomes in a high-volume total joint arthroplasty practice after implementation of a standardized clinical pathway. J Arthroplasty 2017;32(8):2332–8.

37. Curtin BM, Russell RD, Odum SM. Bundled payments for care improvement: boom or bust? J Arthroplasty 2017;32(10):2931–4.

38. Froemke CC, Wang L, DeHart ML, et al. Standardizing care and improving quality under a bundled payment initiative for total joint arthroplasty. J Arthroplasty 2015;30(10):1676–82.

39. Doran JP, Zabinski SJ. Bundled payment initiatives for Medicare and non-Medicare total joint arthroplasty patients at a community hospital: bundles in the real world. J Arthroplasty 2015;30(3):353–5.

40. Whitcomb WF, Lagu T, Krushell RJ, et al. Experience with designing and implementing a bundled payment program for total hip replacement. Jt Comm J Qual Patient Saf 2015;41(9):406–13.

41. Expanded collaboration provides BCBSNC customers with 10-20 percent savings on hip replacement surgeries [press release]. Chapel Hill (NC): BlueCross BlueShield of North Carolina; 2014.

42. Bruch R. A sea change in medicine current shifts in the delivery and payment of medical care. N C Med J 2016;77(4):261–4.

43. Courtney PM, Ashley BS, Hume EL, et al. Are bundled payments a viable reimbursement model for revision total joint arthroplasty? Clin Orthop Relat Res 2016;474(12):2714–21.

44. Tokarski AT, Deirmengian CA, Lichstein PM, et al. Medicare fails to compensate additional surgical time and effort associated with revision arthroplasty. J Arthroplasty 2015;30(4):535–8.

45. Matlock D, Earnest M, Epstein A. Utilization of elective hip and knee arthroplasty by age and payer. Clin Orthop Relat Res 2008;466(4):914–9.

46. Pape B, Thiessen PS, Jakobsen F, et al. Interprofessional collaboration may pay off: introducing a collaborative approach in an orthopaedic ward. J Interprof Care 2013;27(6):496–500.

47. Froimson MI, Rana A, White RE, et al. Bundled payments for care improvement initiative: the next evolution of payment formulations: AAHKS Bundled Payment Task Force. J Arthroplasty 2013;28(8): 157–65.

48. Miller HD. From volume to value: better ways to pay for health care. Health Aff (Millwood) 2009; 28(5):1418–28.

49. Harvey L. Neiman Health Policy Institute. Risk mitigation in bundled payments. 2017. Available at: http://www.neimanhpi.org/ice-t/risk-mitigation-in-bundled-payments/. Accessed March 20, 2017.

50. Centers for Medicare and Medicaid Services. Outlier payments. 2013. Available at: https://www.cms.gov/Medicare/Medicare-Fee-for-Service-Payment/AcuteInpatientPPS/outlier.html. Accessed Mar 20, 2017.

51. Robinow A. The potential of global payment: insights from the field. Commonwealth Fund 2010.

52. Losina E, Walensky RP, Kessler CL, et al. Cost-effectiveness of total knee arthroplasty in the United States: patient risk and hospital volume. Arch Intern Med 2009;169(12):1113.

53. Katz JN, Losina E, Barrett J, et al. Association between hospital and surgeon procedure volume and outcomes of total hip replacement in the United States Medicare population. J Bone Joint Surg Am 2001;83(11):1622–9.

54. Katz JN, Barrett J, Mahomed NN, et al. Association between hospital and surgeon procedure volume and the outcomes of total knee replacement. J Bone Joint Surg Am 2004;86(9): 1909–16.

55. Katz JN, Mahomed NN, Baron JA, et al. Association of hospital and surgeon procedure volume with patient-centered outcomes of total knee replacement in a population-based cohort of patients age 65 years and older. Arthritis Rheum 2007;56(2):568–74.

56. Orlowski JM. Comprehensive care for joint replacement payment model proposed rule, file code CMS–5516–P [press release]. Washington, DC: Association of American Medical Colleges; 2015.

57. Kamath AF, Courtney PM, Bozic KJ, et al. Bundled payment in total joint care: survey of AAHKS membership attitudes and experience with alternative payment models. J Arthroplasty 2015; 30(12):2045–56.

58. Satin DJ, Miles J. Performance-based bundled payments: potential benefits and burdens. Minn Med 2009;92(10):33–5.

59. Courtney PM, Huddleston JI, Iorio R, et al. Socioeconomic risk adjustment models for reimbursement are necessary in primary total joint arthroplasty. J Arthroplasty 2017;32(1):1–5.

60. Tilburt JC, Wynia MK, Sheeler RD, et al. Views of US physicians about controlling health care costs. JAMA 2013;310(4):380–9.

61. Smith A, Blount D, Mitchell J, et al. The bundled payment guide for physicians. Raleigh (NC): Towards Accountable Care Consortium; 2014.

62. Luft HS. Economic incentives to promote innovation in healthcare delivery. Clin Orthop Relat Res 2009;467(10):2497–505.

Trauma

Use of Tourniquets in Limb Trauma Surgery

Yelena Bogdan, MD[a],*, David L. Helfet, MD[b]

KEYWORDS

- Tourniquet • Exsanguination • Orthopedic limb trauma • Tourniquet design • Cuff pressure
- Cuff width

KEY POINTS

- Tourniquets are frequently used in both upper and lower extremities, usually without significant complications.
- Optimal pressure is still unknown, but using limb occlusion pressure rather than systolic blood pressure may be better for decreasing the risk of injury.
- No specific tourniquet design has been proven superior, but recent data points to assessing limb circumference when choosing a tourniquet.
- Protocols and guidelines for tourniquet use, taking patients and the type of procedure into consideration, are needed.
- Tourniquets are not benign and have been associated with fatalities, so the surgeon must remain vigilant and knowledgeable about their risks and benefits.

INTRODUCTION

A tourniquet is a device used to halt blood flow to an extremity. In the modern surgical theater, tourniquets of various designs are used in more than 15,000 procedures every day.[1] The goal of tourniquet application is most often to create a bloodless field; it is, however, also used to assist with limb anesthesia (ie, Bier block), venipuncture (to enlarge blood vessels), and control of catastrophic blood loss in an acute setting.[2]

The historical use of tourniquets dates back to the ancient Romans who used them in amputations,[3] but the actual term was coined in the 1700s by Jean Louis Petit from the French term *tourner* ("to turn").[1] His simple device was a screw-type mechanism that was revolutionary in not requiring an assistant to keep the pressure constant. Lister performed the first nonamputation surgeries with a tourniquet, combined with limb elevation for exsanguination. Later, Esmarch created the flat rubber bandage that now bears his name. In the early 1900s, Cushing developed the pneumatic tourniquet, a variant of which is still used today.[1,3] This design was perfected in the 1980s by McEwen, who invented the modern microcomputer tourniquet, which monitored not only pressure but also leakage, inflation time, and other parameters. It also estimated the limb occlusion pressure (LOP) (the minimal pressure required to halt blood flow) and protected from both depressurization and overpressurization.[2]

Although tourniquets have been in use for many decades, definitive protocols are still lacking; physicians' knowledge of the risks and benefits of this device remains subpar. A study of residents and operating room (OR) assistants used a questionnaire that assessed their knowledge of tourniquet use, including repositioning, correct cuff size and

Disclosure Statement: Neither author reports any relationship with a commercial company that has a direct financial interest in subject matter or materials discussed in the article or with a company making a competing product.

[a] Department of Orthopaedic Trauma, Geisinger Holy Spirit Orthopaedic Surgery, 550 North 12th Street, Suite 140, Lemoyne, PA 17043, USA; [b] Department of Orthopaedic Trauma, Hospital for Special Surgery, 535 East 70th Street, New York, NY 10021, USA

* Corresponding author. Geisinger Holy Spirit Orthopaedic Surgery, 550 North 12th Street, Suite 140, Lemoyne, PA 17043.

E-mail address: ybogdan@geisinger.edu

shape, contraindications, safe inflation time, and other facts. The average test score for residents was 41.3% and 46.7% for assistants. The investigators cautioned that surgeons must be knowledgeable in the application and indications for tourniquets, particularly for medicolegal reasons.[4] It is also important to note that most tourniquets are placed by assistants and not by the surgeons themselves, further divorcing the tourniquet from being an essential part of the case.

Formal protocols on tourniquet use in the United States vary greatly in scope and application, particularly in the prehospital setting. Eighty-four percent of states have statewide emergency medical systems (EMS) exsanguination protocols; only 35% have very clear, detailed instructions on when and how to use tourniquets. This factor likely results in suboptimal and sporadic use.[5] The Eastern Association for the Surgery of Trauma has published a management guideline for penetrating lower extremity trauma that contains a section on tourniquets and states that a tourniquet can be used if direct pressure fails to control bleeding.[6] However, this guideline is listed as level 3, which is defined by a lack of formal evidence.

Generally, no standard exists for tourniquet use; the decision rests with the individual surgeon. This decision is largely based on personal preference and several factors, including procedure duration, technical difficulty, blood loss, and the location of the injury on the body. Recently published articles summarize the various issues in tourniquet application.[1,7] The goal of this work is to review the current literature on indications, technique points, and complications of tourniquets in limb trauma, both in the acute and elective setting.

PREHOSPITAL AND EMERGENCY TOURNIQUET USE

Although most of the literature on tourniquets in trauma focuses on elective procedures, some studies deal specifically with the prehospital setting. Much of what we know of tourniquet use in this setting comes from military experience. In the 1600s, French army surgeon Etienne Morel was one of the first to use tourniquets on the battlefield to treat extremity wounds.[8] In the 1950s and 1960s, Vietnam War casualties often died of massive limb hemorrhage, leading to an increased interest in tourniquets as a lifesaving measure.[9] The explosive weapons of modern warfare in Iraq and Afghanistan also added to the experience of tourniquet use in soldiers.[6,10]

On the battlefield, the Combat Application Tourniquet (CAT; www.combattourniquet.com) involves a simple windlass mechanism that can be applied one-handed with good results. A 4-year study of military prehospital tourniquet use in 550 patients at an average ischemic time of 83 minutes showed 78% overall effectiveness, 94% in upper limbs and 71% in lower limbs. No patient died of hemorrhage.[9] Another prospective observational study of both civilian and military casualties in a Baghdad hospital assessed tourniquet use in the prehospital versus the emergency department (ED) setting. In 232 patients, the mortality rates were 11% in the prehospital group (n = 194) and 24% in the ED group (n = 38). Transient nerve palsies occurred in 1.7%. Prehospital use of the tourniquet was weakly associated with survival; the absence of shock with tourniquet use was also associated with survival. The study also matched a group of patients for the Injury Severity Score and Abbreviated Injury Scale scores. Patients who had a tourniquet placed were matched with those who had compressible limb injuries and would have benefited from a tourniquet but did not get one because of availability or medic decision. All patients in the latter group died (0% vs 77% survival rate).[11]

The frequency of tourniquet use in the military has not translated to the civilian sector, largely because of the faster access to definitive care in the case of civilian trauma.[12] Some investigators state that a tourniquet should never be used as a first-aid measure,[3] but literature exists to counter that position. Civilian settings where tourniquets may be useful include penetrating trauma, such as stab and gunshot wounds, terrorism incidents, rural or wilderness medicine, limb entrapment with an inaccessible bleeding site, industrial or machinery accidents, and extreme or life-threatening situations.[8] One study examined injury patterns and outcomes in 14 civilians who died of exsanguination of an isolated extremity injury. It showed that only one patient had some attempt at bleeding control before EMS arrival, and intravenous (IV) access was not obtained in 71%. This study suggested that aggressive attempts to control limb hemorrhage, such as with a tourniquet, may prevent death from exsanguination.[13]

A retrospective review of 87 civilian patients looked at tourniquet use (primarily with the CAT) in the prehospital, ED, and OR settings. Half of the cohort had tourniquets applied in the prehospital time period, mostly on upper extremities. The Mangled Extremity Severity score and the rate of limb loss did not differ between the groups. No major complications occurred as a result of tourniquet use, except one case of compartment syndrome. In that patient, however, limb ischemia due to arterial transection was documented before tourniquet placement, and the tourniquet's role in precipitating the complication was unclear.[12]

Despite promising data, prehospital tourniquet use remains rare. A study from 2 Canadian centers over a 10-year period of patients with arterial injuries yielded only 8 patients who had tourniquets placed for isolated extremity injury. Only 4 had the tourniquet placed before arrival at the hospital; all of these patients survived, despite being more hypotensive and acidotic than those whose tourniquets were placed in the trauma bay. The investigators compared this group with a group who did not get a tourniquet and who died. All patients who died did so from hemorrhage. The study also showed no statistically significant difference in transfusion rates between the tourniquet and no tourniquet groups but did show a trend toward less transfused blood in the tourniquet group.[14]

Technical points of tourniquet use in the acute limb trauma setting include the understanding that less severe measures, such as direct pressure and pressure dressings, should always comprise the initial attempts to control bleeding.[6] If a tourniquet is applied, it should not be loosened until patients reach the hospital because incremental exsanguination may occur. If bleeding is still not controlled, a second tourniquet can be applied.[8] Frequent reassessment is indicated as the patients are resuscitated; changes in blood pressure may affect tourniquet effectiveness.[10] Pain control is also paramount because a properly applied tourniquet is extremely uncomfortable and will often require IV analgesia.[8] For cases of prolonged transport, limb cooling helps to slow metabolism and protect muscles from ischemia. A study in pigs showed that hypothermic limbs had a faster recovery immediately after tourniquet deflation and 10 days later. The hypothermic pigs also had lower lactate levels, less glycogen breakdown, and a smaller decrease in blood pH, which all served as protection against the inflammatory response.[15]

LIMB TRAUMA SURGERY: GENERAL CONSIDERATIONS
Application
The tourniquet should be placed on the limb as distally as possible, but at least 5 cm proximal to the area of injury, avoiding joints (**Table 1**).[8,10] Prep solutions, such as povidone iodine, can

Table 1 Tips for tourniquet use	
Application	Keep the tourniquet at least 5 cm proximal to area of injury.
	Use a barrier to prevent prep liquid from pooling under tourniquet.
	Curved/wider tourniquets require less pressure to stop the blood flow.
Inflation	Use a fast inflation rate to avoid venous pooling.
	The inflation pressures are 250 mm Hg for the upper extremity and 300 mm Hg for the lower extremity or use LOP + 50–100 mm Hg.
Deflation	Monitor the physiologic changes during deflation.

pool under the tourniquet and cause friction or chemical burns, so a barrier is necessary to prevent liquid from pooling.[16] A surgical glove or another impenetrable drape can be used for this purpose.[17]

Inflation should take place over a short period of time, as slow inflation rates or incorrect application will block venous flow before arterial flow, causing venous congestion and possibly more bleeding.[8,18] Simple elevation is effective in cases when pressure is contraindicated, such as sickle cell anemia.[2] Tourniquet use is also contraindicated in malignancy and infection.[1,19]

The timing of antibiotic administration has been controversial, with some investigators advocating that a period of at least 5 minutes is necessary before tourniquet inflation to allow antibiotics to penetrate the limb.[2] However, a randomized controlled trial of 106 patients compared infection rates in 2 groups: one with antibiotic administration 5 minutes before tourniquet inflation and one with antibiotic administration 1 minute after tourniquet inflation. Contrary to the expected result, the group who had preinflation antibiotics actually had higher infection rates.[20]

Pressure
Published recommendations on tourniquet pressure use a variety of markers to achieve an optimal bloodless field while avoiding high pressures that can lead to nerve injury. These parameters, which can be easily obtained intraoperatively, include systolic blood pressure and mean arterial pressure.[19] A review article

lists the currently accepted parameters; the general recommendation is to stay less than 250 mm Hg in the upper extremity and less than 300 mm Hg in the lower extremity.[7]

Another guide for optimal pressure is the limb LOP, which is the minimum pressure needed to stop arterial blood flow in a given patient or situation. It is calculated before surgery by assessing when a Doppler signal disappears from the distal extremity as the tourniquet is inflated.[1] Many modern tourniquets can calculate the LOP, and a 50- to 100-mm Hg safety margin is frequently added to account for intraoperative physiologic changes. The LOP has been the subject of several studies and is suggested as an alternative in cases when high pressures must be avoided, such as in patients with arterial calcification.[2] Today, however, it remains an infrequently used parameter; a study showed that only 7% of polled physicians (podiatrists) considered the LOP when selecting cuff pressure.[21]

Time

A general recommendation for continuous cuff inflation time ranges from 2.0 to 2.5 hours.[7] The concept of tourniquet time is based on the idea that adenosine triphosphate is depleted during the period of ischemia, and a time limit allows patients' tissues to recover.[22] Despite recommendations, it is important to understand that a safe tourniquet time does not exist and any amount of time can potentially cause damage to the limb.[8] To minimize complications, a deflation interval has been used since the 1950s; its optimal duration, however, remains unclear.[3] One article recommends a 10-minute interval at 2.5 hours of surgery, with further reperfusion intervals at each additional hour.[7] The concept of reperfusion as a means of protection seems to be supported by at least one randomized controlled trial, in which patients undergoing ankle surgery with a tourniquet deflated at the end of the procedure were compared with patients who underwent staggered release (initial tourniquet release followed by 2 cycles of reinflation/deflation, with each cycle occurring over 3 minutes). The staggered-release group experienced decreased metabolic changes reflected in the lactate level and end tidal carbon dioxide. These changes were deemed to be protective to the soft tissues because of less buildup of metabolites indicating tissue damage.[23]

During deflation, it is important to monitor for changes in oxygen parameters, particularly during intramedullary nailing, cementing, or prosthesis insertion. Deflation can release large venous emboli, adding to the patients' already increased clot burden.[1] The surgeon must also balance the need for decreased tourniquet time with the risk of increased bleeding if the tourniquet is released too quickly. Investigators disagree on whether release of the tourniquet before wound closure is recommended.[7]

Cuff Width and Design

Much interest in the type and width of the tourniquet has surfaced in the last decade, particularly with the increase of obesity in the United States. Cuff design becomes important in this population because of the relationship between optimal pressure and limb circumference. A study of healthy volunteers showed an inverse relationship between the LOP and the ratio of the cuff width/limb circumference, meaning that for a given limb, a narrower cuff requires much higher pressure to stop the blood flow.[24] This pressure causes a higher gradient and predisposes to nerve injury. Notably in this study, the relationship of LOP and blood pressure predicts that the LOP will be subsystolic for normotensive patients when the cuff width/limb circumference ratio is greater than 0.3:1.0. Another study of 26 volunteers explored the concept of fitted tourniquets to account for the conical shape of most human limbs. The investigators found that the use of curved and wider tourniquets resulted in lower occlusion pressures: a mean of 183 mm Hg in the arm and 208 mm Hg in the leg. They recommended adding 75 mm Hg to the LOP to account for changes in blood pressure.[25]

With regard to design, the silicone ring tourniquet (SRT) has been introduced to the market as a sterile alternative to the standard pneumatic tourniquet. It consists of a silicone ring encased within a stockinette; the ring is placed over the fingers or toes and rolled up the extremity proximally, achieving compression and exsanguination. A study of 536 patients, with 63% being fracture cases, showed several advantages to the silicone ring design, which was most frequently used on the femur.[26] These advantages include sterility; the ability to access places, such as the groin where a regular tourniquet would not be possible or practical; and a one-step exsanguination process.[27] Limitations of the SRT include injuries that may hinder the roll-on application, including open fractures and the presence of external fixation.[28] No particular design, however, has been 100% proven to be better than another; the choice remains with the surgeon.[7]

UPPER EXTREMITY

Tourniquet Use

The use of tourniquets in the upper extremity has been gaining popularity, both in the hand and trauma literature. One review of 505 patients with upper extremity tourniquets found no immediate or delayed adverse events, even in patients with medical comorbidities. Most of these patients had pressures of 250 mm Hg or less and a tourniquet time of about 30 minutes. This study deemed tourniquets as safe to use in commonly performed hand procedures.[22] However, another study found some disadvantages. In a randomized trial of closed forearm fractures, the pressure ranged from 200 to 250 mm Hg; the visual and verbal pain scores were assessed in patients without a tourniquet, a tourniquet used for less than 1 hour, and a tourniquet used for 1 to 2 hours. The nontourniquet group had less overall pain on postoperative days 1 and 2, particularly in older and male patients.[29]

Technique Points

The optimal position of the tourniquet on the arm is controversial and was evaluated in a study of patients undergoing carpal tunnel release.[30] Either a forearm or upper arm cuff was placed, and outcomes included surgeon assessment of the bloodless field. No major differences stood out in the groups, except the forearm tourniquet often made fingers curl involuntarily and sometimes blocked the surgeon's view. Based on this, upper arm tourniquets were deemed preferable in the study.

In the case of finger tourniquets, the application can be with a rubber catheter held with a hemostat or a finger of a glove rolled up onto the base of the finger.[31] However, such tourniquets provide variable, nonstandard pressures and are often obscure enough to be left in situ accidentally. All-purpose digital tourniquets provide a better option because of their bright colors, but correct sizing is problematic.

The exsanguination method in the upper limb has also been explored, particularly in healthy volunteers. One randomized trial assessed 26 patients who had arm elevation versus esmarch exsanguination before tourniquet inflation at 250 mm Hg for a maximum of 20 minutes. Although there was no difference in recovery after deflation, the pain scores during the time of inflation were in favor of exsanguination.[32] Another randomized study in 100 patients evaluated the elevation for 5 seconds, the squeeze method (manually squeezing the blood out of the limb from distal to proximal), and the esmarch in effectiveness of stopping blood flow. No difference was seen between the latter two, but both were better than elevation.[33] In another study using labeled erythrocytes to assess exsanguination in healthy volunteers, the following reductions in blood volumes were found: elevation 5 seconds, 44% and 4 minutes, 42%; esmarch 69%; gauze bandage 63%; pomidor roll cuff 66%; squeeze method 53%; and Urias bag 57%.[34] This finding suggests that no method is completely effective and that the time of elevation may not be significant beyond 5 seconds.

The tourniquet choice in the upper limb includes the standard pneumatic cuff (PT) or the SRT. The two options do not seem to differ greatly in outcomes. One study of SRT versus a forearm tourniquet in carpal tunnel surgery showed that the mean final pain during the surgery was higher and had a more rapid increase with the conventional tourniquet.[27] However, another randomized study assessed areas of nerve compression in SRT versus PT on the upper arm. Visual analog scale (VAS) pain scores were obtained, and MRI of the radial and ulnar nerves provided the basis for measuring nerve diameters. No differences were found in the two groups.[28] The SRT may have smaller pressure gradients at the cuff edges than the wide tourniquet, causing less chance of nerve injury. This finding seems to be confirmed by another study, in which a wider cuff caused more severe changes in nerve conduction (by 10%) than a narrow cuff.[35]

Complications

Tourniquet nerve injury occurs 2.5 times more commonly in patients with an upper rather than a lower extremity tourniquet,[36] likely because of less soft tissue in that area, with the radial nerve being most susceptible. Complications are mentioned in several published case reports and include arm paralysis lasting 5.5 months after a digital amputation, possibly involving a malfunctioning tourniquet pressure gauge.[37] Posterior interosseous nerve palsy has been known to develop after a forearm tourniquet.[38] Another possible, though rare, complication is upper arm deep venous thrombosis (DVT).[18] Retaining a digital tourniquet after a dressing is more common and has pushed the need for more colorful tourniquets that are removed as part of the postoperative checklist.[39]

LOWER EXTREMITY

Tourniquet Use

The use of tourniquets in the lower extremity during elective trauma surgery has had support in the literature. One retrospective study of 603 patients undergoing ankle open reduction internal fixation (ORIF) with and without a tourniquet looked at opioid use during the first day after surgery. The tourniquet group had a 20% increase in opioid consumption; but in reality, the difference was only 3 mg of opiate, a clinically insignificant amount.[40] Another study randomized 132 patients undergoing ORIF of extra-articular tibia fractures into tourniquet and nontourniquet groups. At the 1-year follow-up, no tourniquet complications were noted. The investigators noted less pain (by one VAS point), less drainage (by 2 mL), and longer OR time (by 6 minutes) in the nontourniquet group, all clinically negligible differences.[41] A systematic review of 4 foot and ankle articles also showed limited differences and few complications with and without the use of tourniquets.[42]

Other investigators, however, are less enthusiastic about tourniquet use in the lower extremity because of concerns about poor visibility of blood vessels, the lack of a cooling effect of circulating blood, time restriction, and other issues.[43] Wound healing problems and erythema with a tourniquet have been documented in at least 3 studies: one in a randomized trial of 54 patients undergoing ankle fixation,[44] another in a randomized trial of tibia fractures,[43] and the third in a randomized trial of distal fibula fractures, which also noted a 1-week longer return to work in the tourniquet group.[45] Another study of thigh tourniquets assessed electromyography (EMG) changes and functional differences in the leg at 6 weeks postoperatively, showing that 71% of patients in the tourniquet group had evidence of denervation on EMG (vs none in control group) and functional capacity of 40% of normal (vs 79% of normal in control group). Interestingly, in the tourniquet group, pressures were similar in patients with and without EMG changes and thigh sizes varied; this suggests that other tourniquet-related factors may be responsible.[46] Lastly, tourniquets in the lower limb are associated with pulmonary morbidity. In a retrospective study of 72 patients undergoing reamed femoral nailing who also had tibia or ankle fractures, patients were grouped according to tourniquet use for the tibia/ankle injury and matched for injury severity. Ventilator-dependent days and intensive-care-unit days increased with increasing tourniquet time. This study suggests that the combination of reamed femoral nailing and tourniquet ischemia may cause increased susceptibility to pulmonary events.[47]

Technique Points

Optimal pressure and the use of thigh tourniquets is contested. In a survey of 140 American Orthopedic Foot and Ankle Society members, common cuff pressures included 301 to 350 mm Hg for the thigh and 201 to 250 mm Hg for the ankle. Only 11% of surgeons used less than 250 mm Hg for the thigh, which, from assessment of the LOP, would be enough for most patients with a safety margin. Only 9% of surgeons used LOP to set pressure. Forty-six percent were concerned with hazards, especially nerve injury, whereas 17% were not concerned at all.[48]

One study attempted to use the LOP to understand optimal pressure in different thigh tourniquets. In this randomized controlled trial, standard versus wide cuffs were used, with LOP set as the pressure in addition to a safety margin. Outcomes included quality of the bloodless field and were acceptable in both types of cuff, although the surgeon was not blinded. Mean pressures that achieved a good bloodless field were 178 mm Hg and 142 mm Hg for narrow and wide cuffs, respectively, far less than the usually used 300 to 350 mm Hg. Using the LOP decreased the average pressure by 33% to 42%. Systolic blood pressure did not correlate well with LOP. The recommendations from this study for the safety margin to be added to LOP were 40 for LOP less than 130, 60 for 131 to 190, and 80 for greater than 190.[49]

Another area of research in leg tourniquets deals with preconditioning of the extremity before tourniquet inflation. This preconditioning requires extra surgical time, but at least one study has shown good results. A randomized trial divided 30 healthy patients scheduled for lower extremity surgery into 2 groups: a control group who had a regular inflated tourniquet and a preconditioning group who had 3 cycles of 5 minutes of ischemia and 5 minutes of reperfusion before inflation of the tourniquet. The outcomes were the levels of inflammatory markers and oxygen exchange up to 24 hours postoperatively. No pulmonary complications occurred in either group, but the preconditioning group had less increase in inflammatory markers and less change in arterial Po_2 and alveolar-arterial oxygen tension ratio. This finding suggests that ischemic preconditioning may decrease pulmonary morbidity in patients at risk.[50]

Complications

Complications specific to lower limb tourniquets are similar to those in the upper extremity. Nerve injury to the femoral[51,52] and saphenous[51] nerves can occur. One study detailed a permanent femoral palsy after patella fracture fixation without prolonged tourniquet time or excessively high pressure, suggesting that our understanding of this phenomenon is still limited.[52] One complication that seems to be more prevalent in the lower limb is compartment syndrome due to ischemia. A case report of 2 patients who developed this complication after a tourniquet warned that tourniquets should be used with caution, particularly in obese and athletic patients. Notably, both patients in the report had high tourniquet pressures, 350 mm Hg and 450 mm Hg.[53] This finding underscores the need for optimal guidelines to reduce excessive pressure.

OTHER CONCERNS

Tourniquet problems not specific to a particular extremity include nerve injury (both transient and permanent),[1] pain, and weakness defined as "post-tourniquet syndrome,"[2] metabolic changes,[54] muscle injury,[2] Volkmann contracture,[3] and systemic complications, such as pulmonary embolism (PE).[55] Fortunately, these remain rare, with an incidence of 0.024% in one Norwegian study.[56]

The highest concern for surgeons is for permanent nerve injury and fatal PE. It is difficult to understand changes to nerves because much of the data used to study nerve function are in animals and uses pressures of 1000 mm Hg, much higher than what is clinically used in humans.[7] However, certain basic science work has improved our understanding of how tourniquets affect nerve tissue. One study assessed conduction of peripheral nerves in baboons. The investigators found that direct pressure on the nerve results in displacement of the node of Ranvier with respect to the Schwann cell junction. Maximal damage occurs at cuff edges, greater at the proximal edge. The study concluded that it is pressure, and not nerve ischemia, that comprises the main issue in nerve injury. Timing is also important, as the number of total affected nodes decreases with less tourniquet time.[57]

Multiple case reports of fatal PE in the setting of tourniquet use have been published,[55,58–61] a rare but grave complication in a routine procedure. A study of clot burden in knee arthroscopy patients using a transesophageal echocardiogram showed that PEs occur within minutes of release and that their number depends on tourniquet time.[62] Another study suggests that rolling and squeezing motions to achieve exsanguination, as with an esmarch

or SRT, can release thrombi and potentially result in fatal consequences.[55] Examination of several trauma case reports of fatal PE show that, in many of these cases, the patients were bedbound for a prolonged period,[58,61] had no DVT prophylaxis[55] or were off their DVT prophylaxis,[60] or were of advanced age.[61] When choosing to use a tourniquet, the surgeon must be aware of this serious complication and weigh the need for a bloodless field against the risk of injury and possibly death.

REFERENCES

1. Noordin S, McEwen J, Kragh JF, et al. Surgical tourniquets in orthopaedics. J Bone Joint Surg Am 2009;91(12):2958–67.
2. Oragui E, Parsons A, White T, et al. Tourniquet use in upper limb surgery. Hand (N Y) 2011;6(2):165–73.
3. Klenerman L. The tourniquet in surgery. J Bone Joint Surg Br 1962;44-B:937–43.
4. Sadri A, Braithwaite IJ, Abdlu-Jabar HB, et al. Understanding of intra-operative tourniquets amongst orthopaedic surgeons and theatre staff - a questionnaire study. Ann R Coll Surg Engl 2010; 92(3):243–5.
5. Ramly E, Runyan G, King DR. The state of the union: nationwide absence of uniform guidelines for the prehospital use of tourniquets to control extremity exsanguination. J Trauma Acute Care Surg 2016;80(5):787–91.
6. Fox N, Rajani RR, Bokhari F, et al. Evaluation and management of penetrating lower extremity arterial trauma: an Eastern Association for the Surgery of Trauma practice management guideline. J Trauma Acute Care Surg 2012;73(5 Suppl 4): S315–20.
7. Fitzgibbons PG, Digiovanni C, Hares S, et al. Safe tourniquet use: a review of the evidence. J Am Acad Orthop Surg 2012;20(5):310–9.
8. Lee C, Porter KM, Hodgetts TJ. Tourniquet use in the civilian prehospital setting. Emerg Med J 2007;24(8):584–7.
9. Lakstein D, Blumenfeld A, Sokolov T, et al. Tourniquets for hemorrhage control on the battlefield: a 4-year accumulated experience. J Trauma 2003; 54(5 Suppl):S221–5.
10. Rush RM, Arrington ED, Hsu JR. Management of complex extremity injuries. Tourniquets, compartment syndrome detection, fasciotomy, and amputation care. Surg Clin North Am 2012; 92(4):987–1007.
11. Kragh JF, Walters TJ, Baer DG, et al. Survival with emergency tourniquet use to stop bleeding in major limb trauma. Ann Surg 2009;249(1):1–7. https://doi.org/10.1097/SLA.0b013e31818842ba.

12. Inaba K, Siboni S, Resnick S, et al. Tourniquet use for civilian extremity trauma. J Trauma Acute Care Surg 2015;79(2):232–3.

13. Dorlac WC, DeBakey ME, Holcomb JB, et al. Mortality from isolated civilian penetrating extremity injury. J Trauma 2005;59(1):217–22.

14. Passos E, Dingley B, Smith A, et al. Tourniquet use for peripheral vascular injuries in the civilian setting. Injury 2014;45(3):573–7.

15. Irving GA, Noakes TD. The protective role of local hypothermia in tourniquet-induced ischaemia of muscle. J Bone Joint Surg Br 1985;67(2):297–301.

16. Ellanti P, Hurson C. Tourniquet-associated povidone-iodine-induced chemical burns. BMJ Case Rep 2015;2015. https://doi.org/10.1136/bcr-2014-208967.

17. Tomlinson PJ, Harries WJ. The use of a surgical glove in the prevention of tourniquet-associated chemical burns. Ann R Coll Surg Engl 2008; 90(3):255.

18. Desai K, Dinh TP, Chung S, et al. Upper extremity deep vein thrombosis with tourniquet use. Int J Surg Case Rep 2015;6:55–7.

19. Cox C, Yao J, Flatt AE, et al. Tourniquet usage in upper extremity surgery. J Hand Surg Am 2010; 35(8):1360–1.

20. Akinyoola AL, Adegbehingbe OO, Odunsi A. Timing of antibiotic prophylaxis in tourniquet surgery. J Foot Ankle Surg 2011;50(4):374–6.

21. Kalla TP, Younger A, McEwen JA, et al. Survey of tourniquet use in podiatric surgery. J Foot Ankle Surg 2003;42(2):68–76.

22. Drolet BC, Okhah Z, Phillips BZ, et al. Evidence for safe tourniquet use in 500 consecutive upper extremity procedures. Hand (N Y) 2014;9(4):494–8.

23. van der Velde J, Serfontein L, Iohom G. Reducing the potential for tourniquet-associated reperfusion injury. Eur J Emerg Med 2013;20(6):391–6.

24. Graham B, Breault MJ, McEwen JA, et al. Occlusion of arterial flow in the extremities at subsystolic pressures through the use of wide tourniquet cuffs. Clin Orthop Relat Res 1993; 286:257–61.

25. Pedowitz RA, Gershuni DH, Botte MJ, et al. The use of lower tourniquet inflation pressures in extremity surgery facilitated by curved and wide tourniquets and an integrated cuff inflation system. Clin Orthop Relat Res 1993;237–44. https://doi.org/10.1097/00003086-199302000-00038.

26. Drosos GI, Ververidis A, Mavropoulos R, et al. The silicone ring tourniquet in orthopaedic operations of the extremities. Surg Technol Int 2013;23:251–7.

27. Drosos GI, Ververidis A, Stavropoulos NI, et al. Silicone ring tourniquet versus pneumatic cuff tourniquet in carpal tunnel release: a randomized comparative study. J Orthop Traumatol 2013; 14(2):131–5.

28. Kovar FM. Nerve compression and pain in human volunteers with narrow vs wide tourniquets. World J Orthop 2015;6(4):394.

29. Omeroğlu H, Uçaner A, Tabak AY, et al. The effect of using a tourniquet on the intensity of postoperative pain in forearm fractures. A randomized study in 32 surgically treated patients. Int Orthop 1998; 22(6):369–73.

30. Odinsson A, Finsen V. The position of the tourniquet on the upper limb. J Bone Joint Surg Br 2002;84(2):202–4.

31. Brewster MBS, Upadhyay PK, Hill CE. Finger tourniquets: a review of National Patient Safety Agency recommendations, available devices and current practice. J Hand Surg Eur Vol 2015;40(2):214–5.

32. Lees DA, Penny JB, Baker P. A single blind randomised controlled trial of the impact on patient-reported pain of arm elevation versus exsanguination prior to tourniquet inflation. Bone Joint J 2016;98-B(4):519–25.

33. Blønd L, Jensen NV, Søe Nielsen NH. Clinical consequences of different exsanguination methods in hand surgery. A double-blind randomised study. J Hand Surg Eur Vol 2008;33(4):475–7.

34. Blønd L, Madsen JL. Exsanguination of the upper limb in healthy young volunteers. J Bone Joint Surg Br 2002;84(4):489–91.

35. Mittal P, Shenoy S, Sandhu JS. Effect of different cuff widths on the motor nerve conduction of the median nerve: an experimental study. J Orthop Surg Res 2008;3:1.

36. Lowe JB 3rd, Sen SK, Mackinnon SE. Current approach to radial nerve paralysis. Plast Reconstr Surg 2002;110(4):1099–113.

37. Aho K, Sainio K, Kianta M, et al. Pneumatic tourniquet paralysis. Case report. J Bone Joint Surg Br 1983;65(4):441–3.

38. Maguiña P, Jean-Pierre F, Grevious MA, et al. Posterior interosseous branch palsy following pneumatic tourniquet application for hand surgery. Plast Reconstr Surg 2008;122(2):97e–9e.

39. Selvan D, Harle D, Fischer J. Beware of finger tourniquets: a case report and update by the National Patient Safety Agency. Acta Orthop Belg 2011; 77(1):15–7.

40. Kruse H, Christensen KP, Møller AM, et al. Tourniquet use during ankle surgery leads to increased postoperative opioid use. J Clin Anesth 2015; 27(5):380–4.

41. Saied A, Zyaei A. Tourniquet use during plating of acute extra-articular tibial fractures: effects on final results of the operation. J Trauma 2010; 69(6):E94–7.

42. Smith TO, Hing CB. The efficacy of the tourniquet in foot and ankle surgery? A systematic review and meta-analysis. Foot Ankle Surg 2010; 16(1):3–8.

43. Salam AA, Eyres KS, Cleary J, et al. The use of a tourniquet when plating tibial fractures. J Bone Joint Surg Br 1991;73(1):86–7.

44. Konrad G, Markmiller M, Lenich A, et al. Tourniquets may increase postoperative swelling and pain after internal fixation of ankle fractures. Clin Orthop Relat Res 2005;(433):189–94.

45. Maffulli N, Testa V, Capasso G. Use of a tourniquet in the internal fixation of fractures of the distal part of the fibula. A prospective, randomized trial. J Bone Joint Surg Am 1993;75(5):700–3.

46. Dobner JJ, Nitz AJ. Postmeniscectomy tourniquet palsy and functional sequelae. Am J Sports Med 1982;10(4):211–4.

47. Pollak AN, Battistella F, Pettey J, et al. Reamed femoral nailing in patients with multiple injuries. Adverse effects of tourniquet use. Clin Orthop Relat Res 1997;(339):41–6.

48. Younger ASE, Kalla TP, McEwen JA, et al. Survey of tourniquet use in orthopaedic foot and ankle surgery. Foot Ankle Int 2005;26:208–17.

49. Younger ASE, McEwen JA, Inkpen K. Wide contoured thigh cuffs and automated limb occlusion measurement allow lower tourniquet pressures. Clin Orthop Relat Res 2004;428(428):286–93.

50. Lin LN, Wang LR, Wang WT, et al. Ischemic preconditioning attenuates pulmonary dysfunction after unilateral thigh tourniquet-induced ischemia-reperfusion. Anesth Analg 2010;111(2):539–43.

51. Kornbluth ID, Freedman MK, Sher L, et al. Femoral, saphenous nerve palsy after tourniquet use: a case report. Arch Phys Med Rehabil 2003;84(6):909–11.

52. Mingo-Robinet J, Castañeda-Cabrero C, Alvarez V, et al. Tourniquet-related iatrogenic femoral nerve palsy after knee surgery: case report and review of the literature. Case Rep Orthop 2013;2013: 368290.

53. Hirvensalo E, Tuominen H, Lapinsuo M, et al. Compartment syndrome of the lower limb caused by a tourniquet: a report of two cases. J Orthop Trauma 1992;6(4):469–72.

54. Murphy CG, Winter DC, Bouchier-Hayes DJ. Tourniquet injuries: pathogenesis and modalities for attenuation. Acta Orthop Belg 2005;71(6): 635–45.

55. Feldman V, Biadsi A, Slavin O, et al. Pulmonary embolism after application of a sterile elastic exsanguination tourniquet. Orthopedics 2015;38(12): e1160–3.

56. Odinsson A, Finsen V. Tourniquet use and its complications in Norway. J Bone Joint Surg Br 2006; 88(8):1090–2.

57. Ochoa J, Fowler TJ, Gilliatt RW. Anatomical changes in peripheral nerves compressed by a pneumatic tourniquet. J Anat 1972;113(Pt 3): 433–55.

58. Pollard BJ, Lovelock HA, Jones RM. Fatal pulmonary embolism secondary to limb exsanguination. Anesthesiology 1983;58(4):373–4.

59. Araki S, Uchiyama M. Fatal pulmonary embolism following tourniquet inflation. A case report. Acta Orthop Scand 1991;62(5):488.

60. Hofmann AA, Wyatt RW. Fatal pulmonary embolism following tourniquet inflation. A case report. J Bone Joint Surg Am 1985;67(4):633–4.

61. Darmanis S, Papanikolaou A, Pavlakis D. Fatal intraoperative pulmonary embolism following application of an Esmarch bandage. Injury 2002;33(9): 761–4.

62. Hirota K, Hashimoto H, Kabara S, et al. The relationship between pneumatic tourniquet time and the amount of pulmonary emboli in patients undergoing knee arthroscopic surgeries. Anesth Analg 2001;93:776–80.

Articular Incongruity in the Lower Extremity
How Much Is Too Much?

Tim R. Beals, DO[a], Robert Harris, MD[b],
Darryl A. Auston, MD, PhD[c],*

KEYWORDS
• Articular reduction • Periarticular fractures • Lower extremity trauma • Posttraumatic arthritis • PTOA • Articular congruity

KEY POINTS
• Posttraumatic arthritis can occur after intraarticular fractures of the lower extremity and is multifactorial in origin. • The threshold of acceptable articular incongruity in each joint varies and is likely related to the particular biology and biomechanics of the joint involved. • Surgical restoration of articular congruity may help to lower the risk of posttraumatic arthritis, but high-quality human studies are lacking in many areas.

INTRODUCTION

Posttraumatic osteoarthritis (PTOA) is a clinical sequela of injury to the articular cartilage most often related to intraarticular fracture. These fractures result in direct injury to the cartilage, articular incongruity, and joint instability, which contribute to altered chondral biology and mechanical function of the limbs. These alterations can result in degeneration of the chondral surface and subsequent PTOA of the joint.

Hyaline cartilage of the articular surface functions to distribute loads and minimize peak stresses on the subchondral bone. Chondrocytes are continually synthesizing matrix proteins to counteract the normal degradation of matrix macromolecules. Loading of the joint results in both mechanical and electrical signaling of chondrocytes to modulate matrix synthesis, and allows the cartilage to adapt to physiologic stress. Hyaline cartilage is composed of cells, macromolecular matrix, and water; there is a distinct lack of nerves, blood vessels, and lymphatics. Owing to this lack of vascularity, chondrocytes rely on diffusion for nutrition and their metabolism is primarily anaerobic, making for a decreased capacity to adapt to injury and heal.

PTOA is a significant contributor to degenerative joint disease burden, at an estimated annual cost in the billions of dollars in the United States.[1] The incidence of PTOA after joint trauma varies depending on the joint and articular surface involved (Table 1).[2–14] These rates have remained relatively constant over time, despite advances in surgical technique and equipment.

Variability in the occurrence of PTOA after articular trauma likely represents a combination of local differences in cartilage structure, loading at the time of injury, and joint biomechanics. The causes of PTOA after joint injury are multifactorial, and include acute mechanical injury to the cartilage, inflammatory response with altered

Conflicts of Interest and Source of Funding: The authors have no conflicts of interest related to this work.
[a] Jack Hughston Memorial Hospital, Department of Orthopedic Surgery, 4401 Riverchase Drive, Phenix City, AL 36867, USA; [b] Hughston Orthopedic Trauma at Midtown Medical Center, Jack Hughston Memorial Hospital, Department of Orthopedic Surgery, 4401 Riverchase Drive, Phenix City, AL 36867, USA; [c] Hughston Trauma at Orange Park Medical Center, 1895 Kingsley Avenue, Suite 300, Orange Park, FL 32073, USA
* Corresponding author.
E-mail address: Darryl.auston@gmail.com

Table 1 Reported rate of posttraumatic arthritis by joint	
Joint	Risk of Posttraumatic Arthritis (%)
Acetabulum[2]	11–38
Femoral head[3]	20
Distal femur[4]	23–35
Tibial plateau[5,6]	23–44
Plafond[7]	70–75
Talar body[8–12]	48–90
Calcaneus[13,14]	100

biologics, and chronic pathologic mechanical loading secondary to joint incongruity, instability, and malalignment.[15]

PATHOGENESIS OF POSTTRAUMATIC OSTEOARTHRITIS

Direct Injury

Direct mechanical injury is the initial contributor to chondral degeneration in PTOA. An extreme supraphysiologic force is required for fracture of the articular surface, with the cartilage tissue initially absorbing sufficient energy to disrupt chondral biology. Chondrocytes at the fracture site experience these loading forces, and demonstrate a significant reduction in viability after simulated tibial plafond fracture, 74.1% versus 91.4% more distant to fracture lines.[16] These differences in chondrocyte viability have been demonstrated in vivo as well, with explanted articular cartilage of the calcaneus after fracture showing a similar 73% versus 95% viability.[17]

Metabolic Injury

After the initial mechanical loading insult, local alterations in metabolism serve to further the cascade toward degeneration and PTOA. Mitochondrial injury to the chondrocyte results in the release of oxygen free radicals, with subsequent matrix disruption, and further chondrocyte death.[18,19]

Articular injury also results in the release of inflammatory mediators, including tumor necrosis factor-alpha, interleukin-1, nitrous oxide, and matrix metalloproteinases.[19–21] These inflammatory mediators play a significant role in further degradation and advancement to PTOA. In an animal model comparing normal mice with a breed that produces decreased interleukin-1, and increased interleukin-4 and -10 (antiinflammatory mediators), the test group demonstrated

significantly reduced joint inflammatory response with a relative protection from PTOA.[22]

Chronic Injury

Chronic mechanical alterations across the articular surface also contribute to further degradation. Joint incongruity, instability, and malalignment all likely play a role, although to what degree has yet to be fully determined, and likely depends on the joint involved.

It is intuitive that articular step off would lead to increased loading through decreased contact surface area, and cadaver models have demonstrated an up to 300% increase in contact stresses.[23] The addition of joint instability can result in a shift of the loading of the joint to an anatomic location not adapted for such stresses, and unable to accommodate these new loads.[24,25] Despite this, other models of joint incongruity demonstrate minimal increases in contact stresses.[26,27] It should be noted that these results came from static loads in a fixed joint position, thus not allowing for the evaluation of transient stresses during physiologic motion and load bearing.

Whereas PTOA is multifactorial in etiology, there is evidence that accurate articular reduction can affect the rate of PTOA. This article addresses the role of articular reduction in fractures of the lower extremity and analyzes the support in orthopedic literature in an attempt to answer the question, "How much is too much incongruity?"

Evaluation of Joint Congruity

One factor that limits our understanding of the influence of articular incongruity on PTOA and outcomes is the accuracy of radiographic evaluation of this incongruity. Interrater reliabilities of plain radiographs for articular incongruity in tibial plateau fractures have been shown to be poor, with differences of up to 12 mm.[28] Computed tomography (CT) allows for a much more accurate evaluation of the articular surface, but with an increased cost and radiation load.[29] Because much of the data on articular reduction and PTOA are based on plain radiographic studies, results should be interpreted with these limitations in mind.

Acetabulum

The acetabulum is a hemispherical recess formed from the triradiate cartilage between the ilium, pubis, and ischium. It is covered with hyaline cartilage, and deepened by the peripheral labrum. The acetabular fossa is fat filled and serves as the attachment for the ligamentum teres; the floor of the acetabular fossa is the quadrilateral surface.

Reports in the 1960s on simple fracture patterns in the younger patient and complex fractures in the elderly could be treated with conservative measures yielding satisfactory outcomes.[30–33] These classic articles demonstrated that incongruence in the weight-bearing portion of the acetabular dome and the femoral head gave poor outcomes, which may be improved with open reduction and internal fixation, anatomic reduction, and appropriate stabilization. Letournel and Judet[34] reported on 350 surgically repaired acetabular fractures. They achieved 77.2% very good, 8.3% good, and 16.5% poor outcomes. These investigators found good correlation with the quality of the reduction and clinical outcomes. Of the 74% with anatomic reductions, 90% had a satisfactory clinical result.

In 1986, Matta and colleagues[35] reported on a retrospective analysis of 204 acetabular fractures and the evaluation of the weight bearing dome. These investigators demonstrated that satisfactory results were achievable when the weight-bearing dome remains intact and that surgical fixation with anatomic reduction improves outcomes in displaced fractures. Matta and colleagues[36] published a separate prospective study of 121 cases of displaced factures. Of the reductions, 63% were considered anatomic (<1 mm displacement on plain radiographs) and 93% of these patients had satisfactory results. These investigators also noted that with experience poor outcomes decline and anatomic reductions increase. In 2012, Matta and colleagues[37] reviewed survivorship in 810 operatively treated acetabular fractures. The cumulative 20-year survival rate was 79%. Negative outcome predictors were nonanatomic reduction, age greater than 40 years, anterior hip dislocation, postoperative incongruence of the acetabular roof, posterior wall involvement, marginal impaction, femoral head cartilage lesion, an initial displacement of greater than 20 mm, and the use of an extended iliofemoral approach.

In certain minimally displaced fractures in the younger patient or elderly patients, minimally invasive techniques have been described using special fluoroscopy views or with computer-assisted acetabular fixation.[38–40] Investigators have demonstrated satisfactory results in selected acetabular fractures with percutaneous and limited open techniques. In 2012, Starr and colleagues[41] reviewed their series of percutaneous screw fixation in elderly patients and found the rate of conversion to total hip arthroplasty was the same as open approaches for fracture fixation.

Elderly patients represent a different operative challenge for treating surgeons. Acetabular fractures in geriatric patients are more likely the result of low-energy trauma and advanced age has been reported as a risk for diminished outcomes.[37] In 2017, Ryan and colleagues[42] performed a retrospective review of 27 patients age 60 years or older who sustained displaced acetabular fractures over an 11-year period. These patients met the criteria for operative treatment but were managed with nonoperative measures. This study reviewed the outcomes with the Short Form-8, Western Ontario and McMaster Universities Osteoarthritis Index scores, 1-year mortality, and conversion to open reduction and internal fixation or hip arthroplasty. Conversion to total hip arthroplasty was 15% and mortality rate at 1 year was 24%. Their results demonstrated surprisingly good outcome scores with nonoperative treatment. The authors concluded there is a role for nonoperative treatment with early mobilization in this patient population when there is an absence of posterior instability.

In the young or physiologically young patient open anatomic reduction of the articular surface with articular incongruity of less than 2 mm is recommended to produce the best long-term outcomes.[34–36] In the elderly, less active patient, the degree of acceptable articular incongruity is unclear. These patients may benefit from a limited approach or nonoperative management.

Femoral Head

Femoral head fractures are often associated with hip dislocations, with about 7% to 16% of traumatic hip dislocations having an associated femoral head fracture.[43,44] This association seems to become more prevalent in anterior dislocations, with 1 series reporting 68% of anterior dislocations having a concomitant femoral head fracture.[45] Given the high-energy nature of these injuries and association with hip dislocations, fractures of the acetabulum and femoral neck are common.

The femoral head is a relative sphere ranging in diameter from about 40 to 60 mm, with deviation from a perfect sphere of up to 1.5 mm.[46] Hyaline cartilage covers the femoral head, and about 70% of the articular surface is involved in load transmission.[47] Loss of congruency with the acetabulum from femoral head fractures decreases the area of load transmission, with a resulting increase in peak compressive forces.

The nonoperative management of a reduced femoral head fracture is limited to small infrafoveal fractures, displaced by less than 1 mm and not associated with intraarticular debris. Owing to the potential debilitating nature of these injuries, most require operative consideration.[48]

There are few long-term reports of hip dislocations with femoral head fractures. Dreinhofer and colleagues[49] reported 15 of 26 patients with fair to poor outcomes at 5 years. Swiontkowski and colleagues[48] reported on their study of 24 patients followed for more than 2 years. One-half were treated with a posterior approach and one-half with an anterior approach. There were no cases of avascular necrosis in the anterior approach group, but there was an increase in heterotopic ossification formation. Stannard and colleagues[50] found a 3.2-fold higher incidence of avascular necrosis with a Kocher–Langenbeck approach versus those repaired though the Smith–Peterson approach.

Percutaneous methods or arthroscopically assisted methods may play a role in surgical management given the potential complications of open approaches. Homma and colleagues[51] provided a case report of Pipkin IV femoral head fracture treat with 2 percutaneous headless compression screws. With 4 years of follow-up, these investigators reported union with a "full Harris Hip Score," as well as no osteonecrosis or PTOA on MRI. Matsuda[52] described the case of Pipkin II fracture without associated dislocation managed with arthroscopic reduction and headless screw fixation. Return to full activity was reported at 4 months postoperatively. Park and colleagues[53] described similar treatment of a Pipkin I fracture. Larger series and long-term outcomes are not yet available.

To date, no studies have evaluated specifically the quality of articular reduction and outcome. Given the large, concentric articulation of the hip joint, it is generally accepted that near anatomic reduction is necessary.

Distal Femur

Distal femoral fractures account for between 4% and 7% of femoral fractures, and 31% of all femoral fractures below the hip.[54–56] The estimated annual incidence in the United States is reported at 31 per million.[57] This incidence follows a bimodal age distribution, with higher energy mechanisms in younger patients and lower energy mechanisms in older populations with bony insufficiency.

Bony insufficiency plays a large role in the incidence of distal femur fractures in general, with the large majority of fractures occurring in patients older than 50, and greater than 80% of these fractures in the elderly population occurring in women.[54,58] In roughly two-thirds of lower energy distal femur fractures, patients have a history of osteopenia and/or insufficiency fractures to the hip, proximal humerus, distal radius, pelvis, or vertebra. However, owing to bony insufficiency often leading to fracture propagation through the metaphyseal bone, there is a lesser incidence of intraarticular involvement than in younger patients with high-energy trauma.[59]

The current body of published data on articular incongruity of the distal femur has been formed entirely from animal model studies. Lefkoe and colleagues[60] created a 5-mm incongruency in the medial femoral condyle of 22 white rabbits, compared with an articular reduction in an additional 12 animals. The step off was created without sacrificing alignment or stability. Gross appearance, histology, radiographs, and chemical analysis of glucose aminoglycan levels were performed at 10 and 20 weeks. Osteophyte formation, fibrillation of the femoral condyle and medial tibial plateau, and decreased cellularity were noted at 10 weeks. These changes progressed significantly at 20 weeks, with the additional observation of decreased glucose aminoglycan levels. These changes were not seen with anatomic reduction. When the experiment was repeated with a 2-mm step off, however, hyaline-appearing repair cartilage was noted.[61] Of the 18 specimens with incongruity, 15 demonstrated congruity of the repair tissue at 20 weeks. These findings suggest a reduction within the thickness of the articular cartilage can allow for a repair and remodeling response.

Llinas and colleagues[62] demonstrated a similar capacity to heal partial thickness incongruences of 0.5 and 1.0 mm. These results were also obtained in a white rabbit model with an articular step off induced in the medial femoral condyle. In the 54 specimens of this study, the capacity to repair and remodel was demonstrated at both levels, with a more rapid healing response noted in the 0.5- mm group.

Lovasz and colleagues[63] further corroborated these findings in their study with 21 white rabbits, using an 0.5-mm step off. Interestingly, these repair and remodel systems were nullified when instability was introduced with an anterior cruciate ligament resection.[64] In those 12 specimens, significant radiographic, gross, and histologic evidence of degeneration were demonstrated at 12 and 24 weeks despite the same 0.5-mm step off tested previously. There was no difference in the degeneration parameters noted between the anterior cruciate ligament–deficient step off group and a control anterior cruciate ligament–deficient group with no step off, suggesting that instability is a major contributor of articular degeneration, regardless of articular surface deformity.

These animal models demonstrate an intriguing possibility for chondral repair and preservation with minimal articular incongruence, but high-quality studies in human subjects are not available. The animal data also serve to further exemplify the interplay between joint congruence and stable kinematics in the survival of native cartilage after articular injury.

Tibial Plateau

The knee is a complex diarthrodial joint with intricate bony morphology, mechanical alignment, and multiple soft tissue interactions contributing to normal joint loading and stability. The anterior cruciate ligament and posterior cruciate ligament resist anterior and posterior translation of the tibia on the femur, respectively. The medial collateral ligament is the primary resistance to valgus force and has intimate connections from the deep medial collateral ligament to the medial meniscus. The lateral collateral ligament is the primary restraint to varus force. The crescent-shaped, fibrocartilaginous menisci serve to deepen the femoral tibial articulation and allow for load dissipation.

The knee demonstrates a complex motion profile beyond simple flexion and extension. Internal and external rotation of the tibia on the femur, known as the "screw home" mechanism, as well as femoral "roll back," result in a knee flexion axis that is not through a fixed point, but along a gradually altered path of instant centers of rotation. This biomechanical motion profile results in changes of local chondral loading during dynamic weightbearing of the joint.

The significant varus and valgus, translational, and impaction forces that cause tibial plateau fractures, as well as the close proximity of the knee ligaments and menisci to the zone of bony injury, result in a high association of these fractures with ligamentous and meniscal injuries. In high-energy mechanisms, more than 70% of these fractures demonstrated MRI evidence of at least 1 ligament tear, with about 50% demonstrating at least 2 knee ligaments damaged. Additionally, about 50% of such fractures had a meniscal injury identified.[65] In 1 study, 18 of 20 patients with nondisplaced or minimally displaced tibial plateau fractures had ligamentous or meniscal injury on MRI.[66]

The interplay between articular injury, displacement, alignment, and stability makes isolating their individual contributions to outcome difficult. In 1 biomechanical study, Brown and colleagues[67] produced tibial plateau fractures in 7 cadaveric specimens, and sequentially altered the articular step off between 0.25 and 3.0 mm, using pressure-sensitive Fuji-film to assess peak pressures during loading. They found a statistically significant increase in peak pressures between the 1.5- and 3.0-mm step off data, with 3.0 mm of incongruity resulting in an increase of peak pressures to about 175% that of no incongruity. The interval from 1.5 to 3.0 mm was also observed to result in no contact between the depressed fragment and the distal femur. It should be noted that their specimens were stripped of all soft tissue attachments about the knee, including ligaments and menisci, and all loading was performed on a static knee.

Blokker and colleagues[68] rated reductions as anatomic, less than 5 mm, and more than 5 mm incongruity in 60 fractures (38 operatively treated). They evaluated rates of "satisfactory" outcome at an average follow-up of 38.6 months (range, 3–108). They found that an articular step off of greater than 5 mm resulted in "unsatisfactory" outcome in 100% of patients. The rate of unsatisfactory outcomes in patients with less than 5 mm of residual incongruity was reported at 25%, and 14.3% in anatomic reductions. They found no correlation between ligamentous injury identified and treated at time of injury with patient outcomes, and concluded that articular reduction was the most important factor for patient outcomes. There was no evaluation of PTOA.

Moore and colleagues[69] performed serial radiographic and clinical evaluations of 165 plateau fractures treated both operatively and nonoperatively. These investigators found a significant drop off in subjective outcomes with greater than 10 mm of incongruity, and a linear relationship between incongruity and objective scoring of knee alignment, stability, and range of motion. There was no analysis of arthrosis, and no subanalysis to separate the effects of incongruity, alignment, and instability on outcomes.

Lansinger and colleagues[70] published a 20 year follow-up on 102 tibial plateau fractures (57 treated operatively), with analysis of outcomes in the 52 of those patients (32 operative) with a component of articular depression, comparing residual step offs of 1 to 5, 6 to 10, and more than 10 mm. The only reported "poor" outcome in their series was associated with a greater than 10-mm incongruity, with an overall rate of 81% "good" or "excellent" outcomes in that cohort. Conversely, less than 10 mm was associated with a 96% rate of "good" or excellent" outcomes. Instability was considered the indication for surgery in this study population, and 5 of the 6 fair or poor results were in the operative arm. The authors concluded that joint instability rather than articular step off should be the primary indication of operative decision making, regardless of articular incongruity.

Su and colleagues[71] compared quality of reduction with patient outcomes in 39 operative tibial plateaus in patients over the age of 55. They demonstrated statistically significant drops in Short Musculoskeletal Function Assessment scores with worsening Rasmussen radiographic scores of reduction. Importantly, the Rasmussen score gives equal weighting to limb alignment and articular incongruity, and there was no breakdown of the individual contribution of these components to the study population's outcomes scores. The authors advocated surgical intervention in displaced fractures for the restoration of alignment and congruity.

Honkonen[72] reviewed 131 fractures (76 operative) at an average follow-up of 7.6 years (range, 3.3–13.4). Articular step off was rated as 0, 1 to 3, 3 to 6, or more than 6 mm. The percentage of "acceptable" outcomes dropped significantly to less than 50% when a step off of at least 3 mm was noted. A stronger correlation was noted with instability and malalignment, as any instability beyond "mild" (1+ anterior or posterior drawer, or <10° varus/valgus instability) was associated with a 70% unsatisfactory outcome rate. Analysis of limb alignment after healing revealed 29 patients in the cohort with varus or valgus alignment of greater than 5°. Ten patients with either varus or valgus malalignment of greater than 10° universally yielded unsatisfactory results. The authors found in the remaining 19 patients with malalignment between 6° and 10°, valgus malalignment was functionally and subjectively well-tolerated. However, they noted increasingly poorer results with increasing varus malalignment. A subanalysis of this same patient cohort for PTOA showed no correlation between articular incongruity and radiographic evidence of degeneration.[73] There was, however, a significant correlation with instability. Late instability noted at follow-up was associated with 69%

PTOA rate, whereas instability at presentation demonstrated a 75% rate, even when repair or reconstruction was performed. Notably, degeneration was heavily correlated with total meniscectomy, with a rate of 74% versus 37% in knees without meniscectomy performed.

Rademakers and colleagues[6] presented similar results in their review of 109 operative fractures with 5 to 27 years of follow-up (average of 14 years). They found a significant contribution of malalignment with greater than 5° deviation increasing the risk of moderate to severe radiographic osteoarthrosis to 27% compared with 9% with more normal alignment. No distinction was made in their study between varus or valgus alignment. No correlation was found between quality of reduction and PTOA rate, although no articular incongruity of more than 4 mm was identified.

In contrast, Decoster and colleagues[74] followed 30 nonoperative tibial plateau fractures treated with cast bracing for 10 to 13 years, with assessment of PTOA on radiographs. Their patient cohort demonstrated a 100% rate of no to minimal arthrosis changes when articular incongruity was less than 4 mm, with an average Iowa knee score of 93. Fractures with greater than 4 mm of step off resulted in a 50% incidence of more significant arthrosis, and a reduction in the average Iowa score to 61. Ligamentous instability was noted in only 4 patients, with one noted to progress to significant arthrosis. They further noted the contribution of fracture pattern, with 70% of bicondylar fractures developing degenerative changes. The authors concluded that depression of less than 4 mm was amenable to nonoperative management with early range of motion, whereas more than 4 mm of displacement and bicondylar fractures may be better served with alternative treatment.

Overall, there are conflicting data regarding absolute tolerances of articular step off in the tibial plateau. Recommendations based on clinical outcomes range from 3 to 10 mm. More consistently found through the literature, however, is the contribution of joint stability, preservation of the menisci, and limb alignment to PTOA and clinical outcomes in displaced tibial plateau fractures.

Tibial Plafond

Tibial plafond fractures account for about 1% of fractures of the lower extremity and up to 10% of fractures of the tibia.[75–82] These fractures represent a spectrum from low-energy simple injuries to high-energy complex injuries, and are most commonly associated with motor vehicle collisions.[76,83,84] The high energies imparted on the distal tibia, along with its subcutaneous location, result in 10% to 50% of these injuries presenting as open fractures.[83,85–98]

The distal tibial articular surface, often referred to as the plafond (French for ceiling), has a quadrilateral shape with attached pyramidal medial malleolus. The distal tibia articulates with the body of the talus, as well as the distal fibula through the incisura fibularis. The ligamentous attachments near the articular surface include the deltoid ligament complex at the medial malleolus, the anterior inferior tibiofibular ligament, and the posterior inferior tibiofibular ligament. The ligaments attach to each of the major fragments classically seen in impaction fractures of the plafond, with the anterior inferior tibiofibular ligament attaching to the anterolateral "Chaput" fragment and the posterior inferior tibiofibular ligament attaching to the posterolateral "Volkmann" fragment.

Fractures of the plafond result from a combination of axial loading and rotational forces. Higher energy mechanisms tend to be associated with more axial loading, and greater comminution and soft tissue injury; low-energy fractures result from pure torsional loading, as seen with skiing injuries. The contribution of axial loading to these fractures is critical to the outcome of the articular surface, because this high level of compression causes cartilage necrosis.

Fractures of the tibia plafond are one of the most challenging fractures that face the orthopedic trauma specialist. Despite the evolution of the management of these injuries, the results can vary because of the nature of the injury, limited soft tissue envelope, and the cellular damage to the cartilage at the time of injury. Before 1963, the operative results of pilon fractures were disappointing, with good results in less than 50% in most studies.[99,100] Ruedi and Allgower[101] reported 74% good to excellent results in 84 pilons with a 4.2-year follow-up. Heim and Nasser[102] reported similar good outcomes and low rates of wound infection. Both studies included lower energy skiing injuries, with only 6% being open in the study by Ruedi and Allgower.[101] Other centers of excellence with experienced surgeons, such as Kellam and Wiss in North America, were not able to replicate this level of success and their series had many high-energy and open fractures.[103,104] Owing to these problems, in the 1990s several authors reported on the use of external fixation and limited internal fixation with good to excellent outcomes in 60% to 71%.[105,106] Some studies used hybrid frames or the Ilizarov technique to avoid the cantilever effect, and reported good outcomes.[83] Beside the inability to completely reduce the articular surface with ligamentotaxis, pin tract issues and ankle stiffness were common until the frame was removed; however, there were fewer total wound complications. Watson and colleagues[107] reported on a staged method with external fixation and a delay of 13 days average for final fixation. In their series of 107 pilon fractures, all patients received immediate calcaneal pin traction or traveling traction external fixation. Tscherne grade 0 and 1 soft tissue injuries underwent open reduction and internal fixation, whereas Tscherne grades 2 and 3 and all open fractures were treated with limited open reduction and internal fixation and stabilization with hybrid ringed external fixators. At an average of 4.9 years of follow-up, good to excellent results were reported in 81% of the hybrid external fixator group and 75% of the open reduction internal fixation group.

Despite early good results, outcomes can degrade over time. Ruedi and Allgöwer[108] followed their study patients for 9 years and found degenerative changes despite good reduction in low-energy fractures. Pollack and colleagues[109] followed their series patients with external fixation or open reduction and internal fixation for 2 years and found significant pain, swelling, and disability with a correlation to the use of an external fixator.

Korkmaz and colleagues[110] demonstrated that the most important factor affecting outcome in surgically treated tibia pilon fractures was the quality of the reduction. Poor functional scores were found independent from the type of surgery and quality of reduction in Rüedi/Allgöwer type 3 fractures, which was characterized with articular surface comminution and metaphyseal impaction.

Sanders and colleagues[111] compared the use of a posterior lateral approach for the posterior malleolus and external fixation followed by delay for definitive fixation to external fixation and a delay for open reduction and internal fixation using a single incision. A total of 116 patients were treated surgically with postoperative CT scans completed. Twenty-six fractures presented as an open injury. Of these 116 patients, 35 underwent staged fixation of the posterior malleolar component at an average of 2 days postinjury, followed by delayed anterior fixation at an average of 14 days postinjury. The remaining 81 patients underwent anterior fixation alone, on average

17 days postinjury. Of the 95 patients with sufficient follow-up (≥12 months), there were 24 nonunions. There was a statistically significant association of nonunion with a staged posterior approach (40% vs 19%). CT reduction for staged posterior versus an anterior-alone approach was not different for any of the 3 categories (63% vs 57% at <1 mm, 31% vs 26% at 1–2 mm, and 6% vs 17% at >2 mm). In this series, there was no benefit to combined surgical approaches to tibial pilon fractures with regard to the quality of articular reduction. It seems, from this investigation, that there may be a significantly greater risk of nonunion associated with the addition of the staged posterior approach. Although articular reduction is of paramount importance, multiple approaches for direct reduction and fixation of all fragments may lead to further complications.

High-energy pilon fractures are challenging injuries. Multiple options are described for the definitive surgical management of these fractures, but there is no level I evidence for optimal management. Anatomic reduction of the fracture, restoration of joint congruence, and reconstruction of the posterior column with a correct limb axis minimizing the soft tissue insult are the key points to a good outcome when treating pilon fractures. Even when these goals are achieved, there is no guarantee that results will be acceptable in the mid term owing to the frequent progression to posttraumatic arthritis.

In high-energy fractures with soft tissue compromise, a staged treatment is generally accepted as the best way to take care of these devastating fractures. The axial cuts from the CT scans are essential to defining the location of the main fracture line, the fracture pattern (sagittal or coronal), and the number of fragments. All of this information is crucial for preoperative planning, incision placement, and articular surface reduction. No single method of fixation is ideal for all pilon fractures, or suitable for all patients. Definitive decision making depends most on the fracture pattern, condition of the soft tissues, the patient's profile, and surgical expertise.

Talar Body

Fractures of the talar body are distinguished from talar neck fractures in that talar body fractures involve both the tibiotalar joint as well as the posterior facet of the subtalar joint, whereas talar neck fractures are considered primarily extraarticular with some involving the middle facet of the subtalar joint.[8,112,113] Isolated talar body fractures are rare, accounting for less than 1% of all fractures.[9,113] Historically, rates of PTOA after talar body fractures are reported between 48% and 90%.[8–12] These published rates may not reflect the true rate of PTOA in isolated talar body fracture because these reports include talar body fractures associated with ipsilateral injuries to the ankle, tibial plafond, hindfoot, and midfoot. Additionally, talar body fractures can occur with simultaneous fracture of the talar neck. As such, some reports include combined talar neck and body fractures, making it difficult to assess the outcomes of talar body fractures in isolation.

Sneppen and colleagues[9] reported on a series of 51 isolated talar body fractures that included 6 subsets of fracture patterns: medial or lateral compression fractures of the talar dome, coronal shear, sagittal shear, fractures of the posterior process, fractures of the lateral tubercle, and comminuted crush fractures involving the tibiotalar and subtalar joints. Additionally, they divided the fractures into groups of nondisplaced, displaced, and displaced with subluxation of the tibiotalar, subtalar, or both joints. However, it was not noted the radiographic requirements for displacement. Three patients underwent surgical fixation, although it is unclear which subtypes were indicated for those procedures. The remainder were treated with closed reduction and casting. The rate of PTOA overall was 55%, with 50% of compression injuries resulting in tibiotalar arthritis, 65% of shear injuries, and 75% of crush injuries with PTOA of the tibiotalar, subtalar, or both joints. Additionally, 43% of injuries rated as healed without displacement were noted to develop PTOA. Clinical evaluation revealed that only 24% of patients had minor or no complaints. The remaining 76% reported moderate (29%) or severe (47%) complaints. Only 37% of patients returned to their previous level of work. The high rate of poor outcomes associated with primarily nonoperative treatment led the authors to recommend surgical fixation of these injuries.

Vallier and colleagues[113] have reported the largest series to date of surgically treated talar body fractures. Fifty-seven patients with talar body fractures were treated surgically; 40% had associated talar neck fracture. Of the 57 patients, 38 were followed for an average of 33 months, with 26 of 38 reported to have a complete sets of radiographs. Reduction of the body fractures was deemed anatomic in 21 of 26 patients. Four patients had articular incongruity of 1 to 2 mm, and 1 patient had 10° of angular malalignment. The authors report radiographic

PTOA in the tibiotalar joint of 65% of patients, in the subtalar joint of 35% of patients. End-stage PTOA was seen in the tibiotalar joint of 6 patients, in the subtalar joint of 2 patients, and in both joints of 6 patients. The incidence of end-stage PTOA was more common in combined talar body and talar neck fractures, open fractures, and comminuted fractures. As expected, end-stage PTOA led to worse functional outcome scores. At the time of last follow-up, 20 of the 30 patients had returned to work. Of those who did not return to work, 5 were unemployed at the time of injury. The authors note that surgical fixation can restore congruity of the tibiotalar and subtalar joints; however, many patients developed PTOA.

A series of 25 patients with 26 isolated talar body and/or talar neck fractures were reported by Lindvall and colleagues.[112] Eight of these were talar body fractures, 16 were talar neck fractures, and 2 were combined talar neck and body fractures. All patients were treated with surgical fixation of the injuries. Reduction was deemed anatomic in 16 fractures, nearly anatomic in 5 fractures, and poor in 5 fractures. Patients were followed for a minimum of 48 months. PTOA of the subtalar joint was found in all 25 patients at the last reported follow-up. Fifteen patients had PTOA of both the tibiotalar and subtalar joints. No tibiotalar PTOA was identified in any patient. Pain scores were recorded, and all patients reported some level of chronic pain. Five patients reported severe, 10 patients reported moderate, and 10 patients reported mild pain.

The authors of these 3 studies universally recommend surgical fixation when treating displaced talar body and/or talar neck fractures. Sneppen and colleagues[9] attributed the high rate of poor outcomes to malunion from nonoperative management and articular damage at the time of injury. They recommend exact anatomic reduction and stable fixation to reduce the impact of malunion on poor patient outcomes. Both surgical series achieve a high rate of anatomic or nearly anatomic reductions in 46 of 52 combined patients (88%) identified as having articular incongruity of 2 mm or less, and 37 (71%) having anatomic reduction. Despite meticulous surgical technique and excellent reductions, a high percentage of patients went on to develop PTOA in either the tibiotalar or subtalar joints, or both, with chronic pain and potentially poor functional outcomes. However, the patient outcomes seem to be improved over nonoperative management for displaced fractures. The authors of the surgical reports continue to recommend anatomic reduction and fixation with recommendations to counsel patients about the potentially devastating outcomes associated with these injuries.

Calcaneus

Treatment of displaced intraarticular calcaneus fractures (DIACFs) remains a subject of debate. Historically, conservative treatment was preferred owing to the poor results of surgical intervention.[114] Advances in imaging modalities, implant design, and surgical techniques have led to an increase in surgical treatment of DIACF. Despite this, prospective studies show inconsistent results with improved patient outcomes in some studies, and no difference in patient outcomes in other studies when comparing nonoperative with operative treatment of DIACF.[115–117] Despite these controversies, it is evident that some patients can benefit from operative treatment of DIACFs. Despite surgical intervention, subtalar PTOA is a recognized complication of this injury with rates reported as high as 100% in some series.[13,14]

Sanders and colleagues[118] reported on 120 DIACFs and established a classification system for DIACFs based on the fracture pattern of the posterior facet. The surgical technique reported by this group prioritizes anatomic reduction of the posterior facet, followed by restoration of Bohler's angle by reduction and fixation of the calcaneal body. Recently, the same group published a long-term follow-up study that included patients from the original series. There were 108 fractures with a minimum of 10-year follow-up that were evaluated after surgical treatment of DIACFs.[14] The mean follow-up for the cohort was 15 years, and 70 fractures were identified as Sanders type II and 38 were identified as Sanders type III fractures. Of these fractures, 95% were deemed to have an anatomic reduction, and 100% of the patients had radiologic evidence of subtalar PTOA. Of the patients, 29% required subtalar fusion. Breakdown of subtalar fusion by fracture classification showed patients with Sanders type III fractures were 4 times more likely to need fusion compared with Sanders type II fractures. Long-term functional outcomes of the remaining patients not requiring fusion showed 77% of patients were at or above the US average for Short From-36 Physical Component Scores, and average visual analog scores were 1.75, with 56% reporting little or no pain. The authors state that anatomic reduction of the posterior facet can improve functional outcomes, allow for normal or slightly modified shoe wear, and return to work in many cases. They caution that, despite anatomic reduction, patients may experience permanent difficulty with uneven ground and experience chronic mild pain.

Makki and colleagues[13] reported on 47 DIACFs treated surgically with an average follow-up of 10 years. There were 26 fractures identified as Sanders type II, 18 as Sanders type III, and 3 as Sanders type IV. The surgical technique included reduction on the posterior facet, but focused on restoration of the Bohler angle. As with the previous study, all patients had some evidence of subtalar PTOA. Five patients required subtalar fusion. Functional outcomes of the remaining patients not requiring fusion were based on American Orthopaedic Foot and Ankle Society scores and Creighton–Nebraska health foundation assessment. Overall, 74.5% of patients reported good to excellent results. The authors recommend surgical treatment with a goal of restoration of hindfoot shape and Bohler's angle.

A prospective, randomized, controlled, multicenter study evaluated operatively and nonoperatively treated DIACFs.[115] Three hundred nine patients (161 operatively treated) were followed for a minimum of 2 years. Posterior facet reductions were characterized in 156 patients. Anatomic reductions were achieved in 31% with an articular incongruity of less than 2 mm in 50%. The remaining 29% were deemed comminuted reductions. As with the previous study, the Bohler's angle was found to be prognostic in patient outcome. With respect to articular congruity, the authors report that patient's with Sanders type II fractures benefit from surgical treatment; operatively treated patients were 2.74 times more likely to score above average on Short Form-36 scores. Additionally, patients with light or moderate workloads benefitted from operative treatment over nonoperative treatment. No advantage was seen in operative treatment of higher energy injuries (Sanders type IV fractures, fractures with low Bohler's angles). The authors conclude that anatomic or near anatomic reduction of the posterior facet improves patient outcomes in carefully selected patients. The authors recommend nonoperative treatment of older men, patients with occupations requiring heavy workloads, and patients receiving worker's compensation.

Csizy and colleagues[119] performed a review of a prospective, randomized trial database of patients with DIACFs that had failed operative or nonoperative treatment and required subtalar fusion for PTOA. There were 44 patients who required subtalar fusion and compared with 417 patients not requiring fusion. Of those 44 patients, 7 had been treated operatively for the initial injury, and 37 were treated nonoperatively. The results are consistent with previous studies. Increasing severity of injury as indicated by Sanders classification increases risk of subtalar fusion with Sanders type IV fractures 5.5 times more likely to receive fusion over Sanders type II fractures. Patients with an initial Bohler angle of 0° were 10 times more likely to undergo subtalar fusion than patients with initial Bohler angles of greater than 15°. Patients receiving worker's compensation were 3 times more likely to need fusion. Consistent with previous studies, the authors concluded that patients receiving worker's compensation, who are heavy laborers, or who have higher energy injuries (Sanders type IV, low Bohler angle) are at high risk of subtalar fusion with nonoperative treatment. However, in contrast with other studies, the authors recommend surgical treatment of these injuries to decrease the possibility of future subtalar fusion.

DIACFs represent a complex injury in patients with a variety of work and lifestyle demands. Consensus has not been reached on the treatment of these injuries despite decades of research with recommendations for surgical intervention varying depending on fracture patterns and patient demographics. Once surgery is indicated, optimal surgical treatment should involve anatomic or near anatomic reconstruction of the posterior facet with restoration of the Bohler angle. Most authors characterize near anatomic reduction of the posterior facet as 2 mm or less of articular incongruity. It seems that nearly all patients with DIACFs can anticipate some degree of PTOA despite surgical intervention. However, there does seem to be some benefit of surgical fixation in certain fracture patterns. Simpler fracture patterns such as Sanders type II seem to benefit from operative management. That benefit then seems to decrease as the complexity of the fracture pattern increases with Sanders type IV fractures leading to high rates of subtalar fusions regardless of treatment.

SUMMARY

Intraarticular fractures carry a significant risk for PTOA, and this risk varies across different joint surfaces of the lower extremity. These differences are likely owing to anatomic and biomechanical specifics of each joint surface. The development of PTOA after trauma is multifactorial, involving acute chondral injury,

Table 2	
Maximum recommended articular incongruity	
Joint	Incongruity (mm)
Acetabulum[34–36]	2
Femoral head[48]	1
Distal femur[58]	2
Tibial plateau[66,67,69]	3–10
Plafond[80,98,99,102,103,105]	2
Talar body[8–12]	2
Calcaneus[13,14]	2

inflammatory response, articular incongruity, mechanical axis deviation, and instability. High-quality human studies are lacking to delineate the threshold articular incongruity that significantly increases risk for PTOA and diminishes clinical outcomes. Available recommendations are noted in Table 2. Available studies must also be analyzed critically, because plain radiographs show poor inter-rater reliabilities for the evaluation of articular step off. Even with anatomic reduction of the articular surface, close attention must be paid to the mechanical axis and joint stability to optimize outcomes.

REFERENCES

1. Brown TD, Johnston RC, Saltzman CL, et al. Post-traumatic osteoarthritis: a first estimate of incidence, prevalence, and burden of disease. J Orthop Trauma 2006;20(10):739–44.
2. Giannoudis PV, Grotz MR, Papakostidis C, et al. Operative treatment of displaced fractures of the acetabulum: a meta-analysis. J Bone Joint Surg Br 2005;87(1):2–9.
3. Giannoudis PV, Kontakis G, Christoforakis Z, et al. Management, complications and clinical results of femoral head fractures. Injury 2009;40(12):1245–51.
4. Rademakers MV, Kerkhoffs GM, Sierevelt IN, et al. Intra-articular fractures of the distal femur: a long-term follow-up study of surgically treated patients. J Orthop Trauma 2004;18(4):213–9.
5. Weigel DP, Marsh JL. High-energy fractures of the tibial plateau: knee function after longer follow-up. J Bone Joint Surg Am 2002;84(9):1541–51.
6. Rademakers MV, Kerkhoffs GM, Sierevelt IN, et al. Operative treatment of 109 tibial plateau fractures: five- to 27-year follow-up results. J Orthop Trauma 2007;21(1):10.
7. Marsh JL, Weigel DP, Dirschl DR. Tibial plafond fractures: how do these ankles function over time? J Bone Joint Surg Am 2003;85(2):287–95.
8. Inokuchi S, Ogawa K, Usami N. Classification of fractures of the talus: clear differentiation between neck and body fractures. Foot Ankle Int 1996;17(12):748–50.
9. Sneppen O, Christensen SB, Krogsoe O, et al. Fracture of the body of the talus. Acta Orthop Scand 1977;48(3):317–24.
10. Elgafy H, Ebraheim NA, Tile M, et al. Fractures of the talus: experience of two level 1 trauma centers. Foot Ankle Int 2000;21(12):1023–9.
11. Kenwright J, Taylor RG. Major injuries of the talus. J Bone Joint Surg Br 1970;52(1):36–48.
12. Mindell ER, Cisek EE, Kartalian G, et al. Late results of injuries to the talus: analysis of forty cases. J Bone Joint Surg 1963;45(2):221.
13. Makki D, Alnajjar HM, Walkay S, et al. Osteosynthesis of displaced intra-articular fractures of the calcaneum: a long-term review of 47 cases. J Bone Joint Surg Br 2010;92(5):693–700.
14. Sanders R, Vaupel ZM, Erdogan M, et al. Operative treatment of displaced intraarticular calcaneal fractures: long-term (10-20 Years) results in 108 fractures using a prognostic CT classification. J Orthop Trauma 2014;28(10):551–63.
15. Anderson DD, Chubinskaya S, Guilak F, et al. Post-traumatic osteoarthritis: improved understanding and opportunities for early intervention. J Orthop Res 2011;29(6):802–9.
16. Tochigi Y, Buckwalter JA, Martin JA, et al. Distribution and progression of chondrocyte damage in a whole-organ model of human ankle intra-articular fracture. J Bone Joint Surg Am 2011;93(6):533–9.
17. Ball ST, Jadin K, Allen RT, et al. Chondrocyte viability after intra-articular calcaneal fractures in humans. Foot Ankle Int 2007;28(6):665–8.
18. Goodwin W, McCabe D, Sauter E, et al. Rotenone prevents impact-induced chondrocyte death. J Orthop Res 2010;28(8):1057–63.
19. Martin JA, Buckwalter JA. Post traumatic osteoarthritis: the role of stress induced chondrocyte damage. Biorheology 2006;43(3–4):517–21.
20. Green DM, Noble PC, Ahuero JS, et al. Cellular events leading to chondrocyte death after cartilage impact injury. Arthritis Rheum 2006;54(5):1509–17.
21. Guilak F, Fermor B, Keefe FJ, et al. The role of biomechanics and inflammation in cartilage injury and repair. Clin Orthop Relat Res 2004;423:17–26.
22. Ward BD, Furman BD, Huebner JL, et al. Absence of posttraumatic arthritis following intraarticular fracture in the MRL/MpJ mouse. Arthritis Rheum 2008;58(3):744–53.
23. McKinley TO, Rudert MJ, Tochigi Y, et al. Incongruity-dependent changes of contact stress rates in human cadaveric ankles. J Orthop Trauma 2006;20(10):732–8.

24. McKinley TO, Tochigi Y, Rudert MJ, et al. The effect of incongruity and instability on contact stress directional gradients in human cadaveric ankles. Osteoarthritis Cartilage 2008;16(11):1363–9.

25. Goreham-Voss CM, McKinley TO, Brown TD. A finite element exploration of cartilage stress near an articular incongruity during unstable motion. J Biomech 2007;40(15):3438–47.

26. Giannoudis PV, Tzioupis C, Papathanassopoulos A, et al. Articular step-off and risk of post traumatic osteoarthritis: evidence today. Injury 2010;41(10): 986–95.

27. Brown TD, Pope DF, Hale JE, et al. Effects of osteochondral defect size on cartilage contact stress. J Orthop Res 1991;9(4):559–67.

28. Martin J, Marsh JL, Nepola JV, et al. Radiographic fracture assessments: which ones can we reliably make? J Orthop Trauma 2000;14(6):379–85.

29. Moed BR, Carr SE, Gruson KI, et al. Computed tomographic assessment of fractures of the posterior wall of the acetabulum after operative treatment. J Bone Joint Surg Am 2003;85(3): 512–22.

30. Rowe CR, Lowell JD. Prognosis of fractures of the acetabulum. J Bone Joint Surg 1961;43A:30.

31. Larson CB. Fracture dislocations of the hip. Clin Orthop 1973;92:147.

32. Carnesale PG, Stewart MJ, Barnes SN. Acetabular disruption and central fracture dislocation of the hip. J Bone Joint Surg 1975;57A:1054.

33. Pennal GF, Davidson J, Garside H, et al. Results of treatment of acetabular fractures. Clin Orthop 1980;15:115.

34. Letournel E, Judet R. Fractures of the acetabulum. 2nd edition. Berlin: Springer-Verlag; 1993.

35. Matta JM, Mehne DK, Roffi R. Fractures of the acetabulum: early results of a prospective study. Clin Orthop 1986;205:241.

36. Matta JM, Merritt PO. Displaced acetabular fractures. Clin Orthop 1988;230:83.

37. Matta JM, Tannast M, Najibi S. Two to twenty –year survivorship of the hip in 810 patients with operatively treated acetabular fractures. J Bone Joint Surg 2012;94:1559.

38. Starr AJ, Walter JC, Harris RM, et al. Percutaneous screw fixation of fractures of the iliac wing and fracture dislocations of the sacro-iliac joint. J Orthop Trauma 2002;16:116–23.

39. Starr AJ, Reinert CM, Jones AL. Percutaneous fixation of the columns of the acetabulum: a new technique. J Orthop Trauma 1998;12:51–8.

40. Kahler DM. Computer-assisted fixation of acetabular fractures and pelvic ring disruptions. Tech Orthop 2000;10(1):20–4.

41. Gary JL, VanHal M, Gibbons SD, et al. Functional outcomes in elderly patients with acetabular fractures treated with minimally invasive reduction and percutaneous fixation. J Ortho Trauma 2012; 26(5):278–83.

42. Ryan SP, Manson TT, Sciadini MF, et al. Functional outcomes of elderly patients with nonoperatively treated acetabular fractures that meet operative criteria. J Orthop Trauma 2017;31(12):644–9.

43. Epstein HC. Posterior fracture-dislocations of the hip; long-term follow-up. J Bone Joint Surg Am 1974;56(6):1103–27.

44. Epstein HC, Wiss DA, Cozen L. Posterior fracture dislocation of the hip with fractures of the femoral head. Clin Orthop Relat Res 1985;201(201):9–17.

45. DeLee JC, Evans JA, Thomas J. Anterior dislocation of the hip and associated femoral-head fractures. J Bone Joint Surg Am 1980;62(6):960–4.

46. Cathcart RF. The shape of the femoral head and preliminary results of clinical use of a nonspherical hip prosthesis. J Bone Joint Surg Am 1971; 53:397.

47. Greenwald AS, Haynes DW. Weight-bearing areas in the human hip joint. J Bone Joint Surg Br 1972; 54(1):157–63.

48. Swiontkowski MF, Thorpe M, Seiler JG, et al. Operative management of displaced femoral head fractures: case matched comparison of anterior versus posterior for Pipkin I and Pipkin II fractures. J Ortho Trauma 1992;6:437–42.

49. Dreinhofer KE, Schwarzkopf SR, Haas NP, et al. Femur head dislocation fractures. Long term outcome of conservative and surgical therapy. Unfallchirurg 1996;99:400–9 [in German].

50. Stannard JP, Harris HW, Volgas DA, et al. Functional outcome of patients with femoral head fractures associated with hip dislocations. Clin Ortho Relat Res 2000;377:44–56.

51. Homma Y, Miyahara S, Mogami A, et al. Percutaneous screw fixation for a femoral head fracture: a case report. Arch Orthop Trauma Surg 2014;134:371.

52. Matsuda DK. A rare fracture, an even rarer treatment: the arthroscopic reduction and internal fixation of an isolated femoral head fracture. Arthroscopy 2009;25(4):408–12.

53. Park MS, Her IS, Cho HM, et al. Internal fixation of femoral head fractures (Pipkin I) using hip arthroscopy. Knee Surg Sports Traumatol Arthrosc 2014; 22:898–901.

54. Kolmert L, Wulff K. Epidemiology and treatment of distal femoral fractures in adults. Acta Orthop Scand 1982;53:957–62.

55. Ostrum R, Geel C. Indirect reduction and internal fixation of supracondylar femur fractures without bone graft. J Orthop Trauma 1995;9:278–84.

56. Ali AM, Villafuerte J, Hashmi M, et al. Judet's quadricepsplasty, surgical technique, and results in limb reconstruction. Clin Orthop Relat Res 2003;415:214–20.

57. Zlowodzki M, Bhandari M, Marek DJ, et al. Operative treatment of acute distal femur fractures: systematic review of 2 comparative studies and 45 case series (1989 to 2005). J Orthop Trauma 2006;20:366–71.

58. Arneson TJ, Melton LJ 3rd, Lewallen DG, et al. Epidemiology of diaphyseal and distal femoral fractures in Rochester, Minnesota, 1965-1984. Clin Orthop Relat Res 1988;234:188–94.

59. Schatzker J, Tile M. The rationale of operative fracture care. New York: Springer-Verlag; 1987.

60. Lefkoe TP, Trafton PG, Ehrlich MG, et al. An experimental model of femoral condylar defect leading to osteoarthrosis. J Orthop Trauma 1993;7:458–67.

61. Lefkoe TP, Walsh WR, Anastasatos J, et al. Remodeling of articular step-offs. Is osteoarthrosis dependent on defect size? Clin Orthop Relat Res 1995;314:253–65.

62. Llinas A, McKellop HA, Marshall GJ, et al. Healing and remodeling of articular incongruities in a rabbit fracture model. J Bone Joint Surg Am 1993;75: 1508–23.

63. Lovasz G, Llinas A, Benya PD, et al. Cartilage changes caused by a coronal surface stepoff in a rabbit model. Clin Orthop Relat Res 1998;354: 224–34.

64. Lovasz G, Park SH, Ebramzadeh E, et al. Characteristics of degeneration in an unstable knee with a coronal surface step-off. J Bone Joint Surg Br 2001;83:428–36.

65. Stannard JP, Lopez R, Volgas D. Soft tissue injury of the knee after tibial plateau fractures. J Knee Surg 2010;23(4):187–92.

66. Shepherd L, Abdollahi K, Lee J, et al. The prevalence of soft tissue injuries in nonoperative tibial plateau fractures as determined by magnetic resonance imaging. J Orthop Trauma 2002;16(9): 628–31.

67. Brown TD, Anderson DD, Nepola JV, et al. Contact stress aberrations following imprecise reduction of simple tibial plateau fractures. J Orthop Res 1988;6(6):851–62.

68. Blokker CP, Rorabeck CH, Bourne RB. Tibial plateau fractures: an analysis of the results of treatment in 60 patients. Clin Orthop Relat Res 1984;182(182):193–9.

69. Moore TM, Patzakis MJ, Harvey JP. Tibial plateau fractures: definition, demographics, treatment rationale, and long-term results of closed traction management or operative reduction. J Orthop Trauma 1987;1(2):97–119.

70. Lansinger O, Bergman B, Korner L, et al. Tibial condylar fractures. A twenty-year follow-up. J Bone Joint Surg Am 1986;68(1):13–9.

71. Su EP, Westrich GH, Rana AJ, et al. Operative treatment of tibial plateau fractures in patients older than 55 years. Clin Orthop Relat Res 2004; 421(421):240–8.

72. Honkonen SE. Indications for surgical treatment of tibial condyle fractures. Clin Orthop Relat Res 1994;302(302):199–205.

73. Honkonen SE. Degenerative arthritis after tibial plateau fractures. J Orthop Trauma 1995;9(4): 273–7.

74. DeCoster TA, Nepola JV, el-Khoury GY. Cast brace treatment of proximal tibia fractures. A ten-year follow-up study. Clin Orthop Relat Res 1988;231(231):196–204.

75. McCann PA, Jackson M, Mitchell ST, et al. Complications of definitive open reduction and internal fixation of pilon fractures of the distal tibia. Int Orthop 2011;35(3):413–8.

76. Calori GM, Tagliabue L, Mazza E, et al. Tibial pilon fractures: which method of treatment? Injury 2010; 41:1183–90.

77. Borrelli J, Ricci WM. Acute effects of cartilage impact. Clin Orthop 2004;423:33–9.

78. Bourne RB. Pylon fractures of the distal tibia. Clin Orthop 1989;240:42–6.

79. Egol KA, Wolinsky P, Koval KJ. Open reduction and internal fixation of tibial pilon fractures. Foot Ankle Clin 2000;5:873–85.

80. Pugh KJ, Wolinsky P, Pienkowski D, et al. Comparative biomechanics of hybrid external fixation. J Orthop Trauma 1999;13:418–25.

81. Raikin S, Froimson MI. Combined limited internal fixation with circular frame external fixation of intra-articular tibial fractures. Orthopedics 1999; 22:1019–25.

82. Ries MD, Meinhard BP. Medial external fixation with lateral plate internal fixation in metaphyseal tibia fractures: a report of eight cases associated with severe soft-tissue injury. Clin Orthop 1990; 256:215–24.

83. Barbieri R, Schenk RS, Koval K, et al. Hybrid external fixation in the treatment of tibial plafond fractures. Clin Orthop 1996;332:16–22.

84. Okcu G, Aktuglu K. Intra-articular fractures of the tibial plafond: a comparison of the results using articulated and ring external fixators. J Bone Joint Surg Br 2004;86:868–75.

85. Ovadia DN, Beals RK. Fractures of the tibial plafond. J Bone Joint Surg Am 1986;68:543–51.

86. Boraiah S, Kemp TJ, Erwteman A, et al. Outcome following open reduction and internal fixation of open pilon fractures. J Bone Joint Surg Am 2010;92(2):346–52.

87. Liporace FA, Yoon RS. Decisions and staging leading to definitive open management of pilon fractures: where have we come from and where are we now? J Orthop Trauma 2012;26:488–98.

88. Beck E. Results of operative treatment of pilon fractures. In: Tscherne H, Schatzker J, editors.

Major fractures of the pilon, the talus, and the calcaneus. Heidelberg (Germany): Springer-Verlag; 1993. p. 49–51.

89. Blauth M, Bastian L, Krettek C, et al. Surgical options for the treatment of severe tibial pilon fractures: a study of three techniques. J Orthop Trauma 2001;15:153–60.

90. Bone L, Stegemann P, McNamara K, et al. External fixation of severely comminuted and open tibial pilon fractures. Clin Orthop 1993;292:101–7.

91. Kim HS, Jahn JS, Kim SS, et al. Treatment of tibial pilon fractures using ring fixators and arthroscopy. Clin Orthop 1997;334:244–50.

92. McFerran MA, Smith SW, Boulas HJ, et al. Complications encountered in the treatment of pilon fractures. J Orthop Trauma 1992;6:195–200.

93. Muhr G, Breitfuss H. Complications after pilon fractures. In: Tscherne H, Schatzker J, editors. Major fractures of the pilon, the talus, and the calcaneus. Heidelberg (Germany): Springer-Verlag; 1993. p. 65–7.

94. Patterson MJ, Cole JD. Two-staged delayed open reduction and internal fixation of severe pilon fractures. J Orthop Trauma 1999;13:85–91.

95. Pugh KJ, Wolinsky PR, McAndrew MP, et al. Tibial pilon fractures: a comparison of treatment methods. J Trauma 1999;47:937–41.

96. Swiontkowski MF, Sands A, Grujic L, et al. Open reduction with screw/plate fixation for pilon fractures: complications and functional outcome. Presented at the 11th Annual Meeting of the Orthopaedic Trauma Association, Tampa, Florida, Sep 29- Oct 10, 1995.

97. Waddell JP. Tibial plafond fractures. In: Tscherne H, Schatzker J, editors. Major fractures of the pilon, the talus, and the calcaneus. Heidelberg (Germany): Springer-Verlag; 1993. p. 43–8.

98. Cannada L. The no-touch approach for operative treatment of pilon fractures to minimize soft tissue complications. Orthopedics 2010;33:734–8.

99. Bonnier P. Les fractures du pilon. Lyon (France): University of Lyon; 1961.

100. Decoulx P, Razeman JP, Rousselle Y. Fractures du pilon tibiale. Rev Chir Orthop Reparatrice Appar Mot 1961;47:563.

101. Ruedi T, Allgöwer M. Fractures of the lower extremity into the ankle joint. Injury 1969;1:92–9.

102. Heim U, Nasser M. Fractures du pilon tibial. Rev Chir Orthop 1977;63:5.

103. Kellum JF, Waddell JP. Fractures of the distal tibial metaphysis with intra-articular extensions the distal explosion fracture. J Trauma 1979;19: 593–601.

104. Teeny SM, Wiss DA. Open reduction and internal fixation of tibial plafond fractures. Variables contributing to poor results and complications. Clin Orthop 1993;292:108–17.

105. Tornetta P, Weiner L, Bergman M. Pilon fractures: treatment with combined internal and external fixation. J Orthop Trauma 1993;7:489–96.

106. Marsh JL, Napola JV, wuest TK, et al. Unilateral external fixation until healing with dynamic axial fixator for severe open tibia fractures. J Orthop Trauma 1991;5:341–8.

107. Watson JET, Moed BR, Karges DE, et al. Pilon fractures: treatment protocol based on severity of the soft tissue. Clin Orthop 2000;375:78–90.

108. Ruedi T, Allgöwer M. The operative treatment of intra-articular fractures of the lower end of the tibia. Clin Orthop 1979;138:105–10.

109. Pollack AN, McCarthy ML, Bess RS, et al. Outcomes after treatment of high-energy tibial plafond injuries. J Bone Joint Surg Am 2003;15:153–60.

110. Korkmaz A, Ciftdemir M, Ozcan M, et al. The analysis of the variables, affecting outcome in surgically treated tibia pilon fractured patients. Injury 2013;44(10):1270–4.

111. Chan DS, Balthrop PM, White B, et al. Does a staged posterior approach have a negative effect on OTA 43C fracture outcomes? J Orthop Trauma 2017;31(2):90–4.

112. Lindvall E, Haidukewych G, DiPasquale T, et al. Open reduction and stable fixation of isolated, displaced talar neck and body fractures. The J Bone Joint Surg 2004;86(10):2229–34.

113. Vallier HA, Nork SE, Benirschke SK, et al. Surgical treatment of talar body fractures. J Bone Joint Surg 2003;85-A(9):1716–24.

114. Lindsay WR, Dewar FP. Fractures of the os calcis. Am J Surg 1958;95(4):555–76.

115. Buckley R, Tough S, McCormack R, et al. Operative compared with nonoperative treatment of displaced intra-articular calcaneal fractures: a prospective, randomized, controlled multicenter trial. J Bone Joint Surg 2002;84-A(10):1733–44.

116. Agren PH, Wretenberg P, Sayed-Noor AS. Operative versus nonoperative treatment of displaced intra-articular calcaneal fractures: a prospective, randomized, controlled multicenter trial. J Bone Joint Surg Am. 2013;95(15):1351–7.

117. Ibrahim T, Rowsell M, Rennie W, et al. Displaced intra-articular calcaneal fractures: 15-year follow-up of a randomised controlled trial of conservative versus operative treatment. Injury 2007;38(7): 848–55.

118. Sanders R, Fortin P, DiPasquale T, et al. Operative treatment in 120 displaced intraarticular calcaneal fractures. Results using a prognostic computed tomography scan classification. Clin Orthop Relat Res 1993;290:87–95.

119. Csizy M, Buckley R, Tough S, et al. Displaced intra-articular calcaneal fractures: variables predicting late subtalar fusion. J Orthop Trauma 2003;17(2): 106–12.

Pediatrics

Hip Surveillance in Children with Cerebral Palsy

Aaron Huser, DO, Michelle Mo, MD, PhD,
Pooya Hosseinzadeh, MD*

KEYWORDS

• Hip displacement • Hip surveillance • Children • Cerebral palsy

---

KEY POINTS

• Hip displacement is seen in more than one-third of children with cerebral palsy, with a higher prevalence in children who do not ambulate.

• Hip displacement in this population is typically progressive, leading to hip subluxation and ultimately dislocation.

• Because early stage of hip displacement can be silent, hip surveillance programs have been recommended for early diagnosis and treatment of hip disorders.

• Treatment of hip disorders depends on the degree of dysplasia, functional status of the patient, and patient age. Surgical treatment options include preventive, reconstructive, and salvage procedures.

• The implementation of hip surveillance programs has resulted in a decrease in the number of salvage procedures in children with cerebral palsy.

INTRODUCTION

Cerebral palsy (CP) refers to a heterogenous group of conditions that leads to a disorder of motor function, movement, and posture. It affects the developing and immature brain, resulting in a permanent and nonprogressive dysfunction of the central nervous system. Despite the presence of a static and nonprogressive encephalopathy, the musculoskeletal involvement in children with CP is typically progressive. Approximately 1 in 323 children are affected with CP, making it one of the most common motor disabilities of childhood.[1,2] The primary motor abnormalities of CP are often accompanied by other symptoms, such as musculoskeletal abnormalities, intellectual disability, seizure disorders, and communication and behavioral difficulties. Of the musculoskeletal abnormalities seen in CP, hip disorders are among the most common abnormalities (second most common after foot and ankle abnormalities), affecting almost one-third of children with CP, with an increased prevalence in patients that have a higher level of involvement (Higher Growth Motor Function Classification System [GMFCS] level). Hip disorders in children with CP cover a wide spectrum of pathology ranging from the hip at risk, to subluxated hips, dislocated hips, and dislocated hips with degenerative arthritis and pain. Progression of hip disorders in children with CP can lead to significant pain and problems with gait, sitting, and hygiene.[3,4] By understanding the pathophysiology, natural history, and outcomes of hip surveillance programs, one can better develop methods to prevent, manage, and treat hip disorders in children with CP.

The authors have no conflicts of interest to disclose and no financial disclosures.
Department of Orthopaedic Surgery, Washington University School of Medicine, St. Louis Children's Hospital, 1 Children's Place, Suite 4S60, St Louis, MO 63110, USA
* Corresponding author.
E-mail address: hosseinzadehp@wustl.edu

This review article provides an overview of the natural history, pathophysiology, physical examination, and radiographic evaluation of hip disorders. It then focuses on the current literature and analyzes the current evidence regarding the hip at risk, outcomes of existing hip surveillance programs, and guidelines and protocols that have been established to diagnose, manage, and treat hip disorders in children with CP.

EPIDEMIOLOGY AND NATURAL HISTORY

Children with CP are at an increased risk for hip displacement and dislocation, with the greatest risk in children with the most severe forms of CP.[5,6] Current estimates of hip dysplasia in children with CP is approximately 35%, with the prevalence of hip subluxation estimated to be between 25% and 60% and the prevalence of dislocation to be 10% to 15%.[3,6–10] The incidence of hip subluxation and dislocation is known to increase with worsening disease severity as defined by the GMFCS level[11]; of note, hip displacement was observed in less than 5% of independent ambulators, whereas it was observed in more than 60% of children with no walking capacity.[12] Additionally, the prognosis and incidence of hip disorders is correlated with the ability of a child to pull to standing by 3 years of age; children with the ability to pull to standing have a lower incidence of hip disorders and a better prognosis.[5,13]

Understanding the natural history of hip dysplasia in CP is crucial, because it provides a framework for intervention and prevention. Studies have demonstrated that hip displacement is more frequent in quadriplegia than in diplegia, with a progression in migration percentage (MP) found to be 4 times as great in children with quadriplegic CP than in children with diplegic CP. Spasticity was also observed to be a critical etiologic factor for hip displacement; more frequent hip displacement occurs in children with GMFCS levels of IV or V with spastic CP compared with children with dyskinetic forms of CP.[5,14]

In general, the progression of hip dysplasia is gradual, and it usually occurs over a period of several years (Fig. 1). It tends to be a permanent process; once a hip begins to subluxate, it frequently requires treatment to correct. Hips that have a migration index of greater than 50% will not reduce spontaneously and one-third of those will progress to dislocation.[3]

Many children with a dysplastic hip progressing to dislocation will develop a painful hip by early adulthood; as hip displacement progresses, the articular cartilage of the femoral head degenerates secondary to pressures from the surrounding soft tissues. Pain from hip dysplasia occurs primarily from dislocated hips, because hips that are subluxated were noted to be only slightly more painful than reduced hips.

In terms of the onset of hip dysplasia in children with CP, subluxation frequently occurs before the age of 5 years, with the mean age of dislocation occurring around the age of 6 to 7 years. Children with CP are at greatest risk of hip dislocation between 4 and 12 years of age.[5,14]

PATHOPHYSIOLOGY AND ANATOMY

Most children with CP have an anatomically normal hip at birth.[15] However, secondary to the natural history of spastic CP, as described

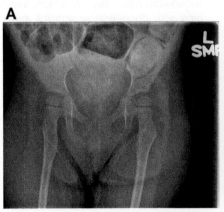 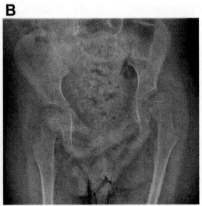

Fig. 1. Progression of hip displacement in a child with Growth Motor Function Classification System level V cerebral palsy. (A) Pelvis radiograph at 3 years of age showing both femoral heads well covered under the acetabulum. (B) Pelvis radiograph at 5 years of age showing left hip subluxation.

in the previous section, there is an increased risk for hip displacement; this process is often referred to as silent subluxation because children frequently are not symptomatic until the hip dislocates.[5,16] The musculoskeletal pathology of CP is progressive, unlike the nonprogressive neurologic processes of CP, leading to an excess in muscle tone and spasticity that worsens with growth. The excess in muscle tone exerts a constant force on the developing hip, causing bony deformity, joint instability, and deformation of the femur and acetabulum. With time, lateral hip displacement occurs, with the hip's center of rotation shifting from the center of the femoral head to the lesser trochanter.[17]

Asymmetric muscle spasticity is thought to be one of the primary drivers of hip displacement in children with CP. Several altered components in dysplastic hips can be observed in the proximal femur and acetabulum. Abnormalities seen with the proximal femur are anteversion of the femoral neck in the transverse plane, coxa valga (increased neck–shaft angle), and dysplastic and degenerative changes. It is thought that femoral neck anteversion and coxa valga may result from delayed walking and limitations in gross motor function, which correlates with the observation that a higher GMFCS level is related to an increased risk of hip displacement. Radiographic and clinical studies have shown that spastic hip adductors and flexors cause the femoral head to be directed into the posterolateral acetabular labrum, leading to deformation of the femoral head by the capsule and superior acetabular rim, and eventual cartilage erosion.[5,18] In addition, the epiphysis displaces superolaterally, becoming wedge shaped, and the lesser trochanter is also observed to enlarge in size. With regard to proximal femoral anteversion, it has been noted that, although children with spastic hip dysplasia have normal femoral anteversion at birth, the normal developmental decrease in anteversion does not occur in those children.[5,16]

Abnormalities seen with the acetabulum are the presence of acetabular deficiency and a high acetabular index. Elevated hip forces, up to 6-fold, in children with spastic hip dysplasia lead to early changes of the acetabulum at around 30 months of age, with higher observed acetabular indices. The deforming hip forces also cause a delay of bony maturation of the acetabulum, with the greatest increase in deformation of the acetabulum occurring with an MP of 52% to 68%. Computed tomography (CT) studies of the hips in children with CP have shown that posterolateral acetabular deficiency is the most common pattern observed. However, the pattern of acetabular deficiency usually depends on the direction of hip subluxation or dislocation.[5,16,18,19]

PHYSICAL EXAMINATION AND RADIOGRAPHIC EVALUATION

Clinical examination is a critical aspect for the conduction of a thorough evaluation of hip disorders in children with CP and spastic hip disease. Important components of assessment include:

1. Assigning the GMFCS level, thus defining risk level;
2. Assessing hip abduction;
3. Assessing hip flexion contracture;
4. Evaluating the child's spine, pelvic obliquity, and knee and ankle range of motion; and
5. Evaluating pain and/or difficulties with sitting, standing, or walking.

When conducting the examination, hip abduction should be measured with the hip and knee extended to thoroughly assess hip adduction contracture and spasticity. Hip abduction is not a primary indicator of the risk for hip displacement, but it has been observed that hip abduction of less than 30° is associated with an increased risk for displacement and with difficulty in perineal care.[20]

The presence of hip flexion contracture can be assessed using the Thomas test, and range of motion is documented for the hips, knees, and ankles. With the Thomas test, the child is placed in the supine position with the uninvolved limb flexed to eliminate lumbar lordosis and the involved extremity flat; the affected hip is then passively ranged into extension until the pelvis tilts anteriorly with hip flexion contracture defined as the angle between the longitudinal axis of the affected thigh and the horizontal line of the examination table.[21] Spasticity and contractures are noted for the knees and ankles for proper planning to occur for patients who may be eligible for single event multilevel surgery.

During the physical examination, pelvic obliquity and an evaluation of the child's spine should be conducted, because pelvic obliquity may be the result of neuromuscular scoliosis, a common finding in nonambulatory children with CP, or it may be the result of unilateral hip dislocation. If a child is able to stand, the examination should be conducted in the standing position, and in the sitting position if the child is nonambulatory.

Leg length discrepancy is also important to note, because a discrepancy could result from unilateral hip dislocation, or an apparent shortening secondary to pelvic obliquity or a windblown hip from a unilateral adduction contracture.[5,16] Briefly, windblown hip (Fig. 2) is caused by an adduction deformity of one hip and an abduction deformity of the other hip. It is a deformity that affects primarily nonambulatory children with severe spasticity owing to asymmetric activity of the abductors, adductors, internal rotators, and external rotators.[5,22] This deformity interferes with the ability of the child to sit properly in a wheelchair.

Although rare, occurring in only 1.5% of dislocations/subluxations, anterior hip dislocations/subluxations are also important to note. It affects predominantly children with severe quadriplegia who have hypotonia or extension posturing. Children who have anterior hip dislocations/subluxations tend to have physical examination findings in which the hip is in extension, external rotation, and adduction with knee extension contractures; or the hip is in extension, external rotation, and abduction with knee flexion contractures; or there is severe hypotonia without any contractures.[5,23]

Although clinical examination is an important aspect of hip surveillance for children with CP, clinical examination alone is insufficient for the adequate evaluation of hip displacement. Radiographic evaluation, primarily with an anteroposterior radiograph of the pelvis in a supine position, is the second crucial component in guiding decisions for the treatment and surveillance of hip disorders. A standardized radiographic technique is followed to ensure consistency between interval radiographs and between patients. The pelvis should be in symmetric position, lumbar spine flat, with both hips in neutral abduction/adduction. Migration index or MP, which measures the lateral displacement of the hip, and acetabular index, which measures the degree of acetabular dysplasia, are then determined (Fig. 3). If the pelvis is tilted or rotated, however, it can cause false values with the acetabular index and MP, and can create difficulties in interpreting the femoral–acetabular relationship.[5,9,14,24] If the hips are abducted or adducted, the MP measurement can be affected. Hip adduction falsely increases the MP and hip abduction decreases the MP.

MP is the most reliable and reproducible measurement of hip displacement in children with CP, and as a result is the primary radiographic measurement used for hip surveillance and treatment planning; the upper limit of a normal MP is 25% at 4 years of age with a measurement error of ±10%.[9,10,14,20,24] Children with CP at skeletal maturity (defined as closure of the triradiate cartilage) can further be evaluated with the Melbourne Cerebral Palsy Hip Classification System, which is a radiographic 6-stage classification of hip morphology.[25] The classification involves both quantitative and qualitative features and is based on status of Shenton's line, deformity of the femoral head, acetabular deformity, pelvic obliquity, and the MP. Grade I is a normal hip with grade V being a dislocated hip. Grade VI was added to denote that the hip joint is lost to some form of salvage surgery.

Additional imaging can also be useful in guiding preoperative assessment. CT scans with 3-dimensional reconstruction can allow surgeons to assess abnormalities of the femoral head, evaluate acetabular morphology to determine area of greatest acetabular deficiency, and assess accurate femoral anteversion. However, it should be noted that adequate alignment of the femur in the CT scanner was needed to have accurate measurement of femoral anteversion.[26] Ultrasound examination can be helpful in cases of coxa valga, where CT scans can be inaccurate.[26,27]

Hip Surveillance

The goal of managing the spastic hip is to maintain a flexible, reduced, and painless hip.[28] The purpose of a hip surveillance program is to identify hips that are at risk for progressive displacement and to allow for early assessment and management by orthopedic surgeons to

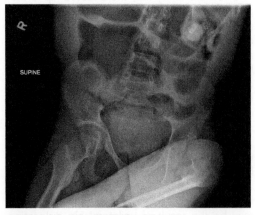

Fig. 2. Pelvis radiograph of a child with windblown hip deformity. The left hip has adducted and internally rotated and the right hip is abducted and externally rotated.

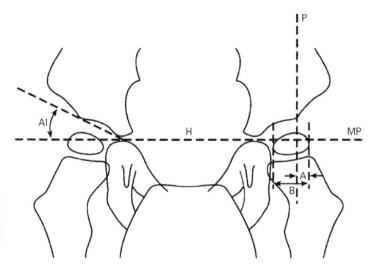

Fig. 3. Migration percentage (MP) is measured by the percentage of the ossified femoral head that is, lateral to the Perkins line (MP = A/D × 100%). AI, acetabular index; H, Hilgenliner's Line; P, Perkins Line. (*From* Dobson F, Boyd RN, Parrott J, et al. Hip surveillance in children with cerebral palsy. Impact on the surgical management of spastic hip disease. J Bone Joint Surg Br 2002;84(5):721; with permission. *Reproduced with permission of* the licensor through PLSclear.)

prevent the possible pain, decreased motion, and decreased quality of life associated with painful dislocated hips.[25] Once hip displacement is diagnosed, potential treatment options include nonoperative treatment, preventative surgeries (soft tissue releases), reconstructive surgeries (proximal femoral and acetabular osteotomies), and salvage procedures (proximal femoral resection, valgus osteotomy, arthrodesis, and arthroplasty).[16]

There are multiple successful surveillance programs reported in the literature.[11,29,30] Most surveillance programs use a combination of MP and GMFCS level to guide screening recommendations. Table 1 summarizes the recommendations

of 2 selected surveillance programs created by Pruszczynski and colleagues[11] (also known as Alfred I. Dupont Hospital protocol) and the Cerebral Palsy Follow-up Programme in Sweden. The recommendations from the Australian Hip Surveillance Program are also described.

The Australian Guidelines recommend a screening anteroposterior pelvis radiograph between 12 and 24 months of age for all children diagnosed with CP. The guidelines then branch, depending on the GMFCS level of the patient. For patients classified as GMFCS level I, the guidelines recommend additional physical screenings at ages 3 and 5 years, but do not suggest additional radiographic follow-up unless

Table 1		
Screening recommendations for hip surveillance programs		
Level	**Age 2–8 y**	**Age 8–18 y**
GMFCS I, II (MP <30%)	One radiograph	None
GMFCS I, II (MP >30%)	Annual radiograph	Every 2 y
GMFCS III, IV, V (MP <30%)	Annual	Every 2 y
GMFCS III, IV, V (MP >30%)	Every 6 mo	Annual
	CPUP	
GMFCS I	None unless clinical deterioration	
GMFCS II	Radiograph at ages 2 and 6; if no deterioration and MP <33% continue to monitor clinically	
GMFCS III–V	Annual to age 8 after confirmation of CP diagnosis, >8 y old, monitor clinically	

Abbreviations: CP, cerebral palsy; CPUP, Cerebral Palsy Follow-up Programme; GMFCS, Growth Motor Function Classification System.

Data from Pruszczynski B, Sees J, Miller F. Risk factors for hip displacement in children with cerebral palsy: systematic review. J Pediatr Orthop 2016;36(8):829–33.

the GMFCS level has changed. The patients classified as GMFCS level II should be seen at 1 year after their initial evaluation according to the Australian Guidelines, and again between the ages of 4 and 5 years and between ages of 8 and 10 years. Repeat clinical examinations and anteroposterior radiographs of the pelvis should be attained at each of these visits. If the MP remains stable (no change >10% over a 12-month period) and the GMFCS level is the same, these patients will continue the aforementioned schedule. However, if the MP is deemed unstable, yearly assessments and pelvic radiographic studies should be performed.

For the GMFCS levels III and IV, population the Australian Guidelines recommend a follow-up evaluation at 6 months after their initial screening. If the GMFCS classification is the same and the MP is stable, repeat pelvic images should be obtained every 12 months. If the MP is unstable, then clinical and radiographic evaluations should be performed every 6 months. At 7 years of age, if the MP is less than 30% and stable and the GMFCS is unchanged, pelvic radiographs may be discontinued until prepuberty (typically age 11 for girls and 13 for boys). For GMFCS level V individuals, repeat radiographic and clinical examinations should occur every 6 months. At 7 years of age if the MP is stable and less than 30%, further radiographic evaluation only needs to occur every 12 months.

The Australian Guidelines also have recommendations based for the Winters–Gage–Hicks gait classification for children with the hemiplegic type of CP. These authors recommend screening for children with a type IV gait (hip adducted and internal rotation, knee flexion, and ankle equinus). They recommend screening at the ages of 5 and 10 years. If, at the 5-year evaluation, the MP is abnormal or unstable, they recommend 12-month follow-up visits with repeat clinical evaluation and pelvic radiographs. If they verified Winters–Gage–Hicks class IV at the 10-year screening, the Australian Guidelines also recommend yearly screening with pelvic radiography. For all patients with GMFCS levels II through V or a Winters–Gage–Hicks class IV gait pattern who have limb length discrepancy, pelvic obliquity, deteriorating gait, or an MP of greater than 30%, surveillance should continue every 12 months after skeletal maturity.

The screening program recommended by Pruszczynski and colleagues based on a systematic review of the literature has to some extent simplified the screening recommendations (see Table 1).

Although few studies have analyzed the results of these surveillance programs, the available evidence supports the implementation of surveillance programs in children with CP. In 2009, Connelly and colleagues[29] retrospectively reviewed 12 years of data from their Tasmanian surveillance group and found that, of the 208 children taking part in the surveillance program, only 15 children had hip dislocation, six of which were secondary to follow-up or surgical failure. The remaining dislocations were found on initial surveillance examination or owing to parental refusal. Of those dislocated hips, only 2 patients underwent salvage procedures (Level IV evidence).

In 2001, Kentish and colleagues[31] published their findings from the Queensland cohort in Australia. They had 1240 patients with CP enrolled in their prospective study. Only 1 patient who participated in the surveillance program developed hip dislocation over their 5-year study period.[31] Two salvage procedures were performed in this cohort owing to previous failed reconstructive procedures (Level II evidence). Hagglund and colleagues[8] published a 20-year retrospective cohort review of 689 children. Their study had 3 cohorts: a historical control (before implementation of a hip surveillance protocol), an initial study group born between 1992 and 1997, and a second study group born between 1998 and 2007. They reported no dislocations in the second study group at the onset of 2014, and 2 dislocations in the initial study group. The control cohort had 9 dislocations. No salvage procedures were performed on the patients in either the initial or the second study groups[8] (Level III evidence).

Treatment

As described, the treatment of the at-risk hip includes nonoperative management, preventative surgery, reconstructive surgery, and salvage procedures. Nonoperative management includes bracing, physical therapy, and injections. A randomized, controlled trial compared the effect of botulinum toxin injections and bracing versus a control group who did not receive the interventions.[32] The botulinum toxin was injected every 6 months in the adductors and medial hamstrings. At 3 years, there was no difference in the change in MP between the 2 groups, and the authors did not recommend the bracing and Botox injection (Level I evidence).[32]

Preventative surgery includes both adductor releases and iliopsoas release. The adductor release may include the adductor longus, gracilis, and adductor brevis. The iliopsoas release may be done at the level of the lesser trochanter or over the brim. Indications for adductor releases have historically been an MP of greater than 25° to 30° and abduction of less than 30° to 45°.[16,33] In 2005, Presedo[33] and his team conducted a retrospective review of a group of 65 patients with CP who underwent adductor tenotomy with or without iliopsoas release with a minimum of 8 years of follow-up. They found that 67% of the patients had a good or fair result and that 46% required either repeat soft tissue release or reconstructive surgery.[33] They also stated that the MP at 1-year after surgery was the best predictor for final outcome, and patients who walked preoperatively had better long-term outcomes. They did not find that age was a significant contributing factor to outcome[33] (Level III evidence).

Another study published by Shore and colleagues[16] in 2012 found that walking ability was a strong predictor of success for adductor release. Their mean postoperative follow-up was 7 years and they defined failure as an MP of more than 50° or the need for an additional reconstructive procedure[16] (Level III evidence).

Reconstructive options for the spastic hip include osteotomies of both the femur and/or pelvis. The proximal femoral osteotomy is indicated in patients with an MP of greater than 50% or a break in Shenton's line.[34] The proximal femoral osteotomy is used to correct the coxa valga and femoral anteversion (**Fig. 4**). When correcting valgus, it is important to remember that the patient will lose abduction motion and that it is important to maximize preosteotomy abduction through the previously described soft tissue releases. In 2010, Canavese and

colleagues[35] published a study looking at the long-term results of unilateral proximal femoral osteotomies and the effect on the ipsilateral and contralateral hip. They found that 44% required operation on the contralateral hip for progressive subluxation[35] (Level IV evidence). Shore and colleagues[34] reviewed their series of 567 proximal femoral osteotomies at a mean of 8.3 years and found that 37% required additional procedures on the hip or had an MP of greater than 50% at the final follow-up. They also found that lower GMFCS level, increase surgical volume, and older age at the time surgery were strong predictors of success (Level III evidence).

In 1997, Kim and Wenger[18] published a study that examined the acetabular deficiency in neuromuscular patients using CT scans. They found that posterior deficiency was the most common type of acetabular deficiency, but there was also anterior, midsuperior, and mixed types of deficiencies as well.[18] Different pelvic osteotomies have been described for the spastic hip. These include the Pemberton osteotomy, Dega osteotomy, and San Diego osteotomy.[36–39] In 1996, Gordon and colleagues[37] published on the success of the Pemberton osteotomy with no redislocations and only 1 subluxation in 52 hips at a mean of 4 years postoperatively (Level IV evidence). In 2014, Mallet and colleagues[40] published their results with single stage reconstruction (both iliac and femoral osteotomy). They performed a Dega osteotomy of the ilium, a proximal femoral osteotomy, and soft tissue release on 20 hips (**Fig. 5**). They followed all patients to skeletal maturity with an average of 9 years of follow-up and found only 1 subluxation and 1 dislocation in their series[40] (Level IV

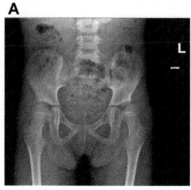
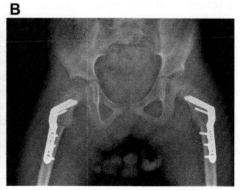

Fig. 4. Pelvis radiograph before and after varus derotational femoral osteotomy in a 6-year-old child with Growth Motor Function Classification System level IV cerebral palsy. (*A*) Preoperative radiograph showing left hip subluxation. (*B*) Radiographs 4 weeks after varus femoral osteotomy showing improvement in femoral head coverage by the acetabulum.

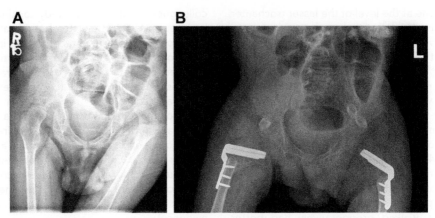

Fig. 5. Single-stage hip reconstruction in a 10-year-old with bilateral hip dislocation. (A) Preoperative radiograph showing bilateral hip dislocation with acetabular dysplasia. (B) Radiograph 2 months after bilateral proximal femoral osteotomy and bilateral Dega osteotomies of the pelvis showing both hip well-covered under the acetabulum.

evidence). The San Diego osteotomy was described by Mubarak and associates in 1992,[41] and is similar to the Dega osteotomy with an additional completion of the osteotomy through the inner table of the ilium at its most posterior extent. They performed a single-stage San Diego osteotomy, femoral osteotomy, and soft tissue release in 18 hips and at their latest follow-up (mean of 6 years and 10 months) only 1 hip with subluxation[41] (Level IV evidence). A recent review of 144 hips treated using hip reconstructive procedures with a mean of 4.9 years of follow-up demonstrated a stable MP in all patients classified as GMFCS levels I through III.[42] However, the authors found an increase of 2% in the MP per year in patients who were GMFCS levels IV and V and cautioned that these patients should be monitored closely for progression of hip displacement[42] (Level III evidence).

With the advent of hip screening programs, the need for salvage procedures has decreased in the regions using these programs.[8,30,32] As mentioned, salvage procedures include resection, valgus osteotomy, arthroplasty, and arthrodesis. Resection is indicated in skeletally mature patients with painful and dislocated hips with degenerative changes. The Girdlestone procedure was used initially for resection arthroplasty; however, it has largely been abandoned owing to recurrence of pain, proximal migration, and skin breakdown.[43] In 1978, Castle and Schneider[44] described an interposition arthroplasty and resection where the 2 heads of the rectus muscle were used to cover the proximal femur and the gluteal muscle bellies were interposed over the acetabulum. In 2009,

Knaus and Terjesen[45] published their results of proximal femoral resection and soft tissue interposition on 20 patients. Of the 20 patients, 14 were satisfied at last follow-up (range, 1–6 years) and all patients were able to sit[45] (Level IV evidence). Valgus osteotomy is another salvage option and indicated for patients with loss of abduction and a painless dislocated hip. The main goal of this procedure is to help with perineal care by increasing hip abduction.

Total hip arthroplasty has also been used as a salvage option in dislocated hips in patients with CP. A recent study using the National Joint Registry for England and Wales showed improvement in pain for patients undergoing total hip arthroplasty; however, this patient cohort had increased revision rates compared with the control group[46] (Level III evidence). Last, hip arthrodesis is an option for a salvage procedure. Fucs and colleagues[47] reviewed hip arthrodesis and found satisfactory results and fusion in all 21 patients, although 4 required construct revisions secondary to the formation of pseudoarthrosis (Level IV evidence). In a 2015 systematic review of articles on salvage procedures, de Souza and colleagues[48] reported that they could not statistically compare the different procedures and concluded that no procedure is superior, but they each have different indications.

SUMMARY

Hip dislocation is common in children with CP especially in children who do not ambulate. Owing to the poor clinical outcomes associated with painful dislocated hips in these children, hip screening programs are recommended.

Level II evidence in the literature supports the effectiveness of these screening programs in decreasing the number of salvage procedures required. The age that screening should be started, discontinued, and the frequency of screening are not well-supported by evidence in the literature and recommendations are mostly expert opinions (Level V evidence). Screening programs typically use radiographic measurement of lateral hip displacement on a supine anteroposterior pelvis radiograph. Based on the clinical and radiographic findings, observation or different treatment options are recommended. Level I evidence suggests that nonoperative treatment with Botox and bracing is not effective, whereas level III evidence supports the effectiveness of adductor tenotomy and femoral and acetabular osteotomy for the treatment of hip displacement in children with CP. The effectiveness of salvage procedures is mainly supported by small retrospective cohorts (Level IV evidence). To address the deficiencies in the current literature in the management of hip problems in children with CP, prospective cohorts comparing different surveillance methods and different hip reconstructive procedures are needed.

REFERENCES

1. Autism, Developmental Disabilities Monitoring Network Surveillance Year Principal Investigators, Centers for Disease Control and Prevention. Prevalence of autism spectrum disorders–autism and developmental disabilities monitoring network, 14 sites, United States, 2008. MMWR Surveill Summ 2012;61:1–19.
2. Maenner MJ, Blumberg SJ, Kogan MD, et al. Prevalence of cerebral palsy and intellectual disability among children identified in two U.S. National Surveys, 2011-2013. Ann Epidemiol 2016;26:222–6.
3. Bagg MR, Farber J, Miller F. Long-term follow-up of hip subluxation in cerebral palsy patients. J Pediatr Orthop 1993;13:32–6.
4. Moreau M, Drummond DS, Rogala E, et al. Natural history of the dislocated hip in spastic cerebral palsy. Dev Med Child Neurol 1979;21:749–53.
5. Flynn JM, Miller F. Management of hip disorders in patients with cerebral palsy. J Am Acad Orthop Surg 2002;10:198–209.
6. Scrutton D, Baird G, Smeeton N. Hip dysplasia in bilateral cerebral palsy: incidence and natural history in children aged 18 months to 5 years. Dev Med Child Neurol 2001;43:586–600.
7. Cooke PH, Cole WG, Carey RP. Dislocation of the hip in cerebral palsy. Natural history and predictability. J Bone Joint Surg Br 1989;71:441–6.
8. Hagglund G, Alriksson-Schmidt A, Lauge-Pedersen H, et al. Prevention of dislocation of the hip in children with cerebral palsy: 20-year results of a population-based prevention programme. Bone Joint J 2014;96-B:1546–52.
9. Hagglund G, Andersson S, Duppe H, et al. Prevention of dislocation of the hip in children with cerebral palsy. The first ten years of a population-based prevention programme. J Bone Joint Surg Br 2005;87:95–101.
10. Soo B, Howard JJ, Boyd RN, et al. Hip displacement in cerebral palsy. J Bone Joint Surg Am 2006;88:121–9.
11. Pruszczynski B, Sees J, Miller F. Risk factors for hip displacement in children with cerebral palsy: systematic review. J Pediatr Orthop 2016;36:829–33.
12. Lonstein JE, Beck K. Hip dislocation and subluxation in cerebral palsy. J Pediatr Orthop 1986;6:521–6.
13. Scrutton D. The early management of hips in cerebral palsy. Dev Med Child Neurol 1989;31:108–16.
14. Terjesen T. The natural history of hip development in cerebral palsy. Dev Med Child Neurol 2012;54:951–7.
15. Beals RK. Developmental changes in the femur and acetabulum in spastic paraplegia and diplegia. Dev Med Child Neurol 1969;11:303–13.
16. Shore B, Spence D, Graham H. The role for hip surveillance in children with cerebral palsy. Curr Rev Musculoskelet Med 2012;5:126–34.
17. Gamble JG, Rinsky LA, Bleck EE. Established hip dislocations in children with cerebral palsy. Clin Orthop Relat Res 1990;(253):90–9.
18. Kim HT, Wenger DR. Location of acetabular deficiency and associated hip dislocation in neuromuscular hip dysplasia: three-dimensional computed tomographic analysis. J Pediatr Orthop 1997;17:143–51.
19. Miller F, Slomczykowski M, Cope R, et al. Computer modeling of the pathomechanics of spastic hip dislocation in children. J Pediatr Orthop 1999;19:486–92.
20. Hagglund G, Lauge-Pedersen H, Wagner P. Characteristics of children with hip displacement in cerebral palsy. BMC Musculoskelet Disord 2007;8:101.
21. Lee KM, Chung CY, Kwon DG, et al. Reliability of physical examination in the measurement of hip flexion contracture and correlation with gait parameters in cerebral palsy. J Bone Joint Surg Am 2011;93:150–8.
22. Nwaobi OM, Sussman MD. Electromyographic and force patterns of cerebral palsy patients with wind-blown hip deformity. J Pediatr Orthop 1990;10:382–8.
23. Selva G, Miller F, Dabney KW. Anterior hip dislocation in children with cerebral palsy. J Pediatr Orthop 1998;18:54–61.

24. Reimers J. The stability of the hip in children. A radiological study of the results of muscle surgery in cerebral palsy. Acta Orthop Scand Suppl 1980; 184:1–100.

25. Wynter M, Gibson N, Willoughby KL, et al. Australian hip surveillance guidelines for children with cerebral palsy: 5-year review. Dev Med Child Neurol 2015;57:808–20.

26. Davids JR, Marshall AD, Blocker ER, et al. Femoral anteversion in children with cerebral palsy. Assessment with two and three-dimensional computed tomography scans. J Bone Joint Surg Am 2003; 85-A:481–8.

27. Pons C, Remy-Neris O, Medee B, et al. Validity and reliability of radiological methods to assess proximal hip geometry in children with cerebral palsy: a systematic review. Dev Med Child Neurol 2013; 55:1089–102.

28. Dobson F, Boyd RN, Parrott J, et al. Hip surveillance in children with cerebral palsy. Impact on the surgical management of spastic hip disease. J Bone Joint Surg Br 2002;84:720–6.

29. Connelly A, Flett P, Graham HK, et al. Hip surveillance in Tasmanian children with cerebral palsy. J Paediatr Child Health 2009;45:437–43.

30. Wynter M, Gibson N, Kentish M, et al. The consensus statement on hip surveillance for children with cerebral palsy: Australian standards of care. J Pediatr Rehabil Med 2011;4:183–95.

31. Kentish M, Wynter M, Snape N, et al. Five-year outcome of state-wide hip surveillance of children and adolescents with cerebral palsy. J Pediatr Rehabil Med 2011;4:205–17.

32. Graham HK, Boyd R, Carlin JB, et al. Does botulinum toxin a combined with bracing prevent hip displacement in children with cerebral palsy and "hips at risk"? A randomized, controlled trial. J Bone Joint Surg Am 2008;90:23–33.

33. Presedo A, Oh CW, Dabney KW, et al. Soft-tissue releases to treat spastic hip subluxation in children with cerebral palsy. J Bone Joint Surg Am 2005;87:832–41.

34. Shore BJ, Zurakowski D, Dufreny C, et al. Proximal femoral varus derotation osteotomy in children with cerebral palsy: the effect of age, gross motor function classification system level, and surgeon volume on surgical success. J Bone Joint Surg Am 2015;97:2024–31.

35. Canavese F, Emara K, Sembrano JN, et al. Varus derotation osteotomy for the treatment of hip subluxation and dislocation in GMFCS level III to V patients with unilateral hip involvement. Follow-up at skeletal maturity. J Pediatr Orthop 2010;30:357–64.

36. Chung CY, Choi IH, Cho TJ, et al. Morphometric changes in the acetabulum after Dega osteotomy in patients with cerebral palsy. J Bone Joint Surg Br 2008;90:88–91.

37. Gordon JE, Capelli AM, Strecker WB, et al. Pemberton pelvic osteotomy and varus rotational osteotomy in the treatment of acetabular dysplasia in patients who have static encephalopathy. J Bone Joint Surg Am 1996;78:1863–71.

38. McNerney NP, Mubarak SJ, Wenger DR. One-stage correction of the dysplastic hip in cerebral palsy with the San Diego acetabuloplasty: results and complications in 104 hips. J Pediatr Orthop 2000;20:93–103.

39. Robb JE, Brunner RA. Dega-type osteotomy after closure of the triradiate cartilage in non-walking patients with severe cerebral palsy. J Bone Joint Surg Br 2006;88:933–7.

40. Mallet C, Ilharreborde B, Presedo A, et al. One-stage hip reconstruction in children with cerebral palsy: long term results at skeletal maturity. J Child Orthop 2014;8:221–8.

41. Mubarak SJ, Valencia FG, Wenger DR. One-stage correction of the spastics dislocated hip. J Bone Joint Surg Am 1992;72:1347–57.

42. Bayusentono S, Choi Y, Chung CY, et al. Recurrence of hip instability after reconstructive surgery in patients with cerebral palsy. J Bone Joint Surg Am 2014;96:1527–34.

43. Baxter MP, D'astous JL. Proximal femoral resection-interposition arthroplasty: salvage hip surgery for the severely disabled child with cerebral palsy. J Pediatr Orthop 1986;6:681–5.

44. Castle ME, Schneider C. Proximal femoral resection-interposition arthroplasty. J Bone Joint Surg Am 1978;60:1051–4.

45. Knaus A, Terjsen T. Proximal femoral resection arthroplasty for patients with cerebral palsy and dislocated hips. Acta Orthop 2009;80:32–6.

46. King G, Hunt LP, Wilkinson JM, et al, National Joint Registry for England Wales, Northern Ireland. Good outcome of total hip replacement in patients with cerebral palsy: a comparison of 389 patients and 425,813 controls from the National Joint Registry for England and Wales. Acta Orthop 2016;87: 93–9.

47. Fucs PM, Yamada HH. Hip fusion as hip salvage procedures in cerebral palsy. J Pediatr Orthop 2014;34:S32–5.

48. de Souza RC, Mansan MV, Bovo M, et al. Hip salvage surgery in cerebral palsy cases: a systematic review. Rev Bras Ortop 2015;50:254–9.

Current Use of Evidence-Based Medicine in Pediatric Spine Surgery

Matthew E. Oetgen, MD, MBA

KEYWORDS

- Evidence-based medicine • Scoliosis • Spondylolysis • Pediatrics • Early onset scoliosis

---

KEY POINTS

- Low-quality data make the use of evidence-based medicine in decisions on scoliosis natural history, treatment, and outcomes difficult.
- Decisions regarding nonoperative management of scoliosis have been investigated using evidence-based medicine, and these studies have shown brace use is successful at controlling spinal deformities.
- The natural history, imaging, treatment, and outcomes of pediatric spondylolysis treatment have been evaluated in the literature using evidence-based techniques.
- Early onset scoliosis lacks quality data to allow evidence-based decisions to be made, but recent work has identified high-impact topics whereby quality studies could help with evidence-based medicine decision-making.

INTRODUCTION

As the focus of medicine has undergone a transformation to more quality-based outcomes, the concept of evidence-based medicine (EBM) has gained importance and acceptance throughout the field. Despite the generic acceptance of EBM, confusion still exists as to exactly what it is and its purpose. In general, EBM is a process of decision-making aimed at making the best decisions for patients as they relate to patients' health care. This process integrates aspects of clinical expertise and experience, patient values, and the best available evidence on a topic to come to these decisions.[1]

Although skeptics of EBM often complain that this is akin to cookie-cutter medicine, there is a real difference between EBM and cookie-cutter medicine. As all 3 of the aforementioned components are necessary for EBM, the inclusion of clinical expertise and experience in this process ensures that clinicians still guide the process of making patient care decisions. The best available evidence is necessary for this process; but this evidence must be evaluated, interpreted in the individual clinical situation, and applied within the bounds of patients' values, thus, leaving clinicians plenty of autonomy in the EBM decision-making process.

In addition, given the rapid pace of medical advancement, often times higher levels of clinical evidence may lag behind clinical standards of care, leaving the clinician the responsibility to interpret the data available and combine this with patients' values and clinical experience to make EBM decisions. Therefore, although the highest levels of clinical evidence are preferred in the EMB process, lower levels of clinical evidence must suffice in times when these are the only data available, leaving patients' values and clinical experience as key components in the EBM process.

Disclosure Statement: The author has no commercial or financial disclosures related to this work, and no funding was received for this work.
Division of Orthopaedic Surgery and Sports Medicine, Children's National Health System, 111 Michigan Avenue, Northwest, Washington, DC 20010, USA
E-mail address: moetgen@childrensnational.org

Orthop Clin N Am 49 (2018) 191–194
https://doi.org/10.1016/j.ocl.2017.11.007

This general lack of high quality data is very much the current status of EBM within the area of pediatric spine surgery. Pediatric spinal deformity surgery is an evolving field because of the constant introduction of new technological advancements as well as the progressive understanding of the cause and clinical course of pediatric spinal deformity. Currently, it seems the use of EBM within this field relies more on patients' values and clinical expertise and less on high-quality evidence for decision-making, due mainly to the paucity of high-quality data generated from large randomized trials and high-quality meta-analyses. Although some high-quality studies do exist, which can and should be integrated in the decision-making process when treating patients with pediatric spinal deformity, there is a dire need for more high-quality data to continue to improve the EBM process within the area of pediatric spinal deformity treatment.

EVIDENCE-BASED MEDICINE AND IDIOPATHIC SCOLIOSIS

Idiopathic scoliosis is a common condition in the pediatric population. Despite the ubiquitous nature of this condition in terms of the number of patients affected and the significant cost to society, there is a real lack of high-quality evidence that drives treatment decisions. Instead, clinical experience seems to be a driving force in much of the decision-making process for idiopathic scoliosis. Much of this clinical decision-making, as it relates to decisions for treatment, lies in the data generated by the classic cohort, the natural history study published by Weinstein and colleagues.[2] Unfortunately, because these data have influenced a standard care pathway for idiopathic scoliosis, there has been little additional study of the natural history of untreated pediatric idiopathic scoliosis, thus, little to guide new evidence-based decisions on the treatment of this condition as they relate to the natural history of the condition.

One of the most well-studied aspects of the treatment of idiopathic scoliosis is the nonoperative treatment of this condition. For many years, bracing has been a mainstay of the treatment of idiopathic scoliosis in growing children with a deformity magnitude between 20° and 45°, despite a relative lack of high-quality data for this treatment. The publication of a multicenter randomized controlled trial by Weinstein and colleagues[3] demonstrating the effectiveness of this treatment generated the first high-quality data to justify this treatment. After this publication, a systematic review of the effect of bracing has been published in the Cochrane Database of Systematic Reviews that found brace treatment did not change patients' quality of life during treatment at the long-term follow-up but did find consistent (although low quality) evidence to suggest brace treatment was able to prevent scoliosis deformity progression.[4] The investigators of this review found significant issues with the quality of the studies included due to high failure rates of randomized controlled trials and difficulties in family acceptance of randomization in these trials. These issues may highlight the difficulties in generating high-quality data in the treatment of scoliosis, as patient acceptance of randomization and participation in randomized controlled trials in the treatment of scoliosis seem to be difficult issues to resolve.

Surgical treatment of idiopathic scoliosis is well accepted, typically for progressive deformities more than 50° to 55° in magnitude. Despite this generally accepted surgical threshold, controversy remains in regard to the optimal surgical approach, optimal target for percentage of deformity correction, and instrumentation construct. Currently no randomized controlled trials exist investigating the surgical treatment of idiopathic scoliosis as compared with nonoperative treatment, leaving the evidence for treatment based on small, nonrandomized, low-quality studies. In their systematic review of the literature as it pertains to the surgical outcomes of patients treated for idiopathic scoliosis, Westrick and Ward[5] found surgical treatment consistently arrests progression of scoliosis, maintains permanent deformity correction, and improves cosmetic appearance; however, definitive evidence that these outcomes were superior to the natural history of this condition was lacking.

As can be appreciated, the treatment of idiopathic scoliosis is based primarily on clinical experience and data from historic studies of low quality in terms of EBM. Difficulties certainly exist, as has been shown in some systematic reviews, in developing and completing high-quality randomized controlled trials of this condition. Despite this lack of high-quality data and these difficulties, given the number of patients affected and the high cost of care associated with idiopathic scoliosis, better efforts are needed to generate high-quality data to improve the ability to apply EBM to this condition.

EVIDENCE-BASED MEDICINE AND SPONDYLOLYSIS

In recent years, the EBM committee for the Scoliosis Research Society (SRS) has performed comprehensive systematic reviews on a range of aspects of pediatric lumbar spondylolysis, generating good-quality evidence regarding the natural history, evaluation, and treatment of this condition. Although wide ranging in scope in regard to spondylolysis, the relatively narrower focus of spondylolysis and smaller volume of published literature, as compared with idiopathic scoliosis, made this task much easier to complete.

The first topics evaluated were the cause, prevalence, natural history, and prognosis of pediatric lumbar spondylolysis.[6] The investigators included a total of 44 articles in their review, with 72% being level I and II evidence. They found good evidence to suggest a high percentage of patients with chronic bilateral pars defects will progress to grade 1 or 2 spondylolisthesis, but typically symptoms of this condition resolve in the short-term. Longer-term, the literature suggested lumbar symptoms are common and lead to later surgical intervention; however, little evidence existed to predict which patients would do well and which would require intervention for symptoms.

The literature regarding imaging of patients with pediatric lumbar spondylolysis was also evaluated by this group, in which 27 studies met their inclusion criteria, of which there were no level I and only 5 level II studies.[7] They found plain radiographs to be widely used as a screening examination but computed tomography (CT) to be the gold standard for imaging in this condition. MRI was determined to be an accurate examination as well, with the benefits of less radiation exposure and the ability to detect early pars stress reactions. Finally, single-photon emission CT (SPECT) was a limited imaging modality due to high false-positive and negative results and high radiation exposure. Tofte and colleagues,[8] examining imaging in terms of diagnostic sensitivity and effective radiation dose exposure to patients, performed a second systematic review on this topic. This group found SPECT to be the most accurate advanced diagnostic modality, with CT and MRI following in effectiveness. Similar to the previous review, these investigators found evidence that a 2-view plain film was the best screening examination in patients suspected of having lumbar spondylolysis.

The results and optimal algorithm for the treatment of spondylolysis is less clear in the literature. The SRS group reviewed this literature and included 58 studies, with none being level I or II evidence.[9] They found pain resolution and return to activity were commonly reported for both nonoperative and operative treatment of lumbar spondylolysis, although little evidence to suggest which patients would benefit from which type of treatment. A more focused review was published investigating the outcome of surgical and nonsurgical treatment in high-grade spondylolisthesis in children as well. This review found no difference in either slip progression or patient-reported outcomes between either group over time but suffered from very limited evidence of data, with only 5 observational studies included in the review.[10] Finally, the evidence for reduction of the deformity compared with fusion in situ when performing a spinal arthrodesis for high-grade spondylolisthesis was evaluated. This review found procedures involving reduction lead to improved spinal alignment and less pseudoarthrosis with no increase in the frequency of neurologic complications; however, this review included a mix of both adult and pediatric studies.[11]

EVIDENCE-BASED MEDICINE AND EARLY ONSET SCOLIOSIS

The development of high-quality evidence within early onset scoliosis (EOS) has been limited. Thus far, most data published consist of relatively small groups of patients or larger cohort series investigating short-term surgical outcomes or complications associated with treatment.[12–15] This lack of high-quality evidence is likely the result of several factors unique to EOS. First, the understanding of disease and surgical techniques are rapidly evolving in this newly appreciated subspecialty. This factor has caused a relative lag in the generation of scientific evidence in regard to these advances. Second, the small patient volumes, as compared with idiopathic scoliosis, and the heterogeneity of the patient population make it difficult to compared populations within this field. Recent work on validated categorization methods of patients may help clinicians develop studies that include a wide variety of patients but can be evaluated in a way that is more useful to the practicing clinician in terms of accurately applying results to similar patient populations.[16] Finally, alternative study methods have predominated the EOS literature to date, resulting in the publication of lower levels of clinical evidence. Methods of structured and validated group consensus have been used in EOS to assess treatment preferences and identify areas of equipoise among surgeon in and attempt to identify high-yield areas of future clinical research.[17,18] This methodical and scientific way of identifying areas in need of study as it pertains to EOS may help focus the limited resources within this field to generate future high-quality data to be used in the process of EBM for this disease.

SUMMARY

The use of EBM in pediatric spinal surgery has been infrequent in the past; however, growing interest in this decision-making technique and improved evidence generation will likely allow it to gain wider use in the future. Traditionally, treatment of children with spinal deformity has relied heavily on clinical expertise; but more recent work into the understanding of patients' values and a coordinated effort to focus future research into clinically high-yield topics will expand the understanding of all stakeholders when clinical decisions are made. Dedication to the development of EBM in pediatric spinal surgery will be needed with work from EBM groups (such as the EBM committee of the SRS) and collaboration of physicians across institutions to generate higher-quality evidence in regard to the cause, natural history, treatment, and outcomes in pediatric spinal surgery.

REFERENCES

1. Evidence Based Medicine Working Group. Evidence based medicine. A new approach to teaching the practice of medicine. JAMA 1992;268: 2420–5.
2. Weinstein SL, Zavala DC, Ponseti IV. Idiopathic scoliosis: long-term follow-up and prognosis in untreated patients. J Bone Joint Surg Am 1981;63: 702–12.
3. Weinstein SL, Dolan LA, Wright JG, et al. Effects of bracing in adolescents with idiopathic scoliosis. N Engl J Med 2013;369(16):1512–21.
4. Negrini S, Minozzi S, Bettany-Saltikov J, et al. Braces for idiopathic scoliosis in adolescents. Cochrane Database Syst Rev 2015;(6):CD006850.
5. Westrick ER, Ward WT. Adolescent idiopathic scoliosis: 5-year to 20-year evidence-based surgical results. J Pediatr Orthop 2011;31(1 Suppl):S61–8.
6. Crawford CH 3rd, Ledonio CG, Bess RS, et al. Current evidence regarding the etiology, prevalence, natural history, and prognosis of pediatric lumbar spondylolysis: a report from the Scoliosis Research Society Evidence-Based Medicine Committee. Spine Deform 2015;3(1):12–29.
7. Ledonio CG, Burton DC, Crawford CH 3rd, et al. Current evidence regarding diagnostic imaging methods for pediatric lumbar spondylolysis: a report from the Scoliosis Research Society Evidence-Based Medicine Committee. Spine Deform 2017;5(2):97–101.
8. Tofte JN, CarlLee TL, Holte AJ, et al. Imaging pediatric spondylolysis: a systematic review. Spine 2017; 42(10):777–82.
9. Crawford CH 3rd, Ledonio CG, Bess RS, et al. Current evidence regarding the surgical and nonsurgical treatment of pediatric lumbar spondylolysis: a report from the Scoliosis Research Society Evidence-Based Medicine Committee. Spine Deform 2015;3(1):30–44.
10. Xue X, Wei X, Li L. Surgical versus nonsurgical treatment for high-grade spondylolisthesis in children and adolescents: a systematic review and meta-analysis. Medicine 2016;95(11):e3070.
11. Longo UG, Loppini M, Romeo G, et al. Evidence-based surgical management of spondylolisthesis: reduction or arthrodesis in situ. J Bone Joint Surg Am 2014;96(1):53–8.
12. Bess S, Akbarnia BA, Thompson GH, et al. Complications of growing-rod treatment for early-onset scoliosis: analysis of one hundred and forty patients. J Bone Joint Surg Am 2010;92(15): 2533–43.
13. Luhmann SJ, Smith JC, McClung A, et al, Growing Spine Study Group. Radiographic outcomes of shilla growth guidance system and traditional growing rods through definitive treatment. Spine Deform 2017;5(4):277–82.
14. Johnston CE, McClung AM, Thompson GH, et al, Growing Spine Study Group. Comparison of growing rod instrumentation versus serial cast treatment for early-onset scoliosis. Spine Deform 2013;1(5):339–42.
15. Farooq N, Garrido E, Altaf F, et al. Minimizing complications with single submuscular growing rods: a review of technique and results on 88 patients with minimum two-year follow-up. Spine 2010; 35(25):2252–8.
16. Williams BA, Matsumoto H, McCalla DJ, et al. Development and initial validation of the classification of early-onset scoliosis (C-EOS). J Bone Joint Surg Am 2014;96(16):1359–67.
17. Vitale MG, Gomez JA, Matsumoto H, et al, Chest Wall and Spine Deformity Study Group. Variability of expert opinion in treatment of early-onset scoliosis. Clin Orthop Relat Res 2011;469(5): 1317–22.
18. Corona J, Miller DJ, Downs J, et al. Evaluating the extent of clinical uncertainty among treatment options for patients with early-onset scoliosis. J Bone Joint Surg Am 2013;95(10):e67.

Pediatric Orthopedic Trauma
An Evidence-Based Approach

Elizabeth W. Hubbard, MD[a], Anthony I. Riccio, MD[b],*

KEYWORDS

- Supracondylar humerus fracture • Medial epicondyle fracture • Femoral shaft fracture
- Clavicle fracture • Evidence-based medicine • Open fracture

KEY POINTS

- Displaced supracondylar humerus fractures should be managed with closed reduction and pin fixation. Pin placement, size, and surgical timing should be selected based on fracture and patient characteristics.
- Femoral shaft fracture management can be guided by patient age, size, and fracture type. Guidelines are available, but have not yet demonstrated that they streamline how patients receive care.
- Grade 1 open fractures can potentially be treated with local wound debridement, antibiotics, and closed reduction, but this method needs to be proven in randomized studies.
- Although there is strong evidence to suggest that anatomic reduction of specific clavicle fractures in adults improves outcomes, this has not been proven in pediatric patients.

INTRODUCTION

Historically, many pediatric injuries were managed nonsurgically. However, with changes in implant selection and outcomes, studies of operative versus nonoperative treatment, orthopedists have moved toward surgical intervention for certain fractures. To streamline surgical decision making and patient care, the American Academy of Orthopaedic Surgeons (AAOS) has developed clinical guidelines for the management of pediatric diaphyseal femur fractures[1,2] and supracondylar humerus fractures.[3] Although helpful, the guidelines are limited by the lack of high-level evidence relating to certain aspects of these injures. Also, there are currently no other guidelines available for other types of pediatric fractures. The growing body of literature regarding grade 1 open fractures, medial epicondyle fractures, and clavicle

fractures has made management of these injuries three of the most controversial topics in pediatric orthopedics today. This article analyzes the available evidence to help guide the management of each of these injury patterns and highlights areas where additional research is needed.

SUPRACONDYLAR HUMERUS FRACTURES

Supracondylar humerus fractures are the most common fractures involving the elbow in pediatric patients.[4] Given the frequency of these injuries, it is important for both pediatric and general orthopedic surgeons to understand the treatment recommendations for different types of supracondylar humerus fractures.

Nonoperative treatment with either splint or cast immobilization is recommended for Gartland type 1 (nondisplaced) supracondylar

Disclosure Statement: The authors do not have any financial relationships with any device or medical company, and did not receive any external research support that is related to this article.
[a] Department of Orthopaedic Surgery, Shriner's Hospital for Children, 110 Conn Terrace, Lexington, KY 40508, USA; [b] Department of Orthopaedic Surgery, Texas Scottish Rite Hospital for Children, 2222 Welborn Street, Dallas, TX 75219, USA
* Corresponding author.
E-mail address: Anthony.riccio@tsrh.org

Orthop Clin N Am 49 (2018) 195–210
https://doi.org/10.1016/j.ocl.2017.11.008

humerus fractures.[3] Studies comparing methods of immobilization have shown that the use of a posterior splint leads to decreased duration of pain, decreased analgesic use, and faster return to normal activity than collar and cuff immobilization.[5,6]

Treatment for type 2 supracondylar humerus fractures is difficult to discern from the current literature. According to the AAOS guidelines, closed reduction and pin fixation is recommended.[3] However, none the studies used to make these recommendations specifically analyzed Gartland type 2 supracondylar humerus fractures in isolation. Five focused only on type 3 supracondylar fractures[7–11] and the remaining included patients with both type 2 and type 3 fractures.[12–17] Moraleda and colleagues[18] specifically analyzed outcomes of patients who sustained type 2 fractures who were treated without attempted reduction or surgery. Compared with the nonoperative side, the total arc of elbow motion was unchanged, but the affected elbows had significantly more extension and significantly less flexion (8° and 7°, respectively).[18] According to the Flynn criteria, results were deemed satisfactory in 80% of patients.[18] This finding would suggest that not all type 2 supracondylar humerus fractures require operative treatment to ensure a satisfactory outcome. However, the increased risk of cubits varus and the altered arc of elbow motion that is seen with unreduced type 2 supracondylar fractures should be discussed with patients and families when considering nonoperative treatment without reduction for these injuries.[18]

The AAOS recommends that type 3 supracondylar humerus fractures be treated with closed reduction and pin fixation.[3] This method is supported by a wide range of studies that examine type 3 supracondylar humerus fractures alone as well as in combination with other types of fractures.[7–17] However, the urgency of closed reduction and pin fixation of type 3 fractures in patients who are neurovascularly intact upon presentation is not well-defined. There are studies that suggest that delayed operative intervention in this setting can increase the need for open reduction and potentially increase the risk of compartment syndrome.[19–21] However, multiple studies have reported no correlation between surgical timing and the need for open reduction or perioperative complications.[22–26] Therefore, surgical timing is left to the discretion of the surgeon. Important considerations include the patient's degree of swelling, status of the soft tissues, the time interval between injury and patient presentation, and

access to an operating room in the morning should treatment be deferred. It is also important to consider that patients left unreduced can have continued swelling, which can cause the neurovascular status to change over time. Ho and colleagues[27] found that 8% of patients who presented to a level 1 pediatric hospital with a neurovascular injury in the setting of a supracondylar humerus fracture had evidence of progressive decline in their neurovascular status between the initial evaluation in the emergency department and the evaluation in the preoperative holding area.

Pin construct for supracondylar fractures has been a point of interest in the literature. Multiple studies support the use of crossed pins for biomechanical strength, especially against torsional stress.[16,28–33] However, 3 well-placed lateral entry pins that have bicortical purchase and adequate spread across the fracture site have been shown to be biomechanically equivalent to 2 crossed pins.[34,35] Increasing the pin size from 1.6 to 2.0 mm also increases construct strength for lateral entry pins.[36–38] An advantage of all lateral entry pins is that they minimize the risk of iatrogenic ulnar nerve injury.[39] The decreased incidence of iatrogenic nerve injury reported in the literature is one reason why the AAOS recommends that all lateral entry pins be placed when possible for supracondylar fractures.[3] However, the actual incidence of ulnar nerve injury in the setting of medial pin placement is highly variable in the literature and fractures with medial comminution are more stable and have less chance of loss of reduction when a medial pin is placed.[34,40] Making an incision has not been shown to be protective against iatrogenic nerve injury during pin placement, but elbow extension during pin placement is protective.[39] When possible, all lateral entry pins are the preferred method of fixation. However, because medial pins are sometimes essential to maintain fracture reduction, we support using a medial pin when it is necessary. In this setting, we recommend placing 1 or 2 lateral pins first with the elbow flexed to obtain control of the fracture, followed by elbow extension for medial pin placement to minimize the risk of nerve injury.

Patients who present with a cool pulseless extremity in the setting of a supracondylar fracture should ideally undergo emergent closed reduction to try to restore perfusion to the extremity.[3] Preoperative angiography is not recommended in this scenario, because it has only been shown to delay time to surgery with no appreciable patient benefit.[41–43] Fracture reduction has been shown to restore perfusion in 53% to 72% of cases.[42,44–46] It is helpful to have access to a vascular surgeon if there is an arterial injury and pulses are not restored after anatomic fracture reduction. Consideration can be given to proceeding toward open reduction in this scenario, but there are no high-level studies to support this decision and the AAOS clinical guidelines are unable to offer any recommendations in this setting.[3] The surgeon must weigh his or her own personal experience with this injury pattern, access to a vascular team, and the effect that a surgical delay would have on the patient outcome if the decision is made to transfer the patient to a higher level of care before proceeding with reduction.

The "pink pulseless hand" remains a point of controversy in the literature. This term refers to those extremities that are pink with good capillary refill but lack a palpable radial pulse after fracture reduction. Some sources argue for immediate vascular exploration in this scenario.[45,47–49] However, there are studies that support careful observation of these patients after fracture reduction and pinning. Scannell and colleagues[50] reviewed the outcomes of 20 patients who presented with type 3 supracondylar humerus fractures and perfused pulseless extremities. Patients were taken to surgery an average of 7 hours after injury (range, 2–15 hours). Five patients had a palpable radial pulse in the operating room after closed reduction and pinning; 2 additional patients had a palpable pulse at the time of discharge. The remaining 13 patients had perfused extremities but no palpable radial pulse at discharge. All patients had a palpable pulse at the time of final follow-up, although the date of the return of the pulse varied from 0 to 233 days postoperatively. None of the patients required vascular reconstruction.[50] Weller and colleagues[51] found that most patients with a pink pulseless extremity after fracture reduction and pinning had a pulse that could be detected using Doppler imaging. The 5% of patients who had neither a palpable or apparent pulse on Doppler imaging required vascular reconstruction owing to brachial artery injuries. These authors recommended using the patient's capillary refill and the presence of a radial artery signal detectable by Doppler imaging after closed reduction and pinning when deciding whether a patient requires emergent surgical exploration.[51] Sabharwal and colleagues[52] demonstrated that early revascularization procedures in this circumstance have a high rate of reocclusion and subsequently recommended that close observation with

multiple neurovascular checks should be performed before going forward with vascular reconstruction. The AAOS handles this discrepancy in the literature through 2 separate recommendations. The guidelines support emergent closed reduction in the setting of a supracondylar humerus fracture with decreased perfusion to the hand. This description includes the spectrum of "pink pulseless hand" to the cool and pulseless hand. However, the guidelines then indicate that, based on the current literature, they cannot recommend for or against open exploration of the antecubital fossa when a patient has absent wrist pulses but a perfused hand after closed reduction and pinning.[3] The current literature suggests that a hand that is perfused but has absent palpable pulses after closed reduction and pinning needs to be observed closely in the postoperative period with frequent neurovascular checks after surgery if the surgeon decides to not explore the antecubital fossa immediately.

The AAOS guidelines do not offer any recommendations regarding the timing of treatment in patients who present with isolated neurologic injury. Barrett and colleagues[53] found that urgent closed reduction and percutaneous pin fixation did not result in faster neurologic recovery among patients who presented with an isolated anterior interosseous nerve palsy. However, only 35 patients from an initial pool of 4409 met inclusion criteria for the study, giving them an overall incidence of less than 1% of anterior interosseous nerve palsy, which is lower than what has been reported in other studies.[26,27,54] It has been shown that the presence of a neurologic injury upon presentation with a supracondylar humerus fracture is associated with more severe soft tissue injury.[27] Based on the current evidence, we cannot offer a recommendation regarding the urgency of surgical timing when a patient presents with an isolated neurologic injury and a palpable pulse. It is important to remember that a percentage of these patients will have progressive loss of neurologic function between emergency department admission and operative treatment, and this factor should be considered when deciding when to take a patient to the operating room.[27]

FEMORAL SHAFT FRACTURES

Femoral shaft fractures account for 1.6% of all fractures in pediatric patients and are among the most common reasons for hospital admissions in this population.[4] In 2009, the AAOS first released clinical guidelines to aid in treatment decisions for these patients; the guidelines were then updated in 2015.[1,2,55] Although studies have shown that clinical practice guidelines can help to standardize patient care based on the best available evidence,[56–58] reviews of the clinical guidelines for femoral shaft fracture management in children have not demonstrated similar effects.[59] A recent multicenter review demonstrated an increase in the use of rigid locked intramedullary nails in adolescents younger than age 11 and increased surgical management of femoral shaft fractures in children younger than 5.[60] These trends counter recommendations made in the clinical guidelines.[55,60] This is potentially due to the limited high-level evidence available for these injuries. Ultimately, of the 14 recommendations listed, only one had sufficient evidence to be truly "recommended" by the committee. Of the remaining recommendations, 50% were either "suggested" or "optional" based on the available evidence and 6 did not have enough supporting evidence to guide treatment.[1–3]

The AAOS recommends that children younger than 36 months who present with a femoral shaft fracture be evaluated for nonaccidental trauma (NAT).[1] This recommendation is based on multiple population studies that have found 12% to 14% of all femoral shaft fractures in children younger than age 3 are related to NAT.[61–63] Studies also suggest that femoral shaft fractures in children who are not ambulatory have a strong association with NAT, with 30% of femoral shaft fractures in children less than 1 year of age attributable to abuse.[64] Orthopedic injuries are among the most common ways for pediatric victims of NAT to present to the emergency department, so orthopedic surgeons need to have a high level of suspicion to ensure the safety of our patients.[64]

Children who sustain femoral shaft fractures between 0 and 6 months of age can be treated in either a Pavlik harness or spica cast.[1] Podeszwa and colleagues[65] found that patients had 100% fracture union with no clinical evidence of malalignment, regardless of whether they were treated in a Pavlik or a spica. However, the spica group did have a greater number of minor complications relating to skin irritation and breakdown in the cast.[65] Stannard and colleagues[66] evaluated 16 patients treated in a Pavlik harness for isolated femoral shaft fractures and all went on to fracture union after an average of 5 weeks of treatment in the brace. Because a Pavlik harness can be applied in a nonsurgical setting, does not require sedation or a general anesthetic, and has been shown to

significantly reduce skin complications in this population, we feel that this age group can reliably be treated in a Pavlik harness.

Although many investigators recommend that children ages 6 months to 5 years be treated in a spica cast, the AAOS clinical guidelines do not offer any recommendations for or against spica casting in this age group.[1,4,67] Some authors have examined whether flexible nails would be a better option in this population. Heffernan and colleagues[68] compared 141 preschool aged patients treated with closed reduction and spica casting for femoral shaft fractures with 74 patients of similar ages treated with titanium elastic intramedullary nails (TENs). Although both groups had similar time to radiographic union with acceptable coronal and sagittal alignment,[69] these authors found that the TENs group returned to walking and full function after injury faster than the spica patients.[68] Complication rates were low in both groups, but the authors did not divulge the number of TENs patients who required a second surgical procedure for implant removal. Also, the study did not differentiate between polytrauma patients and those with isolated femoral shaft fractures. More than one-third of the patients in the TENs group had other associated injuries (32% vs 13% in the spica group; $P = .002$), which potentially influenced the surgeon's decision to treat these patients with TENs rather than a spica cast.[68] Bopst and colleagues[70] also found that preschool children treated with TENs were able to weight bear and mobilize faster than those who were treated with spica casts. However, 12% of this cohort required an early return to the operating room for revision surgery owing to nail migration through the skin. The authors did not state whether any patients treated with casting required a repeat anesthetic. They also did not report the number of patients who underwent another anesthetic for removal of the TENs nails after fracture union.[70] It has previously been shown that elective implant removal after flexible nail placement for a femur fracture has an infrequent but real risk of complications, and this factor is important to consider when weighing treatment options in this population.[71]

Studies have highlighted the potential burden that a spica cast can place on a family. Parents are more likely to report needing to take time off work because daycare facilities and schools are unable to provide care for this patients during the day.[72] A percentage of patients also require alternate modes of transportation owing to the cast, such as the use of an ambulance to get to and from clinic appointments.[69] Leu and colleagues[73] compared single versus double leg spica casting for patients with femoral shaft fractures. Patient in the single leg group were more likely to fit into car seat and chairs, and care givers were able to take less time off work during the treatment period, with no difference in union rates, fracture alignment, or shortening between the groups.[73] Flynn and colleagues[69] have shown that placing a child in a walking spica cast allows children to crawl, stand, and walk faster than patients treated in a traditional spica. Although almost 1 in 4 patients in the walking spica required an in-clinic cast wedge early in the treatment course, fewer of these patients required a second anesthetic for cast revision than the traditional group and there were no differences in the ultimate coronal or sagittal plane alignment between the groups. Family members of the walking spica group reported a reduced care burden compared with the traditional spica group, and none of the patients treated in a walking spica required an ambulance for transportation.[69]

Ramo and colleagues[74] specifically compared outcomes of children ages 4 to 5 years treated with either spica casting or flexible nails. This study examined 262 patients, 158 of whom were treated with immediate spica casting and 104 who were treated with flexible nails. The flexible nail patients were older, weighed more, and more likely to have sustained a high-energy injury compared with the spica group. Four patients in the spica group returned to surgery for cast removal and nail placement owing to either malalignment (n = 3) or family request (n = 1), and 4 patients in the nail group required early implant removal and spica casting owing to nail migration through the skin. There was no difference between the groups with regards to coronal or sagittal angulation or fracture shortening greater than 20 mm at the time of fracture union.[74] A greater percentage of patients treated with flexible nails had complications (16.3% vs 7.6%; P = .04) and 89% underwent a subsequent surgery versus only 5.1% in the spica group (P<.001), mostly for implant removal.[74] Given the high rates of fracture union and acceptable femoral alignment after treatment, this study suggests that spica casting is the preferred treatment for this age group in the setting of an isolated femoral shaft fracture owing to the significantly lower rates of complications and secondary surgeries.

The AAOS states that flexible intramedullary nails are an option when determining the treatment of femoral shaft fractures in children age 5 to 11 years. This approach has become a generally accepted treatment, with benefits including earlier mobilization, return to walking, return to school, and return to full function in this age group compared with other treatment modalities.[75,76] The studies referenced in the guidelines focused specifically on the use of titanium nails and the guidelines highlight reports of malunion and implant failure when TENs nails are used in children who weigh more than 47 kg and/or are greater than 11 years of age.[77–79] The complication rates seen in this subgroup population treated with TENs have led surgeons to try other treatment modalities for this group, including submuscular plating and rigid intramedullary nail placement in older and heavier patients.[80]

Although are popular in the United States, there are multiple studies comparing stainless steel flexible nails with TENs that suggest that the stainless steel implants are a superior choice from both a strength and a cost perspective. Wall and colleagues[81] demonstrated that the malunion rate was 4 times greater and the major complication rate was more than 2 times greater in patients treated with TENs compared with stainless steel implants, whereas the cost of the stainless steel implant was 3 to 6 times lower. Since the publication of these guidelines, Shaha and colleagues[82] have shown that stainless steel flexible nails can be used in patients who weigh more than 100 lbs without any significant increased risk of nonunion, malunion, or implant. Length unstable fractures have less risk of fracture shortening, implant prominence, and minor perioperative complications when treated with locked stainless steel flexible nails.[83] Although studies of TENs have suggested that 80% canal fill needs to be achieved for maximum fracture stability,[84,85] stainless steel implants can have as little as 60% canal fill with no significant effects on fracture union, shortening, or ultimate alignment.[86] The current guidelines do not address whether titanium or stainless steel implants should be used when considering flexible intramedullary nail placement.[1]

Patients 11 years and older are candidates for either flexible or rigid intramedullary fixation.[1] Studies of TENS nails in this group have shown higher rates of complications, although this is potentially related to the weight rather than the age of these patients.[77,78] Garner and colleagues[87] reported reduced operative time, blood loss, and implant-related complications in length stable femur fractures treated with TENs nails with no increased risk for malunion or limb length discrepancy, although their 66% rate of implant-related complications with rigid nails is higher than what has been reported in other studies.[88–90] The superior biomechanical properties of stainless steel over titanium also makes stainless steel flexible intramedullary nails a reasonable treatment option in this patient population, even in length unstable fractures, although the clinical guidelines do not address this issue.[82,83] The guidelines do state that a piriformis start point should be avoided in this population owing to the risk of avascular necrosis.[1]

GRADE 1 OPEN FRACTURES

Surgical treatment of open fractures to remove contamination and devitalized tissue from the wound is well-established in the literature. Work by Gustilo and Anderson has helped to promote this aggressive treatment of open fractures, and has given orthopedics one of the most widely used classification schemes to help guide the treatment of open fractures.[91–97] Studies have suggested that all open fractures should be managed with antibiotics and surgical debridement, and that both antibiotic administration and debridement should occur within a few hours of injury.

The more recent literature has called the timing and need for operative intervention into question for some types of open fractures. Skaggs and colleagues[98] first reported a retrospective review of 104 open fractures in pediatric patients treated at a single center. All patients underwent operative debridement with an overall infection rate of 1.9%. There was no difference in the infection rate between those treated within 6 hours and those treated either 6 to 12 hours or more than 12 hours after injury. A subsequent multicenter study reviewed surgical timing and rate of infection among 544 open fractures in pediatric patients.[99] Fractures involved a wide variety of anatomic locations, with 178 involving the radius and ulna. Just more than 50% of injuries were classified as grade 1, 28% as grade 2%, and 17% as grade 3. Overall, 62% of all fractures were surgically debrided within 6 hours of injury. Timing to surgery did not vary by fracture grade, although there was a trend toward more rapid surgical intervention in the grade 2 and grade 3 injuries compared with the grade 1 fractures. Surgery was delayed more than 6 hours in more than 40% of grade 1 injuries, 25% of grade 2 injuries, and 36% of grade 3 injuries. Despite this delay, there was no difference in the overall rate of infection (3% among those who underwent surgery within 6 hours vs 2% in those in whom surgery was delayed more than 6 hours; $P = .43$).[99]

This study calls into question the significance of early surgical debridement of open fractures.

Antibiotic timing for the treatment of open fractures in pediatric patients has not been well-reviewed. Patzakis and Wilson cited an infection rate of 4.7% when patients received antibiotics within 3 hours of injury, compared with a 7.2% infection rate when antibiotic administration was delayed by more than 3 hours.[100] Although there is no level 1 evidence to support a strict time interval during which antibiotics need to be given, there is universal agreement that antibiotics should be administered as quickly as possible upon patient arrival to the emergency department.

The treatment of grade 1 open fractures has garnered increasing amounts of attention over the past 20 years. Multiple studies promote the maxim that all open fractures be treated operatively. Studies of grade 1 open forearm fractures treated with antibiotics and surgical debridement consistently report high rates of good to excellent outcomes with high rates of healing and very low rates of infection.[101,102] However, some authors have called into question the need for surgical debridement of type 1 open fractures. By definition, these fractures retain their periosteal coverage, which is thicker in children than in adults. The wounds are not grossly contaminated and the muscle layer is intact. These anatomic factors support the idea that there is adequate blood supply to the fracture site to deliver antibiotics to prevent infection and promote fracture healing.

Yang and colleagues[103] first reviewed the treatment of 91 grade 1 open fractures in adult and pediatric patients. All injuries were irrigated urgently in the emergency department but only one-third of patients underwent formal surgical intervention. Cefazolin was administered within 6 hours of the injury and patients were admitted for an additional 48 hours of intravenous antibiotics. There was a 0% incidence of infection, leading the authors to argue that operative intervention may not be indicated for grade 1 open injuries as long as antibiotics, appropriate wound care, and fracture stabilization are performed in a timely manner.[103]

Subsequently, multiple studies specifically analyzing management of grade 1 open fractures in pediatric patients have been performed. Iobst and colleagues[104] reported on 40 pediatric patients with grade 1 open injuries who presented between 1998 and 2003. Patients received intravenous antibiotics in the emergency department and were subsequently admitted for another 48 to 72 hours for additional antibiotics. Only 4 patients received oral antibiotics after discharge and the overall deep infection rate was 2.5%.[104] Doak and colleagues[105] subsequently reviewed their own experience with 25 pediatric patients, 11 of whom were treated exclusively in the emergency department with a single dose of intravenous antibiotics. The discharge protocol was variable, with 20 patients receiving a prescription for oral antibiotics after discharge; the drug type and duration of treatment was also variable. Only 1 patient developed an infection, although this was not culture proven and symptoms resolved with an additional 48 hours of intravenous antibiotics; surgical debridement was not performed. Bazzi and colleagues[106] similarly found no cases of deep infection after nonoperative management of 40 patients with grade 1 open fractures of the forearm or tibia. Godfrey and colleagues[107] compared the outcomes of 49 patients with grade 1 open fractures treated nonoperatively with 170 patients who underwent surgical debridement and reported only 1 deep infection in the nonoperative group. In addition to the single case of infection, 1 patient who was managed nonoperatively had a loss of reduction after initial management. However, 9 patients in the operative group experienced complications, which included compartment syndrome, acute carpal tunnel syndrome, and a delayed fracture union. As with the prior studies, there was no consistency regarding the type of antibiotic chosen, duration of intravenous treatment, decision to administer oral antibiotics after discharge, or duration of antibiotic administration after discharge.

To minimize inconsistency, Iobst and colleagues[108] developed an institutional protocol for the management of grade 1 open forearm fractures in pediatric patients. All patients receive 1 dose of an intravenous cephalosporin in the emergency department and undergo wound irrigation with saline and betadine. Patients subsequently undergo closed reduction and casting, with a window created in the cast to monitor the wound. Patients are then admitted for an additional 3 doses of intravenous antibiotics and discharged home without further medical treatment. Wound checks and in cast radiographs are obtained 1 week after discharge. In reviewing their experience with 45 patients with open forearm fractures, they had no deep infections, and only 3 of 45 patients lost reduction in the cast and required surgery for repeat reduction.[108] The duration of admission ranged from 26 to 41 hours, and the average time to radiographic fracture healing was 50.5 days. Patients were followed for a minimum of 5 years and there were no known delayed infections.

Currently, there is no level 1 or 2 evidence to support the nonoperative management of grade 1 open fractures in pediatric patients. However, there are a growing number of level 3 studies that suggest this is a safe treatment approach that spares children from surgery and general anesthetic exposure while being cost effective for both the families and the health care system. The existing level 3 and 4 studies advocating nonoperative management are consistent in that each patient received intravenous antibiotics, usually a cephalosporin, in a timely fashion upon arrival in the emergency department. Patients also underwent local wound debridement in the emergency department and fracture reduction with subsequent casting or splinting. The studies vary on the type and duration of antibiotics subsequently administered and the route of administration. No firm treatment recommendations can be made based on the current evidence, but these studies indicate that larger level 1 and 2 studies need to be performed using firm treatment protocols regarding antibiotic administration.

MEDIAL EPICONDYLE FRACTURES

The treatment of acute medial epicondyle fractures in pediatric patients is potentially one of the most debated trauma topics in the literature today. Classically, this is an injury that has been treated nonoperatively with immobilization in a long arm cast for approximately 4 weeks, regardless of the amount of displacement.[109,110] There is consistent agreement that open fractures and medial epicondyle fractures that are incarcerated in the ulnohumeral joint after an elbow dislocation should be treated operatively.[111–116] Possible surgical indications have been extended to include fractures associated with ulnar neuropathy, citing the concern for possible nerve entrapment in the joint, as well as fractures associated with elbow dislocations or documented valgus instability.[111] More recently, there has been an increasing interest in extending surgical treatment to fractures that are more displaced, with some authors citing as little as 2 mm displacement as an indication for surgery.[117,118] Finally, there is growing interest in treating patients based on their level of physical activity, citing that high-demand and/or overhead athletes require an anatomic reduction of the fracture fragment to impart stability and tension the flexor pronator mass.[119–121]

The medial epicondyle is both the attachment point for the anterior bundle of the ulnar collateral ligament as well as the flexor–pronator mass.[111] Biomechanical studies of the ulnar collateral ligament have shown that it plays a crucial role in resisting valgus stress, acting as a static stabilizer of the ulnohumeral joint.[122,123] The anterior bundle is uniquely important, because it plays a role in stability in elbow flexion and extension.[124] The flexor–pronator mass is a dynamic stabilizer of the elbow and it functions as a protective force for the ulnocollateral ligament when the elbow is exposed to torsional stress.[111] Advocates of surgical treatment for medial epicondyle fractures argue that the resulting displacement of the attachment points of both the anterior bundle of the ulnocollateral ligament and the flexor–pronator mass in nonoperatively treated fractures leave the ulnohumeral joint at risk for valgus instability. Those who care for high-level athletes argue that even slight instability to valgus loads place the athletes at risk for cartilage degeneration and long-term arthritis.[125]

Evidence to guide the treatment of medial epicondyle fractures is limited. Josefsson and Danielsson[110] followed patients with medial epicondyle fractures treated nonoperatively for 35 years. These authors cited a high rate of nonunion, although the patients did well functionally. Farsetti and colleagues[126] offered long-term follow-up of both operatively and nonoperatively treated patients, with an average follow-up of approximately 30 years. Regardless of whether patients were treated nonoperatively or surgically, patients were equally likely to have good or fair outcomes at the final follow-up. Patients treated with anatomic reduction through surgery were significantly more likely to go on to osseous union, whereas 17 of 19 patients treated nonoperatively had documented nonunion at follow-up. However, patients had equal results in terms of strength, muscle mass, and elbow stability.[126] The only patients who had poor results where those who underwent fragment excision with suture repair of the soft tissue structures. Because nonunion was so common in the nonoperative group and also seemingly asymptomatic, the authors argued that this should be seen as an expected outcome rather than a complication and that nonoperative treatment should be the accepted treatment for these injuries.[126] Stepanovich and colleagues[127] reported similar findings in a smaller study of only 12 patients, with no difference in elbow stability or strength regardless of treatment. They also found a higher rate of union among surgically treated patients. However, surgically treated patients were significantly more likely to complain of medial elbow pain, although this was not severe enough to require implant removal.

Because classification schemes have been based on amount of fracture displacement, there is increasing interest on how accurately fracture displacement can be measured on radiographs. Pappas and colleagues[128] showed low rates of interobserver reliability when measuring fracture displacement on routine anteroposterior, lateral, and oblique radiographs. Edmonds[129] supported this finding in 2010, which demonstrated that anteroposterior and lateral radiographs consistently underestimated the degree of fracture displacement compared with computed tomography studies. computed tomography scans of 9 patients with displaced medial epicondyle fractures showed that the maximum trajectory of displacement was anterior, which is difficult to measure on pure anteroposterior or lateral radiographs. These images showed minimal medial fracture displacement, which radiographs typically overestimated. Internal oblique radiographs were slightly, but not significantly, better at assessing the displacement, although only 6 of the 9 patients had this image taken as a part of their initial series.

A major argument for treating displaced but closed and nonincarcerated fractures in adolescent patients is that restoring the normal anatomic alignment of the medial collateral ligament will result in less risk of symptomatic valgus instability and improved overall elbow function. However, the current literature does not consistently support this argument. Biggers and colleagues[130] compared operatively and nonoperatively treated medial epicondyle fractures among 31 adolescent patients and cited equally high functional outcome scores in each group, although patients managed nonoperatively were more likely to have radiographic evidence of fracture nonunion, valgus instability of the elbow, and medial epicondyle hypertrophy. One study comparing operative and nonoperative treatment among athletes found that all patients, regardless of treatment, were able to return to their desired sporting activities at the appropriate level for their age and skill.[131] Seven patients were active in baseball and the 3 nonoperatively treated patients had no issues with valgus instability or elbow pain that limited them from play. All patients were followed for a minimum of 2 years.

Surgical stabilization of displaced medial epicondyle fractures makes anatomic sense when the importance of the medial collateral ligament for elbow stability is considered. However, there are no large, high-level studies that document improved function among pediatric patients who undergo operative intervention for medial epicondyle fractures. At this time, the literature continues to support treating open and/or incarcerated fragments operatively and treating nondisplaced or minimally displaced fractures nonoperatively. There is a trend toward operative intervention for medial epicondyle fractures that are displaced by more than 5 mm, but there is no strong evidence to suggest that this results in improved patient outcomes. An understanding of the ideal treatment for this injury would benefit substantially from a well-designed, large, prospective, randomized study.

CLAVICLE FRACTURES

Clavicle fractures account for anywhere from 10% to 15% of all pediatric fractures.[132,133] Ninety percent of these are middiaphyseal injuries.[134] Historically, these fractures were treated nonoperatively with general agreement they have a high rate of union and patients do well clinically with no significant loss of function.[109] However, there has been an increasing trend toward operative intervention for displaced clavicle fractures in pediatric patients in recent years.[135–137] This trend has coincided with recent literature advocating for more aggressive treatment of adults with certain clavicle fractures.

In 2004, Robinson and colleagues[138] prospectively reviewed 886 adults who sustained closed, acute, traumatic, displaced clavicle fractures that were treated nonoperatively. These investigators reported a 4.5% incidence of nonunion with age, female gender, fracture displacement, and comminution each increasing the risk of nonunion. McKee and colleagues[139] then reported that patients who went on to union but who had shortening of 2 cm or more sustained a significant loss of both maximum and endurance strength of the affected shoulder in abduction, forward flexion, and rotation. These studies helped to pave the way for a large, multicenter, randomized, level 1 trial of operative versus nonoperative management of closed clavicle fractures in adults. This study demonstrated that patients with displaced diaphyseal clavicle fractures who were treated operatively had significantly shorter time to union, a decreased risk of nonunion and symptomatic malunion,

improved Disability of Arm Shoulder and Hand scores, and overall increased patient satisfaction compared with those who were treated nonoperatively.[140] To be included in the study, patients were required to have closed fractures that were completely displaced with no cortical contact; patients younger than 16 years of age were not included. These studies have changed acceptable operative criteria for diaphyseal clavicle fractures in adults to include open fractures, threatened skin, presence of an ipsilateral humerus fracture resulting in a floating shoulder, diaphyseal fracture comminution, and/or shortening of 2 cm or more. Relative indications reported include fracture shortening of 15 mm or more and presence of a "z-deformity" in the fracture pattern.[133,141–143]

Because treatment recommendations for management of adults with clavicular fractures have changed, many surgeons are becoming more surgically aggressive in pediatric patients despite the absence of similar high-level studies in this population. Studies of postnatal clavicular growth have shown that females achieve 80% of clavicular growth by age 9 and males achieve 80% of clavicular growth by age 12; neither gender has significant clavicular growth remaining after age 12.[144] This finding suggests that there is limited clavicular remodeling potential in adolescents who are older than 12 years at the time of injury. With this in mind, some surgeons have started to use the operative indications for adult patients in their pediatric population.[142]

Kubiak and Slongo[134] first reported their results on adolescents who underwent operative fixation of their clavicle fractures in 2002. Of 939 patients who presented between 1980 and 2000, only 15 required operative intervention, which accounts for only 1.6% of the affected population in the study period. Indications for surgery included soft tissue impingement with threatened skin, and impingement on surrounding structures, including the trachea. Although there were no major postoperative complications, 13 of the 15 had minor complications, which included numbness at the surgical site, implant prominence, skin irritation, and 1 refracture after healing. Although this study supports the idea that patients can do well postoperatively, surgery is not without risk, the minor complication rate is high, and the authors argue that they continue to treat most of their patients nonoperatively.

Vander Have and colleagues[145] reported on 42 consecutive adolescent patients with closed diaphyseal clavicular fractures, 17 of whom underwent surgical intervention. There was 100% union in the operative group with no reported major complications and only 3 patients went on to have implant removal owing to prominence. In contrast, 5 patients in the nonoperative group reported pain with prolonged overhead activity, easy fatigability, and pain at the fracture union site. Four of these patients underwent surgery for corrective osteotomy and plate fixation with resolution of symptoms. Although the high rate of union and low rate of major complication in the operative group are similar to other studies, the 20% incidence of symptomatic malunion and 16% incidence of corrective osteotomy after union is an outlier in the pediatric literature. Randsborg and colleagues[146] reported on 62 adolescent patients, 9 of whom underwent surgical correction. In contrast with the study by Vander Have and colleagues,[145] 95% of patients in Randsborg's cohort who were treated nonoperatively reported good to excellent long-term results on the Quick Disability of Arm Shoulder and Hand score and the Oxford Shoulder Score. Also unlike the study done by Vander Have and colleagues,[145] 66% of the operative group reported by Randsborg and colleagues required a second surgery for implant removal owing to prominence. Hagstrom and colleagues[147] reported a trend toward better Disability of Arm Shoulder and Hand scores and faster return to play among patients treated nonoperatively, although neither outcome achieved statistical significance. The variability in patient outcomes seen when comparing these studies is likely reflective of the small patient cohort in each study.

One of the driving factors for surgical intervention in adult patients is the increased risk of nonunion when displaced fractures are treated nonoperatively. Extending the adult operative indications to pediatric patients would mean that nonunion could be similarly high in this population when displaced fractures are treated conservatively. However, the current literature does not support this assumption. Hagstrom and colleagues[147] and Vander Have and colleagues[145] reported no nonunions in their nonoperative cohorts, and Randsborg and colleagues[146] reported only 1 nonunion out of 185 patients. Nogi and colleagues[148] submitted a case report of a single nonunion in a 12-year-old patient with a displaced clavicle fracture. The current literature, therefore, suggests that nonunion is uncommon after nonoperative treatment of clavicle fractures in pediatric patients.

Another important consideration in treatment selection is whether pediatric patients have

diminished strength or function when displaced fractures are treated nonoperatively. Although Randsborg and colleagues[146] reported a high rate of patient satisfaction and high functional scores in 95% of patients treated nonoperatively, patients with completely displaced or comminuted clavicular fractures reported significantly worse scores with regard to pain and cosmetic results. Fracture shortening had a small but significant negative effect on the Oxford Shoulder Score, as well as patient cosmetic and overall satisfaction scores. Parry and colleagues[149] sought to determine whether patients who sustained clavicle fractures that healed in a shortened position had lasting deficits in strength and function. This study compared 8 patients treated nonoperatively with 8 patients who underwent operative intervention for similar fracture patterns and found no difference in range of motion, strength or self-reported function. One patient from each group reported dissatisfaction with the cosmetic result, reminiscent of the question, "Would you rather have a bump or a scar?" Similarly, Bae and colleagues[150] identified 21 adolescents who had clavicular fractures treated nonoperatively that healed with more than 2 cm of shortening. No significant loss of strength was seen when comparing the affected side with the nonoperative extremity. Patients lost an average of 7.5° of forward flexion and 6.5° of abduction, which was significant although it is unclear if this loss is of actual clinical relevance. No difference was seen regarding strength.

Surgical treatment is not without risk of complication. Li and colleagues[151] reported an 86% postoperative implication rate in 36 adolescent patients treated surgically for clavicle fractures. The majority of the complications were related to implant prominence and/or irritation, but 16% also reported anterior chest wall numbness, 5% had problems with superficial wound dehiscence, and 1 patient sustained a fracture adjacent to the plate. Luo and colleagues[152] reported a 21.7% complication rate among operatively treated adolescents versus a less than 1% complication rate in 130 adolescents treated nonoperatively.

Although high level studies in adult patients support operative intervention for specific fracture patterns, the current literature in pediatric patients does not demonstrate the same risks of nonunion or loss of function when patients are treated nonoperatively.[138–140,149,150] The current literature suggests that pediatric patients do equally well from a healing and functional standpoint when treated nonoperatively, even in the setting of a shortened and/or displaced fracture. However, the literature is lacking in large, high-level studies. At this time, operative treatment for closed, displaced clavicle fractures in the absence of threatened skin cannot be recommended, but further research is needed in this area.

SUMMARY

The number of studies examining treatment options for pediatric fractures have exploded in recent years, perhaps complicating rather than simplifying surgical decision making and patient care. Although clinical guidelines are available in limited circumstances, these also have shortcomings. There is strong evidence to support closed reduction and pinning of type 3 supracondylar fractures, especially in the cool and pulseless extremity, but surgical timing and management recommendations are less well-defined in the setting of severe soft tissue injury, isolated neurologic injury, and the "pink, pulseless" hand. Similarly, whereas strong evidence supports evaluating young children with femoral shaft fractures for NAT, there is limited high-level evidence available for almost every other clinical scenario involving pediatric femoral shaft fractures. Level 1 and level 2 multicenter studies with firm treatment protocols are needed to better understand how grade 1 open fractures, medial epicondyle fractures, and clavicle fractures in pediatric patients should be managed.

REFERENCES

1. American Academy of Orthopaedic Surgeons (AAOS). Treatment of pediatric diaphyseal femur fractures: evidence-based clinical practice guidelines. 2015. Available at: https://www.aaos.org/research/guidelines/PDFF_Reissue.pdf. Accessed July 7, 2017.
2. Kocher MS, Sink EL, Blasier RD, et al. Treatment of pediatric diaphyseal femur fractures. J Am Acad Orthop Surg 2009;17(11):718–25.
3. American Academy of Orthopaedic Surgeons (AAOS). The treatment of pediatric supracondylar humerus fractures: evidence-based guideline and evidence report. 2011. Available at: https://www.aaos.org/uploadedFiles/PreProduction/Quality/Guidelines_and_Reviews/PSHF_CPG_10.31.16.pdf. Accessed July 7, 2017.
4. Rockwood CA, Beaty JH, Kasser JR. Rockwood and Wilkins' fractures in children. 7th edition. Philadelphia: Wolters Kluwer/Lippincott, Williams & Wilkins; 2010.
5. Oakley E, Barnett P, Babl FE. Backslab versus non-backslab for immobilization of undisplaced supracondylar fractures: a randomized trial. Pediatr Emerg Care 2009;25(7):452–6.
6. Ballal MS, Garg NK, Bass A, et al. Comparison between collar and cuffs and above elbow back slabs in the initial treatment of Gartland type I supracondylar humerus fractures. J Pediatr Orthop B 2008;17(2):57–60.
7. Almohrij SA. Closed reduction with and without percutaneous pinning on supracondylar fractures of the humerus in children. Ann Saudi Med 2000;20(1):72–4.
8. France J, Strong M. Deformity and function in supracondylar fractures of the humerus in children variously treated by closed reduction and splinting, traction, and percutaneous pinning. J Pediatr Orthop 1992;12(4):494–8.
9. Ozkoc G, Gonc U, Kayaalp A, et al. Displaced supracondylar humeral fractures in children: open reduction vs. closed reduction and pinning. Arch Orthop Trauma Surg 2004;124(8):547–51.
10. Kaewpornsawan K. Comparison between closed reduction with percutaneous pinning and open reduction with pinning in children with closed totally displaced supracondylar humeral fractures: a randomized controlled trial. J Pediatr Orthop B 2001;10(2):131–7.
11. Sutton WR, Greene WB, Georgopoulos G, et al. Displaced supracondylar humeral fractures in children. A comparison of results and costs in patients treated by skeletal traction versus percutaneous pinning. Clin Orthop Relat Res 1992;(278):81–7.
12. Khan MS, Sultan S, Ali MA, et al. Comparison of percutaneous pinning with casting in supracondylar humeral fractures in children. J Ayub Med Coll Abbottabad 2005;17(2):33–6.
13. Ababneh M, Shannak A, Agabi S, et al. The treatment of displaced supracondylar fractures of the humerus in children. A comparison of three methods. Int Orthopaedics 1998;22(4):263–5.
14. Padman M, Warwick AM, Fernandes JA, et al. Closed reduction and stabilization of supracondylar fractures of the humerus in children: the crucial factor of surgical experience. J Pediatr Orthop B 2010;19(4):298–303.
15. Pandey S, Shrestha D, Gorg M, et al. Treatment of supracondylar fracture of the humerus (type IIB and III) in children: a prospective randomized controlled trial comparing two methods. Kathmandu Univ Med J (KUMJ) 2008;6(23):310–8.
16. Pirone AM, Graham HK, Krajbich JI. Management of displaced extension-type supracondylar fractures of the humerus in children. J Bone Joint Surg Am 1988;70(5):641–50.

17. Kennedy JG, El Abed K, Soffe K, et al. Evaluation of the role of pin fixation versus collar and cuff immobilisation in supracondylar fractures of the humerus in children. Injury 2000;31(3):163–7.

18. Moraleda L, Valencia M, Barco R, et al. Natural history of unreduced Gartland type-II supracondylar fractures of the humerus in children: a two to thirteen-year follow-up study. J Bone Joint Surg Am 2013;95(1):28–34.

19. Gupta N, Kay RM, Leitch K, et al. Effect of surgical delay on perioperative complications and need for open reduction in supracondylar humerus fractures in children. J Pediatr Orthop 2004;24(3):245–8.

20. Walmsley PJ, Kelly MB, Robb JE, et al. Delay increases the need for open reduction of type-III supracondylar fractures of the humerus. J Bone Joint Surg Br 2006;88(4):528–30.

21. Ramachandran M, Skaggs DL, Crawford HA, et al. Delaying treatment of supracondylar fractures in children: has the pendulum swung too far? J Bone Joint Surg Br 2008;90(9):1228–33.

22. Mehlman CT, Strub WM, Roy DR, et al. The effect of surgical timing on the perioperative complications of treatment of supracondylar humeral fractures in children. J Bone Joint Surg Am 2001;83-A(3):323–7.

23. Iyengar SR, Hoffinger SA, Townsend DR. Early versus delayed reduction and pinning of type III displaced supracondylar fractures of the humerus in children: a comparative study. J Orthop Trauma 1999;13(1):51–5.

24. Carmichael KD, Joyner K. Quality of reduction versus timing of surgical intervention for pediatric supracondylar humerus fractures. Orthopedics 2006;29(7):628–32.

25. Sibinski M, Sharma H, Bennet GC. Early versus delayed treatment of extension type-3 supracondylar fractures of the humerus in children. J Bone Joint Surg Br 2006;88(3):380–1.

26. Garg S, Weller A, Larson AN, et al. Clinical characteristics of severe supracondylar humerus fractures in children. J Pediatr Orthop 2014;34(1):34–9.

27. Ho CA, Podeszwa DA, Riccio AI, et al. Soft tissue injury severity is associated with neurovascular injury in pediatric supracondylar humerus fractures. J Pediatr Orthop 2016. [Epub ahead of print].

28. Zionts LE, McKellop HA, Hathaway R. Torsional strength of pin configurations used to fix supracondylar fractures of the humerus in children. J Bone Joint Surg Am 1994;76(2):253–6.

29. Lee SS, Mahar AT, Miesen D, et al. Displaced pediatric supracondylar humerus fractures: biomechanical analysis of percutaneous pinning techniques. J Pediatr Orthop 2002;22(4):440–3.

30. Nacht JL, Ecker ML, Chung SM, et al. Supracondylar fractures of the humerus in children treated by closed reduction and percutaneous pinning. Clin Orthop Relat Res 1983;(177):203–9.

31. Flynn JC, Matthews JG, Benoit RL. Blind pinning of displaced supracondylar fractures of the humerus in children. Sixteen years' experience with long-term follow-up. J Bone Joint Surg Am 1974;56(2):263–72.

32. Weiland AJ, Meyer S, Tolo VT, et al. Surgical treatment of displaced supracondylar fractures of the humerus in children. Analysis of fifty-two cases followed for five to fifteen years. J Bone Joint Surg Am 1978;60(5):657–61.

33. Abdel Karim M, Hosny A, Nasef Abdelatif NM, et al. Crossed wires versus 2 lateral wires in management of supracondylar fracture of the humerus in children in the hands of junior trainees. J Orthop Trauma 2016;30(4):e123–8.

34. Larson L, Firoozbakhsh K, Passarelli R, et al. Biomechanical analysis of pinning techniques for pediatric supracondylar humerus fractures. J Pediatr Orthop 2006;26(5):573–8.

35. Skaggs DL, Cluck MW, Mostofi A, et al. Lateral-entry pin fixation in the management of supracondylar fractures in children. J Bone Joint Surg Am 2004;86-A(4):702–7.

36. Pradhan A, Hennrikus W, Pace G, et al. Increased pin diameter improves torsional stability in supracondylar humerus fractures: an experimental study. J Child Orthop 2016;10(2):163–7.

37. Gottschalk HP, Sagoo D, Glaser D, et al. Biomechanical analysis of pin placement for pediatric supracondylar humerus fractures: does starting point, pin size, and number matter? J Pediatr Orthop 2012;32(5):445–51.

38. Srikumaran U, Tan EW, Belkoff SM, et al. Enhanced biomechanical stiffness with large pins in the operative treatment of pediatric supracondylar humerus fractures. J Pediatr Orthop 2012;32(2):201–5.

39. Skaggs DL, Hale JM, Bassett J, et al. Operative treatment of supracondylar fractures of the humerus in children. The consequences of pin placement. J Bone Joint Surg Am 2001;83-A(5):735–40.

40. Silva M, Knutsen AR, Kalma JJ, et al. Biomechanical testing of pin configurations in supracondylar humeral fractures: the effect of medial column comminution. J Orthop Trauma 2013;27(5):275–80.

41. Schoenecker PL, Delgado E, Rotman M, et al. Pulseless arm in association with totally displaced supracondylar fracture. J Orthop Trauma 1996;10(6):410–5.

42. Shaw BA, Kasser JR, Emans JB, et al. Management of vascular injuries in displaced supracondylar

humerus fractures without arteriography. J Orthop Trauma 1990;4(1):25–9.

43. Shah AS, Waters PM, Bae DS. Treatment of the "pink pulseless hand" in pediatric supracondylar humerus fractures. J Hand Surg Am 2013;38(7): 1399–403 [quiz:1404].

44. Omid R, Choi PD, Skaggs DL. Supracondylar humeral fractures in children. J Bone Joint Surg Am 2008;90(5):1121–32.

45. White L, Mehlman CT, Crawford AH. Perfused, pulseless, and puzzling: a systematic review of vascular injuries in pediatric supracondylar humerus fractures and results of a POSNA questionnaire. J Pediatr Orthop 2010;30(4):328–35.

46. Griffin KJ, Walsh SR, Markar S, et al. The pink pulseless hand: a review of the literature regarding management of vascular complications of supracondylar humeral fractures in children. Eur J Vasc Endovasc Surg 2008;36(6):697–702.

47. Korompilias AV, Lykissas MG, Mitsionis GI, et al. Treatment of pink pulseless hand following supracondylar fractures of the humerus in children. Int Orthopaed 2009;33(1):237–41.

48. Noaman HH. Microsurgical reconstruction of brachial artery injuries in displaced supracondylar fracture humerus in children. Microsurgery 2006; 26(7):498–505.

49. Mangat KS, Martin AG, Bache CE. The 'pulseless pink' hand after supracondylar fracture of the humerus in children: the predictive value of nerve palsy. J Bone Joint Surg Br 2009;91(11):1521–5.

50. Scannell BP, Jackson JB 3rd, Bray C, et al. The perfused, pulseless supracondylar humeral fracture: intermediate-term follow-up of vascular status and function. J Bone Joint Surg Am 2013; 95(21):1913–9.

51. Weller A, Garg S, Larson AN, et al. Management of the pediatric pulseless supracondylar humeral fracture: is vascular exploration necessary? J Bone Joint Surg Am 2013;95(21):1906–12.

52. Sabharwal S, Tredwell SJ, Beauchamp RD, et al. Management of pulseless pink hand in pediatric supracondylar fractures of humerus. J Pediatr Orthop 1997;17(3):303–10.

53. Barrett KK, Skaggs DL, Sawyer JR, et al. Supracondylar humeral fractures with isolated anterior interosseous nerve injuries: is urgent treatment necessary? J Bone Joint Surg Am 2014;96(21): 1793–7.

54. Muchow RD, Riccio AI, Garg S, et al. Neurological and vascular injury associated with supracondylar humerus fractures and ipsilateral forearm fractures in children. J Pediatr Orthop 2015;35(2):121–5.

55. Jevsevar DS, Shea KG, Murray JN, et al. AAOS clinical practice guideline on the treatment of pediatric diaphyseal femur fractures. J Am Acad Orthop Surg 2015;23(12):e101.

56. Mittal V, Hall M, Morse R, et al. Impact of inpatient bronchiolitis clinical practice guideline implementation on testing and treatment. J Pediatr 2014; 165(3):570–6.e573.

57. Ross RK, Hersh AL, Kronman MP, et al. Impact of Infectious Diseases Society of America/Pediatric Infectious Diseases Society guidelines on treatment of community-acquired pneumonia in hospitalized children. Clin Infect Dis 2014;58(6):834–8.

58. Roussy JP, Bessette L, Bernatsky S, et al. Rates of non-vertebral osteoporotic fractures in rheumatoid arthritis and postfracture osteoporosis care in a period of evolving clinical practice guidelines. Calcif Tissue Int 2014;95(1):8–18.

59. Oetgen ME, Blatz AM, Matthews A. Impact of clinical practice guideline on the treatment of pediatric femoral fractures in a pediatric hospital. J Bone Joint Surg Am 2015;97(20):1641–6.

60. Roaten JD, Kelly DM, Yellin JL, et al. Pediatric femoral shaft fractures: a multicenter review of the AAOS clinical practice guidelines before and after 2009. J Pediatr Orthop 2017. [Epub ahead of print].

61. Miettinen H, Makela EA, Vainio J. The incidence and causative factors responsible for femoral shaft fractures in children. Ann Chir Gynaecol 1991; 80(4):392–5.

62. Rewers A, Hedegaard H, Lezotte D, et al. Childhood femur fractures, associated injuries, and sociodemographic risk factors: a population-based study. Pediatrics 2005;115(5):e543–52.

63. Hinton RY, Lincoln A, Crockett MM, et al. Fractures of the femoral shaft in children. Incidence, mechanisms, and sociodemographic risk factors. J Bone Joint Surg Am 1999;81(4):500–9.

64. Sink EL, Hyman JE, Matheny T, et al. Child abuse: the role of the orthopaedic surgeon in nonaccidental trauma. Clin Orthop Relat Res 2011; 469(3):790–7.

65. Podeszwa DA, Mooney JF 3rd, Cramer KE, et al. Comparison of Pavlik harness application and immediate spica casting for femur fractures in infants. J Pediatr Orthop 2004;24(5):460–2.

66. Stannard JP, Christensen KP, Wilkins KE. Femur fractures in infants: a new therapeutic approach. J Pediatr Orthop 1995;15(4):461–6.

67. Mansour AA 3rd, Wilmoth JC, Mansour AS, et al. Immediate spica casting of pediatric femoral fractures in the operating room versus the emergency department: comparison of reduction, complications, and hospital charges. J Pediatr Orthop 2010;30(8):813–7.

68. Heffernan MJ, Gordon JE, Sabatini CS, et al. Treatment of femur fractures in young children: a multicenter comparison of flexible intramedullary nails to spica casting in young children aged 2 to 6 years. J Pediatr Orthop 2015;35(2):126–9.

69. Flynn JM, Garner MR, Jones KJ, et al. The treatment of low-energy femoral shaft fractures: a prospective study comparing the "walking spica" with the traditional spica cast. J Bone Joint Surg Am 2011;93(23):2196–202.

70. Bopst L, Reinberg O, Lutz N. Femur fracture in preschool children: experience with flexible intramedullary nailing in 72 children. J Pediatr Orthop 2007;27(3):299–303.

71. Levy JA, Podeszwa DA, Lebus G, et al. Acute complications associated with removal of flexible intramedullary femoral rods placed for pediatric femoral shaft fractures. J Pediatr Orthop 2013; 33(1):43–7.

72. Hughes BF, Sponseller PD, Thompson JD. Pediatric femur fractures: effects of spica cast treatment on family and community. J Pediatr Orthop 1995; 15(4):457–60.

73. Leu D, Sargent MC, Ain MC, et al. Spica casting for pediatric femoral fractures: a prospective, randomized controlled study of single-leg versus double-leg spica casts. J Bone Joint Surg Am 2012;94(14):1259–64.

74. Ramo BA, Martus JE, Tareen N, et al. Intramedullary nailing compared with spica casts for isolated femoral fractures in four and five-year-old children. J Bone Joint Surg Am 2016;98(4):267–75.

75. Shemshaki HR, Mousavi H, Salehi G, et al. Titanium elastic nailing versus hip spica cast in treatment of femoral-shaft fractures in children. J Orthop Traumatol 2011;12(1):45–8.

76. Flynn JM, Luedtke LM, Ganley TJ, et al. Comparison of titanium elastic nails with traction and a spica cast to treat femoral fractures in children. J Bone Joint Surg Am 2004;86-A(4):770–7.

77. Sink EL, Gralla J, Repine M. Complications of pediatric femur fractures treated with titanium elastic nails: a comparison of fracture types. J Pediatr Orthop 2005;25(5):577–80.

78. Moroz LA, Launay F, Kocher MS, et al. Titanium elastic nailing of fractures of the femur in children. Predictors of complications and poor outcome. J Bone Joint Surg Br 2006;88(10):1361–6.

79. Lascombes P, Haumont T, Journeau P. Use and abuse of flexible intramedullary nailing in children and adolescents. J Pediatr Orthop 2006;26(6): 827–34.

80. Sink EL, Faro F, Polousky J, et al. Decreased complications of pediatric femur fractures with a change in management. J Pediatr Orthop 2010; 30(7):633–7.

81. Wall EJ, Jain V, Vora V, et al. Complications of titanium and stainless steel elastic nail fixation of pediatric femoral fractures. J Bone Joint Surg Am 2008;90(6):1305–13.

82. Shaha J, Cage JM, Black S, et al. Flexible intramedullary nails for femur fractures in pediatric patients heavier than 100 pounds. J Pediatr Orthop 2016. [Epub ahead of print].

83. Ellis HB, Ho CA, Podeszwa DA, et al. A comparison of locked versus nonlocked Enders rods for length unstable pediatric femoral shaft fractures. J Pediatr Orthop 2011;31(8):825–33.

84. Mahar A, Sink E, Faro F, et al. Differences in biomechanical stability of femur fracture fixation when using titanium nails of increasing diameter. J Child Orthop 2007;1(3):211–5.

85. Lascombes P, Huber H, Fay R, et al. Flexible intramedullary nailing in children: nail to medullary canal diameters optimal ratio. J Pediatr Orthop 2013;33(4):403–8.

86. Shaha JS, Cage JM, Black SR, et al. Redefining optimal nail to medullary canal diameter ratio in stainless steel flexible intramedullary nailing of pediatric femur fractures. J Pediatr Orthop 2017; 37(7):e398–402.

87. Garner MR, Bhat SB, Khujanazarov I, et al. Fixation of length-stable femoral shaft fractures in heavier children: flexible nails vs rigid locked nails. J Pediatr Orthop 2011;31(1):11–6.

88. Keeler KA, Dart B, Luhmann SJ, et al. Antegrade intramedullary nailing of pediatric femoral fractures using an interlocking pediatric femoral nail and a lateral trochanteric entry point. J Pediatr Orthop 2009;29(4):345–51.

89. Reynolds RA, Legakis JE, Thomas R, et al. Intramedullary nails for pediatric diaphyseal femur fractures in older, heavier children: early results. J Child Orthop 2012;6(3):181–8.

90. Sutphen SA, Mendoza JD, Mundy AC, et al. Pediatric diaphyseal femur fractures: submuscular plating compared with intramedullary nailing. Orthopedics 2016;39(6):353–8.

91. Gustilo RB. Interobserver agreement in the classification of open fractures of the tibia. The results of a survey of two hundred and forty-five orthopaedic surgeons. J Bone Joint Surg Am 1995; 77(8):1291–2.

92. Gustilo RB. Current concepts in the management of open fractures. Instr Course Lect 1987;36: 359–66.

93. Gustilo RB. Management of open fractures and complications. Instr Course Lect 1982;31:64–75.

94. Gustilo RB. Use of antimicrobials in the management of open fractures. Arch Surg 1979;114(7): 805–8.

95. Gustilo RB. Management of open fractures. An analysis of 673 cases. Minn Med 1971;54(3): 185–9.

96. Gustilo RB, Anderson JT. Prevention of infection in the treatment of one thousand and twenty-five open fractures of long bones: retrospective and prospective analyses. J Bone Joint Surg Am 1976;58(4):453–8.

97. Gustilo RB, Simpson L, Nixon R, et al. Analysis of 511 open fractures. Clin Orthop Relat Res 1969; 66:148–54.

98. Skaggs DL, Kautz SM, Kay RM, et al. Effect of delay of surgical treatment on rate of infection in open fractures in children. J Pediatr Orthop 2000;20(1):19–22.

99. Skaggs DL, Friend L, Alman B, et al. The effect of surgical delay on acute infection following 554 open fractures in children. J Bone Joint Surg Am 2005;87(1):8–12.

100. Patzakis MJ, Wilkins J. Factors influencing infection rate in open fracture wounds. Clin Orthop Relat Res 1989;(243):36–40.

101. Haasbeek JF, Cole WG. Open fractures of the arm in children. J Bone Joint Surg Br 1995;77(4): 576–81.

102. Luhmann SJ, Schootman M, Schoenecker PL, et al. Complications and outcomes of open pediatric forearm fractures. J Pediatr Orthop 2004; 24(1):1–6.

103. Yang EC, Eisler J. Treatment of isolated type I open fractures: is emergent operative debridement necessary? Clin Orthop Relat Res 2003;(410):289–94.

104. Iobst CA, Tidwell MA, King WF. Nonoperative management of pediatric type I open fractures. J Pediatr Orthop 2005;25(4):513–7.

105. Doak J, Ferrick M. Nonoperative management of pediatric grade 1 open fractures with less than a 24-hour admission. J Pediatr Orthop 2009;29(1): 49–51.

106. Bazzi AA, Brooks JT, Jain A, et al. Is nonoperative treatment of pediatric type I open fractures safe and effective? J Child Orthop 2014;8(6):467–71.

107. Godfrey J, Choi PD, Shabtai L, et al. Management of pediatric type I open fractures in the emergency department or operating room: a multicenter perspective. J Pediatr Orthop 2017. [Epub ahead of print].

108. Iobst CA, Spurdle C, Baitner AC, et al. A protocol for the management of pediatric type I open fractures. J Child Orthop 2014;8(1):71–6.

109. Rang M, Pring ME, Wenger DR. Rang's children's fractures. 3rd edition. Philadelphia: Lippincott Williams & Wilkins; 2006.

110. Josefsson PO, Danielsson LG. Epicondylar elbow fracture in children. 35-year follow-up of 56 unreduced cases. Acta Orthop Scand 1986;57(4): 313–5.

111. Gottschalk HP, Eisner E, Hosalkar HS. Medial epicondyle fractures in the pediatric population. J Am Acad Orthop Surg 2012;20(4):223–32.

112. Fowles JV, Kassab MT, Moula T. Untreated intra-articular entrapment of the medial humeral epicondyle. J Bone Joint Surg Br 1984;66(4): 562–5.

113. Fowles JV, Slimane N, Kassab MT. Elbow dislocation with avulsion of the medial humeral epicondyle. J Bone Joint Surg Br 1990;72(1):102–4.

114. Dias JJ, Johnson GV, Hoskinson J, et al. Management of severely displaced medial epicondyle fractures. J Orthop Trauma 1987;1(1):59–62.

115. Wilson NI, Ingram R, Rymaszewski L, et al. Treatment of fractures of the medial epicondyle of the humerus. Injury 1988;19(5):342–4.

116. Patel NM, Ganley TJ. Medial epicondyle fractures of the humerus: how to evaluate and when to operate. J Pediatr Orthop 2012;32(Suppl 1):S10–3.

117. Lee HH, Shen HC, Chang JH, et al. Operative treatment of displaced medial epicondyle fractures in children and adolescents. J Shoulder Elbow Surg 2005;14(2):178–85.

118. Hines RF, Herndon WA, Evans JP. Operative treatment of medial epicondyle fractures in children. Clin Orthop Relat Res 1987;(223):170–4.

119. Kamath AF, Baldwin K, Horneff J, et al. Operative versus non-operative management of pediatric medial epicondyle fractures: a systematic review. J Child Orthop 2009;3(5):345–57.

120. Kamath AF, Cody SR, Hosalkar HS. Open reduction of medial epicondyle fractures: operative tips for technical ease. J Child Orthop 2009;3(4): 331–6.

121. Cruz AI Jr, Steere JT, Lawrence JT. Medial epicondyle fractures in the pediatric overhead athlete. J Pediatr Orthop 2016;36(Suppl 1):S56–62.

122. Fuss FK. The ulnar collateral ligament of the human elbow joint. Anatomy, function and biomechanics. J Anat 1991;175:203–12.

123. Schwab GH, Bennett JB, Woods GW, et al. Biomechanics of elbow instability: the role of the medial collateral ligament. Clin Orthop Relat Res 1980;(146):42–52.

124. Munshi M, Pretterklieber ML, Chung CB, et al. Anterior bundle of ulnar collateral ligament: evaluation of anatomic relationships by using MR imaging, MR arthrography, and gross anatomic and histologic analysis. Radiology 2004;231(3): 797–803.

125. Woods GW, Tullos HS. Elbow instability and medial epicondyle fractures. Am J Sports Med 1977;5(1):23–30.

126. Farsetti P, Potenza V, Caterini R, et al. Long-term results of treatment of fractures of the medial humeral epicondyle in children. J Bone Joint Surg Am 2001;83-A(9):1299–305.

127. Stepanovich M, Bastrom TP, Munch J 3rd, et al. Does operative fixation affect outcomes of displaced medial epicondyle fractures? J Child Orthop 2016;10(5):413–9.

128. Pappas N, Lawrence JT, Donegan D, et al. Intraobserver and interobserver agreement in the measurement of displaced humeral medial

epicondyle fractures in children. J Bone Joint Surg Am 2010;92(2):322–7.

129. Edmonds EW. How displaced are "nondisplaced" fractures of the medial humeral epicondyle in children? Results of a three-dimensional computed tomography analysis. J Bone Joint Surg Am 2010;92(17):2785–91.

130. Biggers MD, Bert TM, Moisan A, et al. Fracture of the medial humeral epicondyle in children: a comparison of operative and nonoperative management. J Surg Orthop Adv 2015;24(3):188–92.

131. Lawrence JT, Patel NM, Macknin J, et al. Return to competitive sports after medial epicondyle fractures in adolescent athletes: results of operative and nonoperative treatment. Am J Sports Med 2013;41(5):1152–7.

132. Caird MS. Clavicle shaft fractures: are children little adults? J Pediatr Orthop 2012;32(Suppl 1):S1–4.

133. Namdari S, Ganley TJ, Baldwin K, et al. Fixation of displaced midshaft clavicle fractures in skeletally immature patients. J Pediatr Orthop 2011;31(5):507–11.

134. Kubiak R, Slongo T. Operative treatment of clavicle fractures in children: a review of 21 years. J Pediatr Orthop 2002;22(6):736–9.

135. Yang S, Werner BC, Gwathmey FW Jr. Treatment trends in adolescent clavicle fractures. J Pediatr Orthop 2015;35(3):229–33.

136. Carry PM, Koonce R, Pan Z, et al. A survey of physician opinion: adolescent midshaft clavicle fracture treatment preferences among POSNA members. J Pediatr Orthop 2011;31(1):44–9.

137. Suppan CA, Bae DS, Donohue KS, et al. Trends in the volume of operative treatment of midshaft clavicle fractures in children and adolescents: a retrospective, 12-year, single-institution analysis. J Pediatr Orthop B 2016;25(4):305–9.

138. Robinson CM, Court-Brown CM, McQueen MM, et al. Estimating the risk of nonunion following nonoperative treatment of a clavicular fracture. J Bone Joint Surg Am 2004;86-A(7):1359–65.

139. McKee MD, Pedersen EM, Jones C, et al. Deficits following nonoperative treatment of displaced midshaft clavicular fractures. J Bone Joint Surg Am 2006;88(1):35–40.

140. Canadian Orthopaedic Trauma Society. Nonoperative treatment compared with plate fixation of displaced midshaft clavicular fractures. A multicenter, randomized clinical trial. J Bone Joint Surg Am 2007;89(1):1–10.

141. McIntosh AL. Surgical treatment of adolescent clavicle fractures: results and complications. J Pediatr Orthop 2016;36(Suppl 1):S41–3.

142. Pandya NK, Namdari S, Hosalkar HS. Displaced clavicle fractures in adolescents: facts, controversies, and current trends. J Am Acad Orthop Surg 2012;20(8):498–505.

143. Frye BM, Rye S, McDonough EB, et al. Operative treatment of adolescent clavicle fractures with an intramedullary clavicle pin. J Pediatr Orthop 2012;32(4):334–9.

144. McGraw MA, Mehlman CT, Lindsell CJ, et al. Postnatal growth of the clavicle: birth to 18 years of age. J Pediatr Orthop 2009;29(8):937–43.

145. Vander Have KL, Perdue AM, Caird MS, et al. Operative versus nonoperative treatment of midshaft clavicle fractures in adolescents. J Pediatr Orthop 2010;30(4):307–12.

146. Randsborg PH, Fuglesang HF, Rotterud JH, et al. Long-term patient-reported outcome after fractures of the clavicle in patients aged 10 to 18 years. J Pediatr Orthop 2014;34(4):393–9.

147. Hagstrom LS, Ferrick M, Galpin R. Outcomes of operative versus nonoperative treatment of displaced pediatric clavicle fractures. Orthopedics 2015;38(2):e135–8.

148. Nogi J, Heckman JD, Hakala M, et al. Non-union of the clavicle in a child. A case report. Clin Orthop Relat Res 1975;(110):19–21.

149. Parry JA, Van Straaten M, Luo TD, et al. Is there a deficit after nonoperative versus operative treatment of shortened midshaft clavicular fractures in adolescents? J Pediatr Orthop 2017;37(4):227–33.

150. Bae DS, Shah AS, Kalish LA, et al. Shoulder motion, strength, and functional outcomes in children with established malunion of the clavicle. J Pediatr Orthop 2013;33(5):544–50.

151. Li Y, Helvie P, Farley FA, et al. Complications after plate fixation of displaced pediatric midshaft clavicle fractures. J Pediatr Orthop 2016. [Epub ahead of print].

152. Luo TD, Ashraf A, Larson AN, et al. Complications in the treatment of adolescent clavicle fractures. Orthopedics 2015;38(4):e287–91.

Hand and Wrist

Evidence-Based Review of Distal Radius Fractures

Benjamin M. Mauck, MD[a], Colin W. Swigler, MD[b],*

KEYWORDS

- Distal radius • Distal radius fracture • Wrist fracture • Wrist fracture treatment • Colle fracture
- Barton fracture • Smith fracture

KEY POINTS

- Distal radius fractures are one of the most commonly treated fractures in the United States. The highest rates are seen among the elderly, second only to hip fractures. With the increasing aging population these numbers are projected to continue to increase.
- Distal radius fractures include a spectrum of injury patterns encountered by general practitioners and orthopedists alike.
- This evidence-based review of distal radius fractures incorporates current and available literature on the diagnosis, management, and treatment of fractures of the distal radius.

INTRODUCTION

Distal radius fractures are one of the most common occurring in the United States, second only to hip fractures in elderly, with an estimated incidence of 643,000 per year.[1,2] This carries a large financial burden in the elderly alone, with an estimated Medicare system expenditure of $385 to $535 million dollars annually.[3,4] Treatment of distal radius fractures historically has been predominantly by inexpensive means including casting or limited percutaneous fixation. Following the release of the volar locking plate in the early 2000s, and early reports of success with internal fixation, popularity has steadily increased for treatment of distal radius fractures in younger populations.[5–8] Multiple studies have demonstrated good outcomes following internal plate fixation, yet prospective randomized controlled trials are limited in quantity and study design.[9–11] Among the elderly, rates of internal fixation increased from 3% in 1997 to 16% in 2005.[12] Other studies have demonstrated increases of 39% from 1999 to 2007.[13] Given the high rate of distal radius fractures in the elderly,

and the higher cost of internal fixation, this has profound economic implications. Studies of Medicare expenditures for treatment of distal radius fractures found that $170 million in Medicare funds were spent in 2007, a total of 32% of which were toward internal fixation. If physician preference continues to follow progressive trends toward internal fixation, this implies large increases in Medicare expenditure.[14]

In addition, one must also consider the hidden costs, such as loss of productivity, because these injuries average least 1 or more day off work to see a physician, radiographic/routine follow-up, and prescribed days of restricted activity regardless of treatment type. Recent American Academy of Orthopedic Surgeons (AAOS) guidelines recommend weekly radiographic surveillance for 3 weeks following reduction and at cessation of immobilization.[15] Rates of return to work following distal radius fractures have been found to be highly variable and those who have high self-reported pain/disability at baseline are at risk for prolonged loss of work days.[16] Although the highest rate (351.5 per 100,000) of distal radius fractures incurred

Disclosure Statement: None.
[a] Department of Orthopaedic Surgery, Campbell Clinic Orthopaedics, 1211 Union Avenue, Suite 510, Memphis, TN 38104, USA; [b] PGY4, Orthopaedic Surgery Residency, Campbell Clinic, University of Tennessee, 1211 Union Avenue, Suite 510, Memphis, TN 38104, USA
* Corresponding author.
E-mail address: colinswig@campbellclinic.com

annually are in the 75 to 84 year age range, there are still substantial rates (up to 189.3 per 100,000 ages 25–34, 104.5 ages 35–44, and 179.8 ages 45–54) incurred within the working population.[1]

In 2009, AAOS released guidelines for distal radius fractures. However, there still exist large geographic variations in preference for internal fixation over traditional closed treatment methods (ranging from 4.6% to 42.1% for open reduction internal fixation [ORIF]).[17] The lack of prospective level I or II studies leaves treatment decisions largely based on respective review and clinician experience. Koval and colleagues[13] found that hand-fellowship surgeons were significantly more likely to treat with internal fixation than nonfellowship-trained surgeons. Current trends toward ORIF are thought to be related to surgeon's belief that ORIF and locked volar plating are associated with lower complication rates, better function, and better satisfaction than percutaneous or external fixation; however, these have not been completely substantiated in the literature. It is generally accepted that ORIF provides more stable fixation and facilitates earlier range of motion but the clinical significance of this has not been proven. Given the commonality of the distal radius fracture, and surprising inconsistencies in treatment practices, this indicates the need for a better understanding of current treatment methods, outcomes, and the need for more prospective randomized controlled trials. This article serves to review the pertinent and available literature available regarding distal radius fractures.

BONY ANATOMY

There are three independent articulating surfaces of the distal radius: (1) the scaphoid facet, (2) lunate facet, and (3) sigmoid notch. The carpal articulations of the distal radius are concave relative to the carpus. The radioscaphoid articulation occurs on the radial aspect of the distal radius, including the radial styloid. The radiolunate articulation and the sigmoid notch compose the ulnar aspect of the distal radius. The sigmoid notch is oriented in a perpendicular fashion to the lunate facet to comprise the distal radioulnar joint (DRUJ). The sigmoid notch is semicylindrical, providing a saddle for the distal ulna, and forming the DRUJ, a trochoid joint that facilitates a combination of translation and rotation.[18] The distal ulna is thought of as the pivot point for pronation/supination of the wrist, around which the distal radius and carpus pivots. Translation occurs because of the larger radius of curvature of the

sigmoid notch (shallow) and the ulnar head. This results in dorsal and volar translation during pronation and supination, respectively.[18] There are differing degrees of bone density in the distal radius, and as discussed later, are implicated in fracture propagation between the scaphoid and lunate facets.[19–21]

LIGAMENTOUS ANATOMY

Stout ligamentous complexes provide essential stabilization to the articulations of the wrist. Extrinsic ligaments bridge carpal bones to the distal radius or metacarpals. Intrinsic ligaments originate and insert on carpal bones. The radioscapholunate, radiolunotriquetral, radioscaphocapitate, and dorsal radiotriquetral ligaments attach at the articular margin of the distal radius and the respective carpals. The combination of the intrinsic and extrinsic ligaments function to form stable articulations and guide force vectors to the radiocarpal joint. The triangular fibrocartilage complex (TFCC) and it's palmar and dorsal radioulnar ligaments are the prime stabilizers of the DRUJ.[22,23] The robust ligaments of the lunate facet in combination with the TFCC play a large role in stabilization of the ulnar wrist. This exceptionally strong ligamentous complex is why the carpus is virtually always displaced with the volar/dorsal medial fragment of the fractured distal radius.[24]

THREE-COLUMN MODEL

As described by Rikli and Regazzoni,[25] the distal radius and ulna, radiocarpal articulation, and DRUJ can conceptually be divided anatomically into a model with three distinct columns: (1) radial column, (2) intermediate column, and (3) ulnar column.[26] The radial column and intermediate column are supported by the "shaft" or "pedestal" formed by the metadiaphyseal distal radius. The radial column is formed by the radial styloid, scaphoid facet, and attachments of radiolunate ligament, radioscaphocapitate ligament, and brachioradialis. The radial column serves as a buttress for the carpus in radioulnar deviation, the ligamentous attachments of the radioscaphocapitate and radial collateral ligaments prevent translation of the carpus, and has little weight bearing function.[27] The deforming pull of the brachioradialis, with its insertion on the radial column, can cause loss of radial height, inclination, and radial translation. The intermediate column is the primary load-bearing component of the three-column model, which must be assessed for articular congruity and alignment of the mechanical axis of the wrist.[25,27] It is formed by the lunate facet and sigmoid notch. Ligamentous attachments to the lunate (volar) and triquetrum (dorsal) provide important translational restriction of the carpus. Ligamentous attachments between the distal radius and distal ulnar (dorsal/volar radioulnar ligaments) are important in stabilization of the DRUJ and in forearm rotation. The ulnar column serves as the rotational axis for pronosupination of the wrist.[25] It is composed of the distal ulna and TFCC critical for DRUJ stability and forearm rotation. Biomechanical studies have demonstrated that loss of radial height (as little as 5 mm) can cause significant distortion of the TFCC, and to a lesser degree by loss of inclination, or loss of volar tilt.[28]

RADIOGRAPHIC EVALUATION

There are five radiographic measurements to evaluate the distal radius: (1) radial height, (2) radial inclination, (3) ulnar variance, (4) volar tilt, and (5) radial shift.[29] One should also assess for articular step-off, sigmoid notch step-off, DRUJ congruity, and for presence of ulnar styloid fractures.[24] Radial height and ulnar variance are two described methods for assessing the relationship of the articular surfaces of the radius and ulna at the DRUJ. Radial height is the distance between a perpendicular line drawn at the tip of the radial styloid and a second line at the articular surface of the distal ulna, normally approximately 11°.[30] Ulnar variance is typically measured as the distance between a line drawn perpendicular to the long axis of the radius at the sigmoid notch and measuring the amount of ulnar head distal to this line. Comparison imaging of the contralateral (uninjured) wrist should be obtained to account for anatomic variations in DRUJ relationships among individuals. Radial inclination is measured by the angle formed by a line perpendicular to the long axis of the radius and a line connecting the most distal aspect of the ulnar styloid and lunate facet. It is normally approximately 11°.[30] Volar tilt is assessed on lateral imaging of the wrist and is measured by the angle formed by a line connecting the dorsal and volar lip of the articular surface to the long axis of the radius. Volar tilt is normally approximately 11°.[30]

ROLE OF COMPUTED TOMOGRAPHY SCAN

Computed tomography (CT) has evolved as a useful tool for evaluating articular involvement. Cole and colleagues[31] reported improved assessment articular congruity when compared with plain film radiograph. Identification of articular involvement is imperative in the evaluation of distal radius fractures from an operative planning standpoint and prognostic indicator. A study emphasizing the importance of articular evaluation demonstrated any degree of articular incongruity can lead to post-traumatic arthrosis in 91% of patients and 100% if more than 2 mm.[32] Cross-sectional imaging is helpful when the fracture pattern is not clear on plain radiographs and particularly with die-punch patterns.[33] CT scans have also been shown to improve detection of DRUJ involvement and occult scaphoid fractures.[33,34] A study by Harness and colleagues[35] found that three-dimensional imaging, in combination with two-dimensional imaging, significantly changed treatment plans, including operative approach. CT scans, with added radiation and costs, should not be ordered for all distal radius fractures and the utility of the CT scan as an adjunct is best left to the treating surgeon's discretion.[36]

CLASSIFICATION SYSTEMS

Multiple classification systems have been developed to describe distal radius fracture patterns to better guide treatment, although significant amounts of interobserver and intraobserver variability exist among the early classification system.[37] Colles[38] first described the most common fracture pattern of the distal radius in 1814, the dorsally angulated and displaced extra-articular fracture of the distal radius, after which the fracture was named and classic eponym coined. This first description, before development of the roentgen, was based on clinical features only. Multiple eponyms would follow to include Smith fracture (or reverse Colles), Barton fracture, reverse Barton, die-punch, and Chauffer's fracture (Table 1). Following the roentgen, classification systems continued to develop in the 1930s; Nissen-lie, followed by Gartland and Werley in 1951 and Lidstrom in 1959 better describe fracture patterns and radiocarpal articular involvement.[39,40] Frykman[41] expanded this to include the radioulnar articulation and ulnar styloid. The work of Melone in 1984 described the extent of injury to the articular surface by displacement, degree of comminution, and fracture propagation; and as some suggest, an early reference to a column-type model later described by Rikli.[19,25] Fernandez and Geissler[42] subsequently expanded on mechanism of injury correlated with anatomic fracture patterns.

Table 1
Eponym and fracture description
Colle fracture	Dorsally angulated, dorsally displaced fracture of the distal radius
Smith fracture (reverse Colle)	Volar angulation of distal fragment
Barton fracture (volar or dorsal)	Fracture/dislocation of articular rim (volar or dorsal) with associated displacement of the carpus
Die-punch fracture	Fracture of the articular surface with depression of the lunate facet
Chauffer's fracture	Avulsion fracture of the radial styloid

The most comprehensive description, the AO classification system, was developed by Muller and colleagues[43] in 1986 and included 27 descriptions. This was later modified and included three categories based on articular involvement (extra-articular, partially articular, and complete articular) with three subtypes further describing fracture patterns, propagation, and comminution. Although the simplified version improved interobserver and intraobserver agreement, some argued the modification limited clinical usefulness.[37] Multiple studies have looked at reliability of the most common classification systems with variable results.[37,44,45] The best classification system to guide clinical treatment remains controversial and varies among practitioners.

ASSOCIATED INJURIES

Multiple injuries can occur in combination with distal radius fractures. Tears of the TFCC is the most frequently associated injury and has been found in 39% to 84% of unstable distal radius fractures.[46,47] TFCC tears should be considered when associated with resultant DRUJ instability.[48] Radiographs should be assessed for widening of the DRUJ gap distance (radial translation ratio) and the presence of ulnar styloid base fractures (along with displacement) because they have been associated with increased rates of DRUJ instability and should prompt further investigation.[49,50] In a study of 68 patients with intra-articular fractures of the distal radius, Geissler and coworkers[51] found that 68% had associated soft tissue injuries of the wrist including the TFCC (26), scapholunate interosseous ligament [SLIL] (19), and Lunotriquetral interosseous ligament [LTIL] (9). Failure to recognize

such soft tissue injuries can result in decreased functional outcomes, decreased grip strength, and recalcitrant pain following distal radius fractures. Injury of the extensor pollicis longus tendon is a well-known complication associated with distal radius fractures with multiple reports in the literature.[52–55] Exact incidence is unknown but has been reported up to 5.0% in some studies occurring more commonly with fractures with minimal to no displacement.[52,54–56]

Distal radius fractures have been suggested as the most frequent cause of traumatic acute carpal tunnel syndrome (ACTS).[57] Similarly, acute compartment syndrome of the forearm has been a complication of distal radius fractures.[58,59] All patients presenting with distal radius fractures should undergo a clearly documented, thorough neurovascular examination. In those requiring reduction, greater displacement/deformity and presence of a displaced volar fragment have been found to be at risk for developing ACTS.[60,61] In addition, practitioners should be cognizant of the position of the hand and wrist after immobilization because hyperflexion or extension can decrease the volume available in the carpal tunnel and predispose to ACTS.[62] In patients presenting with sensory disturbance, they should be carefully monitored for progression of symptoms, which can help distinguish contusion neuropraxia from ACTS.[63] Patients with ACTS complain of progressive pain and sensory disturbances in the median nerve distribution and should prompt immediate surgical intervention. Transient and delayed carpal tunnel syndromes have been described and warrant observation and appropriate investigation but do not require immediate surgical intervention. There remain no indications for prophylactic release in the asymptomatic patient.[64,65]

Complex regional pain syndrome (CRPS) is a difficult condition to treat, and has been associated with distal radius fractures. Many early studies identified pathology following distal radius fractures and historically it has been described as causalgia, algodysytrophy, Sudeck atrophy, reflex sympathetic dystrophy syndrome, and shoulder-hand syndrome.[41,66–69] The exact incidence of prevalence of CRPS following distal radius fractures remains unclear and has been demonstrated in 22% to 39% of fractures.[70] There has been recent interest in the role of vitamin C supplementation following distal radius fractures to prevent development of CRPS. Although limited because of lack of objective diagnostic criteria for CRPS, two studies have demonstrated significant reduction in incidence of CRPS after distal radius fractures with vitamin C supplementation.[71,72] AAOS 2009 Clinical Practice Guidelines recommended (moderate level of recommendation) adjuvant treatment with vitamin C following distal radius fractures. Unfortunately, a recent meta-analysis of randomized controlled trials failed to demonstrate a significant clinical difference.[73]

McKay and colleagues[74] reviewed the incidence of complications of distal radius fractures, physician- and patient-reported, with a comprehensive list from minor to severe (Tables 2 and 3).

Elderly

Distal radius fractures are the second most common fracture experienced by individuals 65 and older second only to hip fractures.[12,14,17] Higher rates, up to six-fold, have been identified among women compared with men between the age of 64 and 94 years.[75] The relationship between distal radius fractures and low-energy trauma has been related to decreased bone mineral density, and this decrease in bone density typically occurs earlier in men than in women because of menopause.[76] There is consensus that stable fractures are treated successfully by

Table 2 Physician-reported complications	
Complication	**%**
Median nerve compression/carpal tunnel syndrome	22
Radial nerve compression/neuropathy	11
Ulnar nerve compression	6
Complex regional pain syndrome (reflex sympathetic dystrophy)	20
Post-traumatic arthritis	1
Carpal instability/subluxation	1
Delayed union	1
Distal radioulnar joint pathology	5
Tendon adhesions/scarring	7
Rupture extensor pollicis longus	2
Tendon rupture, other	2
Tendinitis, tenosynovitis	14
Trigger finger	2
Dupuytren contracture	2
Compartment syndrome	1

Adapted from McKay SD, MacDermid JC, Roth JH, et al. Assessment of complications of distal radius fractures and development of a complication checklist. J Hand Surg Am 2001;26(5):919; with permission.

Table 3 Patient-reported complications	
Complication	**%**
Median nerve compression/carpal tunnel syndrome	2
Radial nerve compression/neuropathy	4
Ulnar nerve compression	0
Complex regional pain syndrome	21
Post-traumatic arthritis	4
Carpal instability/subluxation	0
Delayed union	0
Distal radioulnar joint pathology	0
Tendon adhesions/scarring	2
Rupture extensor pollicis longus	4
Tendon rupture, other	4
Tendinitis, tenosynovitis	6
Trigger finger	4
Dupuytren contracture	2
Compartment syndrome	1

Adapted from McKay SD, MacDermid JC, Roth JH, et al. Assessment of complications of distal radius fractures and development of a complication checklist. J Hand Surg Am 2001;26(5):919; with permission.

closed means. With regards to unstable fractures, however, studies have correlated decreased bone mineral density with difficulty in maintaining closed reduction and increased risk for further displacement despite adequate immobilization.[77–79]

Further complicating conservative treatment efforts, studies have demonstrated high rates of failure of "remanipulation" after loss of reduction.[80] Such findings have led to subsequent studies identifying risk factors for redisplacement. A study by Lafontaine and colleagues[81] identified five factors as predictors of instability: (1) initial dorsal angulation greater than 20°, (2) dorsal metaphyseal comminution, (3) intra-articular involvement, (4) associated ulna fracture, and (5) age greater than 60 years.

Further investigations have failed to correlate these parameters and suggest that age alone is the only significant risk factor for failure of closed treatment.[77] Despite these findings, many elderly patients still do well with conservative treatment. Multiple studies have demonstrated that outcomes and self-reported disability are not correlated with radiographic appearance or malunion.[82–84] Malunion rates of 50% have been reported in elderly patients with unstable distal radius fractures treated by closed means.[85] Clinical deformity may persist in such cases but in most elderly patients, especially low-demand individuals, this is generally well tolerated.[86] However, with increasing life-expectancy of the aging population, trends have been moving toward anatomic reduction with internal fixation, but this remains controversial.[12,14,17]

Recent literature has explored distal radius as a harbinger of future fragility fractures with conflicting results and variable sensitivity.[87–91] Distal radius fractures are still, however, an osteoporosis-related fracture, and although this may not predict future fragility fractures, patients remain at risk for other fractures of vertebrae and proximal femur. This should prompt clinicians to address the issue, and if necessary, refer to primary care physician or endocrinologists for appropriate work-up and/or treatment.

TREATMENT

The goal of successful treatment, by conservative or operative means, is to restore alignment. Restoration of anatomic alignment in displaced fractures is ideal, but radiographic criteria have been established and subsequently refined for acceptable alignment including less than 2 mm of radial shortening, radial inclination no less than 10 degrees, 10* dorsal to 20* volar tilt, and intra articular step-off less than 2 mm.[24,29] Studies have demonstrated alteration in mechanical loads across the radiocarpal joint, and resultant accelerated degenerative change, with dorsal tilt 20 to 30*.[92] Increased dorsal angulation, along with radial shortening, can lead DRUJ incongruity and resultant loss of pronosupination.[22,28,93] Any articular step-off greater than 2 mm can increase probability of post-traumatic arthrosis, by almost 100%.[32]

Closed Reduction and Casting

Treatment of distal radius fractures by closed reduction and immobilization in a splint or cast has historically been, and remains, the mainstay of treatment of nondisplaced and most stable distal radius fractures. Closed reduction is performed under procedural sedation/monitored anesthesia care, hematoma block, regional nerve block, intravenous regional (Bier block), or general anesthesia. Complications are associated with each method of sedation/analgesia, and studies comparing efficacy and safety have, because of lack of available literature, recommended one method over another.[94] At our institution, after undergoing closed reduction, patients are placed into a molded sugar tong

splint to prevent pronosupination at the elbow. Stable fractures are immobilized in short arm splint, leaving the elbow free. Studies have demonstrated no difference in splinting method for stable distal radius fractures.[95] Recent AAOS clinical treatment guidelines recommend weekly radiographs for the first 3 weeks following immobilization and then again at cessation of immobilization.

Percutaneous fixation

The use of Kirschner wires as a minimally invasive form of fracture stabilization has been described for use in extra-articular fractures by multiple authors.[96–98] Glickel and colleagues[99] demonstrated good long-term outcomes in treatment of two- and three-part fractures. A randomized controlled trial by Kreder and colleagues[100] demonstrated more rapid return of function and better functional outcomes with indirect versus open reduction at 2-year follow-up, although this study did not attempt to compare methods of fixation. Successful use requires good bone quality and limited comminution. However, they only provide limited internal fixation, requiring further immobilization, and fracture "settling" has been described during the healing process.[101] Pins are commonly placed distal to proximal from the radial styloid to the ulnar aspect of the proximal radial diaphysis. Kapandji (intrafocal) technique has been described, inserting Kirschner wires into the fracture site and levering into a better reduced position.[102] A Cochrane database meta-analysis review cautioned their use with only low-level evidence supporting the use of Kirschner wire fixation despite high rates of associated complications.[103] Complications include tendon tethering, tendon injury/rupture, pin migration, vascular injury, verve injury, and pin site infection.

External fixation

External fixation is indicated in the treatment of distal radius fractures, but popularity has declined with improvements in plating techniques. External fixation relies on ligamentotaxis to maintain reduction of the fracture fragments, primarily through the radioscaphocapitate and radiolunate ligaments.[104] Its use has been advocated to temporize patients with polytrauma before transfer to a tertiary referral center, and for initial management for open fractures with severe soft tissue loss.[105] It has also been indicated as supplemental fixation for suboptimal internal fixation.[106] It does require placement of distal pins in either the index or middle finger metacarpal, and associated fractures may preclude its use. Multiple studies have demonstrated a wide range of complications including pin track infection (up to 30%), pin loosening, and higher rates of CRPS caused by overdistraction of the carpus.[104,107] A prospective randomized study by Egol and colleagues[108] compared bridging external fixation and supplemental Kirschner wire fixation versus volar locked plating for unstable distal radius fractures and found similar function at 1 year and similar rates of complications. Another study comparing dorsal Pi plating and external fixation of intraarticular distal radius fractures found significantly higher complications in the dorsal plate group, such that enrollment in that treatment arm was terminated.[109]

Open Reduction Internal Fixation (Dorsal/Volar/Fragment Specific)
Dorsal
Internal fixation of distal radius fractures has traditionally been used in cases of significant dorsal comminution and/or dorsal displacement. Because of high rates of tendon irritation and reported extensor pollicis longus attritional rupture, in original and modified low-profile designs, the plating method become less desirable.[110,111] As a result, virtually all dorsal bridge plates warrant routine removal to avoid tendon complications. At our institution the indications of dorsal plating are limited to fractures with significant dorsal comminution that would limit fracture stabilization with volar plating.

Volar
Following the release of the volar locking plate in the early 2000s, much attention has been focused on the role of internal fixation in treating distal radius fractures. Multiple studies have demonstrated these trends despite high-level evidence supporting the use and justifying the increased costs. Advocates of internal fixation believe the volar plates are superior to dorsal plates for multiple reasons. The surgical approach is thought to be more biologically friendly to extrinsic tendons and is thought to better preserve metaphyseal blood supply.[10,112] Drawbacks of volar fixation include flexor pollicis longus attritional rupture (prominence of plates placed distal to the watershed line), intraarticular screw penetration, and extensor tendon irritation caused by prominent screws in the dorsal cortex.[113–115]

High-level studies reviewing the role of volar plating in treatment of distal radius fractures are limited. Multiple retrospective and comparative studies have demonstrated success in the treatment of unstable distal radius fractures with volar plate fixation.[9–11,112,116,117] Rozental and colleagues[7] compared functional outcomes for unstable distal radius fractures treated with ORIF versus percutaneous treatment and found satisfactory results in both forms of treatment but better functional results for the ORIF group in the early perioperative period suggesting its role in patients desiring a faster return to function. Similar results were shown by Karantana and colleagues[6] in a randomized controlled trial of 130 patients treated with ORIF versus CRPP. Conversely a meta-analysis by Margaliot, and colleagues[107] failed to demonstrate any data to support the use of plate fixation over external fixation. Recent AAOS guidelines failed to find evidence to form conclusive recommendations for or against any treatment type. Although popularity of volar locking plate fixation continues to grow, there are limited high-powered, quality studies comparing their use with other treatment modalities.

Fragment-specific fixation
Fragment-specific fixation involves a variable combination of low-profile small plates and clips that provide customizable construct combinations depending on needs of the individual fracture pattern and fragments involved. Such combinations obviate external fixation in highly comminuted fractures making standard plating techniques difficult or where limited internal fixation would require augmentation. These techniques are technically demanding, relying on surgeon experience, and they are generally more time consuming. In addition, they often require more than one incision or approach. A biomechanical study by Dodds and colleagues[118] found fragment fixation provided superior construct fixation when compared with external fixation of four-part distal radius fractures. Initial clinical results were promising with respect to fixation in a study by Konrath and Bahler[119]; however 8 of 25 patients experienced sensory nerve disturbances (seven were transient). These findings were corroborated in a retrospective study of fragment-specific fixation in 81 patients by Benson and colleagues[120] who also reported good functional outcomes, and 10 patients with radial sensory nerve disturbances. Both studies by Konrath and Benson identified the need for symptomatic plate removal in 12% and 3%, respectively (the latter limited because of 25% drop out). In a prospective comparison of fragment-specific fixation

and volar plate fixation, a study Sammer and colleagues[121] suggested improved subjective and objective outcomes in addition to fewer complications with the use of a volar plate.

OUTCOMES/SUMMARY

The optimal method of fixation for unstable distal radius fractures remains a topic of debate, and is often a result of a surgeon's clinical experience. As this review of the literature demonstrates, there remain few high-quality, randomized controlled clinical trials comparing different forms of fixation. This remains a difficult task, because such a study would require standardizing fracture pattern and available classification systems have variable interobserver agreement even with the addition of CT scanning.[37,44,45] In younger patients the parameters for acceptable reduction remain clear, with a low threshold for operative fixation with any deviation from these, but the optimal method of fixation is inconclusive. The growing elderly population has been clearly shown to tolerate moderate degrees of malunion without significant decrease in self-reported function; however, trends are increasing toward operative fixation of these fractures.[12,14,17,82–84]

With an ever-changing medical economy, and increased scrutiny on the judicious use of resources, physicians are faced with a climate where treatment decisions should be based on gold standard medical literature. In the case of comparing current methods of operative treatment of distal radius fractures, this simply does not exist on a large scale. In addition, the unique patient factor must be accounted for. Paternalistic medicine is a thing of the past, and patient education is paramount to prevent outcomes from falling short of patient-perceived expectations. Patients nowadays have often researched their injury and are exposed to several questionable, if at all, valid resources prompting expectations before even entering the examination room. Such premanagement (operative and nonoperative) expectations may differ from the natural course of any orthopedic injury, and inevitably these expectations will soon translate into tangible patient-based satisfaction metrics. Current literature guiding physicians, and thus patients, to choose the optimal treatment method is inconclusive. More randomized controlled trials directly comparing different operative and nonoperative treatment methods is clearly needed to validate these decisions. These should include relevant standardized clinical outcome metrics because patient satisfaction cannot be measured based on radiographic outcomes. At present, the choice of treatment of the vast spectrum of distal radius fractures must be based on a two-way conversation between the patient, with transparency to limitations of available data, ultimately relying on surgeon experience and patient preference.

REFERENCES

1. Chung KC, Spilson SV. The frequency and epidemiology of hand and forearm fractures in the United States. J Hand Surg Am 2001;26(5):908–15.
2. Larsen CF, Lauritsen J. Epidemiology of acute wrist trauma. Int J Epidemiol 1993;22(5):911–6.
3. Ray NF, Chan JK, Thamer M, et al. Medical expenditures for the treatment of osteoporotic fractures in the United States in 1995: report from the National Osteoporosis Foundation. J Bone Miner Res 1997;12(1):24–35.
4. Burge R, Dawson-Hughes B, Solomon DH, et al. Incidence and economic burden of osteoporosis-related fractures in the United States, 2005-2025. J Bone Miner Res 2007;22(3):465–75.
5. Abramo A, Kopylov P, Geijer M, et al. Open reduction and internal fixation compared to closed reduction and external fixation in distal radial fractures: a randomized study of 50 patients. Acta Orthop 2009;80(4):478–85.
6. Karantana A, Downing ND, Forward DP, et al. Surgical treatment of distal radial fractures with a volar locking plate versus conventional percutaneous methods: a randomized controlled trial. J Bone Joint Surg Am 2013;95(19):1737–44.
7. Rozental TD, Blazar PE, Franko OI, et al. Functional outcomes for unstable distal radial fractures treated with open reduction and internal fixation or closed reduction and percutaneous fixation. A prospective randomized trial. J Bone Joint Surg Am 2009;91(8):1837–46.
8. Koenig KM, Davis GC, Grove MR, et al. Is early internal fixation preferred to cast treatment for well-reduced unstable distal radial fractures? J Bone Joint Surg Am 2009;91(9):2086–93.
9. Fok MW, Klausmeyer MA, Fernandez DL, et al. Volar plate fixation of intra-articular distal radius fractures: a retrospective study. J Wrist Surg 2013;2(3):247–54.
10. Orbay JL. The treatment of unstable distal radius fractures with volar fixation. Hand Surg 2000;5(2):103–12.
11. Orbay JL, Fernandez DL. Volar fixed-angle plate fixation for unstable distal radius fractures in the elderly patient. J Hand Surg Am 2004;29(1):96–102.
12. Chung KC, Shauver MJ, Birkmeyer JD. Trends in the United States in the treatment of distal radial

fractures in the elderly. J Bone Joint Surg Am 2009;91(8):1868–73.

13. Koval KJ, Harrast JJ, Anglen JO, et al. Fractures of the distal part of the radius. The evolution of practice over time. Where's the evidence? J Bone Joint Surg Am 2008;90(9):1855–61.

14. Shauver MJ, Yin H, Banerjee M, et al. Current and future national costs to Medicare for the treatment of distal radius fracture in the elderly. J Hand Surg Am 2011;36(8):1282–7.

15. Lichtman DM. AAOS clinical practice guideline summary: treatment of distal radius fractures. J Am Acad Orthop Surg 2009;18:180–9.

16. MacDermid JC, Roth JH, McMurtry R. Predictors of time lost from work following a distal radius fracture. J Occup Rehabil 2007;17(1):47–62.

17. Chung KC, Shauver MJ, Yin H, et al. Variations in the use of internal fixation for distal radial fracture in the United States Medicare population. J Bone Joint Surg Am 2011;93(23):2154–62.

18. af Ekenstam F, Hagert CG. Anatomical studies on the geometry and stability of the distal radio ulnar joint. Scand J Plast Reconstr Surg 1985;19(1):17–25.

19. Melone CP Jr. Articular fractures of the distal radius. Orthop Clin North Am 1984;15(2):217–36.

20. Melone CP Jr. Open treatment for displaced articular fractures of the distal radius. Clin Orthop Relat Res 1986;(202):103–11.

21. Melone CP Jr. Distal radius fractures: patterns of articular fragmentation. Orthop Clin North Am 1993;24(2):239–53.

22. Adams BD, Lawler E. Chronic instability of the distal radioulnar joint. J Am Acad Orthop Surg 2007;15(9):571–5.

23. Palmer AK, Werner FW. The triangular fibrocartilage complex of the wrist–anatomy and function. J Hand Surg Am 1981;6(2):153–62.

24. Nana AD, Joshi A, Lichtman DM. Plating of the distal radius. J Am Acad Orthop Surg 2005;13(3):159–71.

25. Rikli DA, Regazzoni P. Fractures of the distal end of the radius treated by internal fixation and early function. A preliminary report of 20 cases. J Bone Joint Surg Br 1996;78(4):588–92.

26. Kennedy SA, Hanel DP. Complex distal radius fractures. Orthop Clin North Am 2013;44(1):81–92.

27. Rikli DA, Honigmann P, Babst R, et al. Intra-articular pressure measurement in the radioulnocarpal joint using a novel sensor: in vitro and in vivo results. J Hand Surg Am 2007;32(1):67–75.

28. Adams BD. Effects of radial deformity on distal radioulnar joint mechanics. J Hand Surg Am 1993;18(3):492–8.

29. Graham TJ. Surgical correction of malunited fractures of the distal radius. J Am Acad Orthop Surg 1997;5(5):270–81.

30. Friberg S, Lundstrom B. Radiographic measurements of the radio-carpal joint in normal adults. Acta Radiol Diagn (Stockh) 1976;17(2):249–56.

31. Cole RJ, Bindra RR, Evanoff BA, et al. Radiographic evaluation of osseous displacement following intra-articular fractures of the distal radius: reliability of plain radiography versus computed tomography. J Hand Surg Am 1997;22(5):792–800.

32. Knirk JL, Jupiter JB. Intra-articular fractures of the distal end of the radius in young adults. J Bone Joint Surg Am 1986;68(5):647–59.

33. Arora S, Grover SB, Batra S, et al. Comparative evaluation of postreduction intra-articular distal radial fractures by radiographs and multidetector computed tomography. J Bone Joint Surg Am 2010;92(15):2523–32.

34. Katz MA, Beredjiklian PK, Bozentka DJ, et al. Computed tomography scanning of intra-articular distal radius fractures: does it influence treatment? J Hand Surg Am 2001;26(3):415–21.

35. Harness NG, Ring D, Zurakowski D, et al. The influence of three-dimensional computed tomography reconstructions on the characterization and treatment of distal radial fractures. J Bone Joint Surg Am 2006;88(6):1315–23.

36. Kleinlugtenbelt YV, Madden K, Groen SR, et al. Can experienced surgeons predict the additional value of a CT scan in patients with displaced intra-articular distal radius fractures? Strategies Trauma Limb Reconstr 2017;12(2):91–7.

37. Andersen DJ, Blair WF, Steyers CM Jr, et al. Classification of distal radius fractures: an analysis of interobserver reliability and intraobserver reproducibility. J Hand Surg Am 1996;21(4):574–82.

38. Colles A. Historical paper on the fracture of the carpal extremity of the radius (1814). Injury 1970;2(1):48–50.

39. Gartland JJ Jr, Werley CW. Evaluation of healed Colles' fractures. J Bone Joint Surg Am 1951;33-A(4):895–907.

40. Lidstrom A. Fractures of the distal end of the radius. A clinical and statistical study of end results. Acta Orthop Scand Suppl 1959;41:1–118.

41. Frykman G. Fracture of the distal radius including sequelae–shoulder-hand-finger syndrome, disturbance in the distal radio-ulnar joint and impairment of nerve function. A clinical and experimental study. Acta Orthop Scand 1967;108:1–155.

42. Fernandez DL, Geissler WB. Treatment of displaced articular fractures of the radius. J Hand Surg Am 1991;16(3):375–84.

43. Müller ME, Nazarian S, Koch P. Classification AO des fractures. Tome I. Les os longs. 1st edition. Berlin: Springer-Verlag. p. 106–115.

44. Kreder HJ, Hanel DP, McKee M, et al. Consistency of AO fracture classification for the distal radius. J Bone Joint Surg Br 1996;78(5):726–31.

45. Kural C, Sungur I, Kaya I, et al. Evaluation of the reliability of classification systems used for distal radius fractures. Orthopedics 2010;33(11):801.

46. Lindau T, Adlercreutz C, Aspenberg P. Peripheral tears of the triangular fibrocartilage complex cause distal radioulnar joint instability after distal radial fractures. J Hand Surg Am 2000;25(3):464–8.

47. Richards RS, Bennett JD, Roth JH, et al. Arthroscopic diagnosis of intra-articular soft tissue injuries associated with distal radial fractures. J Hand Surg Am 1997;22(5):772–6.

48. Ruch DS, Yang CC, Smith BP. Results of acute arthroscopically repaired triangular fibrocartilage complex injuries associated with intra-articular distal radius fractures. Arthroscopy 2003;19(5):511–6.

49. Fujitani R, Omokawa S, Akahane M, et al. Predictors of distal radioulnar joint instability in distal radius fractures. J Hand Surg Am 2011;36(12):1919–25.

50. Omokawa S, Iida A, Fujitani R, et al. Radiographic predictors of DRUJ instability with distal radius fractures. J Wrist Surg 2014;3(1):2–6.

51. Geissler WB, Freeland AE, Savoie FH, et al. Intracarpal soft-tissue lesions associated with an intra-articular fracture of the distal end of the radius. J Bone Joint Surg Am 1996;78(3):357–65.

52. Smith FM. Late rupture of extensor policis longus tendon following Colles's fracture. J Bone Joint Surg Am 1946;28:49–59.

53. Christophe K. Rupture of the extensor pollicis longus tendon following Colles fracture. J Bone Joint Surg Am 1953;35-A(4):1003–5.

54. Engkvist O, Lundborg G. Rupture of the extensor pollicis longus tendon after fracture of the lower end of the radius: a clinical and microangiographic study. Hand 1979;11(1):76–86.

55. Bonatz E, Kramer TD, Masear VR. Rupture of the extensor pollicis longus tendon. Am J Orthop (Belle Mead NJ) 1996;25(2):118–22.

56. Roth KM, Blazar PE, Earp BE, et al. Incidence of extensor pollicis longus tendon rupture after nondisplaced distal radius fractures. J Hand Surg Am 2012;37(5):942–7.

57. Bauman TD, Gelberman RH, Mubarak SJ, et al. The acute carpal tunnel syndrome. Clin Orthop Relat Res 1981;(156):151–6.

58. Duckworth AD, Mitchell SE, Molyneux SG, et al. Acute compartment syndrome of the forearm. J Bone Joint Surg Am 2012;94(10):e63.

59. McQueen MM, Gaston P, Court-Brown CM. Acute compartment syndrome. Who is at risk? J Bone Joint Surg Br 2000;82(2):200–3.

60. Dyer G, Lozano-Calderon S, Gannon C, et al. Predictors of acute carpal tunnel syndrome associated with fracture of the distal radius. J Hand Surg Am 2008;33(8):1309–13.

61. Paley D, McMurtry RY. Median nerve compression by volarly displaced fragments of the distal radius. Clin Orthop Relat Res 1987;(215):139–47.

62. Mackinnon SE. Pathophysiology of nerve compression. Hand Clin 2002;18(2):231–41.

63. McDonald AP 3rd, Lourie GM. Complex surgical conditions of the hand: avoiding the pitfalls. Clin Orthop Relat Res 2005;(433):65–71.

64. Pope D, Tang P. Carpal tunnel syndrome and distal radius fractures. Hand Clin 2018;34(1):27–32.

65. Niver GE, Ilyas AM. Carpal tunnel syndrome after distal radius fracture. Orthop Clin North Am 2012;43(4):521–7.

66. Atkins RM, Duckworth T, Kanis JA. Features of algodystrophy after Colles' fracture. J Bone Joint Surg Br 1990;72(1):105–10.

67. Bacorn RW, Kurtzke JF. Colles' fracture; a study of two thousand cases from the New York State Workmen's Compensation Board. J Bone Joint Surg Am 1953;35-A(3):643–58.

68. Green JT, Gay FH. Colles' fracture; residual disability. Am J Surg 1956;91(4):636–42 [discussion: 642–6].

69. Plewes LW. Sudeck's atrophy in the hand. J Bone Joint Surg Br 1956;38-B(1):195–203.

70. Li Z, Smith BP, Tuohy C, et al. Complex regional pain syndrome after hand surgery. Hand Clin 2010;26(2):281–9.

71. Zollinger PE, Tuinebreijer WE, Breederveld RS, et al. Can vitamin C prevent complex regional pain syndrome in patients with wrist fractures? A randomized, controlled, multicenter dose-response study. J Bone Joint Surg Am 2007;89(7):1424–31.

72. Zollinger PE, Tuinebreijer WE, Kreis RW, et al. Effect of vitamin C on frequency of reflex sympathetic dystrophy in wrist fractures: a randomised trial. Lancet 1999;354(9195):2025–8.

73. Evaniew N, McCarthy C, Kleinlugtenbelt YV, et al. Vitamin C to prevent complex regional pain syndrome in patients with distal radius fractures: a meta-analysis of randomized controlled trials. J Orthop Trauma 2015;29(8):e235–41.

74. McKay SD, MacDermid JC, Roth JH, et al. Assessment of complications of distal radius fractures and development of a complication checklist. J Hand Surg Am 2001;26(5):916–22.

75. Singer BR, McLauchlan GJ, Robinson CM, et al. Epidemiology of fractures in 15,000 adults: the influence of age and gender. J Bone Joint Surg Br 1998;80(2):243–8.

76. Hung LK, Wu HT, Leung PC, et al. Low BMD is a risk factor for low-energy Colles' fractures in women before and after menopause. Clin Orthop Relat Res 2005;(435):219–25.

77. Nesbitt KS, Failla JM, Les C. Assessment of instability factors in adult distal radius fractures. J Hand Surg Am 2004;29(6):1128–38.

78. Porter M, Stockley I. Fractures of the distal radius. Intermediate and end results in relation to radiologic parameters. Clin Orthop Relat Res 1987;(220):241–52.

79. Leone J, Bhandari M, Adili A, et al. Predictors of early and late instability following conservative treatment of extra-articular distal radius fractures. Arch Orthop Trauma Surg 2004;124(1):38–41.

80. McQueen MM, MacLaren A, Chalmers J. The value of remanipulating Colles' fractures. J Bone Joint Surg Br 1986;68(2):232–3.

81. Lafontaine M, Delince P, Hardy D, et al. Instability of fractures of the lower end of the radius: apropos of a series of 167 cases. Acta Orthop Belg 1989;55(2):203–16 [in French].

82. Young BT, Rayan GM. Outcome following nonoperative treatment of displaced distal radius fractures in low-demand patients older than 60 years. J Hand Surg Am 2000;25(1):19–28.

83. Anzarut A, Johnson JA, Rowe BH, et al. Radiologic and patient-reported functional outcomes in an elderly cohort with conservatively treated distal radius fractures. J Hand Surg Am 2004;29(6):1121–7.

84. Jaremko JL, Lambert RG, Rowe BH, et al. Do radiographic indices of distal radius fracture reduction predict outcomes in older adults receiving conservative treatment? Clin Radiol 2007;62(1):65–72.

85. Mackenney PJ, McQueen MM, Elton R. Prediction of instability in distal radial fractures. J Bone Joint Surg Am 2006;88(9):1944–51.

86. Arora R, Gabl M, Erhart S, et al. Aspects of current management of distal radius fractures in the elderly individuals. Geriatr Orthop Surg Rehabil 2011;2(5–6):187–94.

87. Barrett-Connor E, Sajjan SG, Siris ES, et al. Wrist fracture as a predictor of future fractures in younger versus older postmenopausal women: results from the National Osteoporosis Risk Assessment (NORA). Osteoporos Int 2008;19(5):607–13.

88. Schousboe JT, Fink HA, Taylor BC, et al. Association between self-reported prior wrist fractures and risk of subsequent hip and radiographic vertebral fractures in older women: a prospective study. J Bone Miner Res 2005;20(1):100–6.

89. Gunnes M, Mellstrom D, Johnell O. How well can a previous fracture indicate a new fracture? A questionnaire study of 29,802 postmenopausal women. Acta Orthop Scand 1998;69(5):508–12.

90. Mallmin H, Ljunghall S, Persson I, et al. Fracture of the distal forearm as a forecaster of subsequent hip fracture: a population-based cohort study with 24 years of follow-up. Calcif Tissue Int 1993;52(4):269–72.

91. Gardsell P, Johnell O, Nilsson BE, et al. The predictive value of fracture, disease, and falling tendency for fragility fractures in women. Calcif Tissue Int 1989;45(6):327–30.

92. Pogue DJ, Viegas SF, Patterson RM, et al. Effects of distal radius fracture malunion on wrist joint mechanics. J Hand Surg Am 1990;15(5):721–7.

93. Kihara H, Palmer AK, Werner FW, et al. The effect of dorsally angulated distal radius fractures on distal radioulnar joint congruency and forearm rotation. J Hand Surg Am 1996;21(1):40–7.

94. Handoll HH, Madhok R, Dodds C. Anaesthesia for treating distal radial fracture in adults. Cochrane Database Syst Rev 2002;(3):CD003320.

95. Bong MR, Egol KA, Leibman M, et al. A comparison of immediate postreduction splinting constructs for controlling initial displacement of fractures of the distal radius: a prospective randomized study of long-arm versus short-arm splinting. J Hand Surg Am 2006;31(5):766–70.

96. Clancey GJ. Percutaneous Kirschner-wire fixation of Colles fractures. A prospective study of thirty cases. J Bone Joint Surg Am 1984;66(7):1008–14.

97. Mah ET, Atkinson RN. Percutaneous Kirschner wire stabilisation following closed reduction of Colles' fractures. J Hand Surg Br 1992;17(1):55–62.

98. Munson GO, Gainor BJ. Percutaneous pinning of distal radius fractures. J Trauma 1981;21(12):1032–5.

99. Glickel SZ, Catalano LW, Raia FJ, et al. Long-term outcomes of closed reduction and percutaneous pinning for the treatment of distal radius fractures. J Hand Surg Am 2008;33(10):1700–5.

100. Kreder HJ, Hanel DP, Agel J, et al. Indirect reduction and percutaneous fixation versus open reduction and internal fixation for displaced intra-articular fractures of the distal radius: a randomised, controlled trial. J Bone Joint Surg Br 2005;87(6):829–36.

101. Barton T, Chambers C, Lane E, et al. Do Kirschner wires maintain reduction of displaced Colles' fractures? Injury 2005;36(12):1431–4.

102. Kapandji A. Intra-focal pinning of fractures of the distal end of the radius 10 years later. Ann Chir Main 1987;6(1):57–63 [in French].

103. Handoll HH, Vaghela MV, Madhok R. Percutaneous pinning for treating distal radial fractures in adults. Cochrane Database Syst Rev 2007;(3):CD006080.

104. Slutsky DJ. External fixation of distal radius fractures. J Hand Surg Am 2007;32(10):1624–37.

105. Bindra RR. Biomechanics and biology of external fixation of distal radius fractures. Hand Clin 2005;21(3):363–73.

106. Bales JG, Stern PJ. Treatment strategies of distal radius fractures. Hand Clin 2012;28(2):177–84.

107. Margaliot Z, Haase SC, Kotsis SV, et al. A meta-analysis of outcomes of external fixation versus plate osteosynthesis for unstable distal radius fractures. J Hand Surg Am 2005;30(6):1185–99.

108. Egol K, Walsh M, Tejwani N, et al. Bridging external fixation and supplementary Kirschner-wire fixation versus volar locked plating for unstable fractures of the distal radius: a randomised, prospective trial. J Bone Joint Surg Br 2008; 90(9):1214–21.

109. Grewal R, Perey B, Wilmink M, et al. A randomized prospective study on the treatment of intra-articular distal radius fractures: open reduction and internal fixation with dorsal plating versus mini open reduction, percutaneous fixation, and external fixation. J Hand Surg Am 2005;30(4):764–72.

110. Axelrod TS, McMurtry RY. Open reduction and internal fixation of comminuted, intraarticular fractures of the distal radius. J Hand Surg Am 1990; 15(1):1–11.

111. Ring D, Jupiter JB, Brennwald J, et al. Prospective multicenter trial of a plate for dorsal fixation of distal radius fractures. J Hand Surg Am 1997; 22(5):777–84.

112. Orbay JL, Touhami A. Current concepts in volar fixed-angle fixation of unstable distal radius fractures. Clin Orthop Relat Res 2006;445:58–67.

113. Tanaka Y, Aoki M, Izumi T, et al. Effect of distal radius volar plate position on contact pressure between the flexor pollicis longus tendon and the distal plate edge. J Hand Surg Am 2011;36(11): 1790–7.

114. Limthongthang R, Bachoura A, Jacoby SM, et al. Distal radius volar locking plate design and associated vulnerability of the flexor pollicis longus. J Hand Surg Am 2014;39(5):852–60.

115. Soong M, Earp BE, Bishop G, et al. Volar locking plate implant prominence and flexor tendon rupture. J Bone Joint Surg Am 2011;93(4):328–35.

116. Wright TW, Horodyski M, Smith DW. Functional outcome of unstable distal radius fractures: ORIF with a volar fixed-angle tine plate versus external fixation. J Hand Surg Am 2005;30(2): 289–99.

117. Orbay JL, Fernandez DL. Volar fixation for dorsally displaced fractures of the distal radius: a preliminary report. J Hand Surg Am 2002;27(2):205–15.

118. Dodds SD, Cornelissen S, Jossan S, et al. A biomechanical comparison of fragment-specific fixation and augmented external fixation for intra-articular distal radius fractures. J Hand Surg Am 2002;27(6):953–64.

119. Konrath GA, Bahler S. Open reduction and internal fixation of unstable distal radius fractures: results using the trimed fixation system. J Orthop Trauma 2002;16(8):578–85.

120. Benson LS, Minihane KP, Stern LD, et al. The outcome of intra-articular distal radius fractures treated with fragment-specific fixation. J Hand Surg Am 2006;31(8):1333–9.

121. Sammer DM, Fuller DS, Kim HM, et al. A comparative study of fragment-specific versus volar plate fixation of distal radius fractures. Plast Reconstr Surg 2008;122(5):1441–50.

Carpal Tunnel Syndrome
Making Evidence-Based Treatment Decisions

James H. Calandruccio, MD*,
Norfleet B. Thompson, MD

KEYWORDS

- Carpal tunnel syndrome • Treatment • Outcomes • Complications • Costs

---

KEY POINTS

- CTS is one of the most common musculoskeletal disorders of the upper extremity.
- Although a high rate of repetitive hand/wrist motions is a risk factor, there is insufficient evidence to implicate computer use in the development of CTS.
- Initial treatment generally is nonoperative, with the strongest evidence supporting bracing/splinting.
- Strong evidence supports operative treatment, regardless of technique, as superior to nonoperative treatment.
- Complications are infrequent and most are minor and transient.

According to the clinical practice guideline (CPG) from the American Academy of Orthopedic Surgeons[1] (AAOS), carpal tunnel syndrome (CTS) is "a symptomatic compression neuropathy of the median nerve at the level of the wrist, characterized physiologically by evidence of increased pressure within the carpal tunnel and decreased function of the nerve at that level." It is the most common compressive neuropathy affecting the upper extremity, present in approximately 3% to 6% of adults in the United States.[2] A study of a "working population" of adults (mostly industrial workers) identified CTS in 8%.[3] CTS also is the most expensive upper extremity musculoskeletal disorder, with an estimated cost of medical care in the United States of more than $2 billion annually. Nonmedical costs, such as workers' compensation costs, lost wages, lost productivity, and disability, are even higher; the median time lost by US workers with CTS is 28 days.[4]

RISK FACTORS FOR CARPAL TUNNEL SYNDROME

Reported risk factors for the development of CTS include age, smoking, obesity, rheumatoid arthritis, diabetes, lupus, hypothyroidism, and multiple sclerosis.[5] Women, especially those taking birth control pills, going through menopause, or taking estrogen, have the highest risk of developing CTS. Working with vibrating tools or on an assembly line that requires prolonged or repetitive flexion of the wrist has been suggested as a risk factor, but scientific evidence is conflicting. The AAOS CPG notes strong evidence that body mass index and a high rate of hand/wrist repetition are associated with an increased risk of developing CTS. A widely held idea is that CTS is associated with computer use,[6,7] but evidence is insufficient to support this; in fact, several articles have disputed it altogether.[8–10] A systematic review and

---

Department of Orthopaedic Surgery and Biomedical Engineering, University of Tennessee-Campbell Clinic, 1211 Union Avenue, Suite 510, Memphis, TN 38104, USA
* Corresponding author.
E-mail address: jcalandruccio@campbellclinic.com

Orthop Clin N Am 49 (2018) 223–229
https://doi.org/10.1016/j.ocl.2017.11.009

meta-analysis that involved 25 studies (92,564 individuals) suggested that type 1 and type 2 diabetes are risk factors for CTS.[11] Another meta-analysis of 58 studies (1,379,372 individuals) determined that high body mass index markedly increases the risk of CTS; obesity increased the risk two-fold, and each one-unit increase in body mass index increased the risk of CTS by 7%.[12]

DIAGNOSIS, PHYSICAL EXAMINATION

CTS is primarily a clinical diagnosis. Symptoms usually include numbness and pain or paresthesia in the median nerve distribution. Commonly used provocative tests include wrist flexion (Phalen), nerve percussion (Tinel), and carpal compression (Durkan) tests. The carpal compression test was found to be more specific (90%) and more sensitive (87%) than either the Tinel or Phalen test (Table 1).[13] No single test in isolation is sufficient to make a definitive diagnosis of CTS. The key elements of a diagnosis of CTS are medial nerve distribution numbness, nocturnal wakening, thenar atrophy, a positive Phalen test, loss of two-point discrimination, and a positive Tinel sign.[14]

Electrodiagnostic studies (EDS) and imaging studies generally are reserved for patients in whom the diagnosis is questionable, but this remains an area of controversy. A survey of members of the American Society for Surgery of the Hand (ASSH) determined that 72% would advise carpal tunnel release (CTR) based on a classic history and examination and complete relief

Table 1
Commonly used provocative tests for carpal tunnel syndrome

Test	Sensitivity (%)	Specificity (%)
Phalen (wrist flexion)	68–70	73–83
Tinel (nerve percussion)	20–50	76–77
Durkan (carpal compression)	87	90
Electrodiagnostic studies	49–84	95–99
Ultrasonography	82	92
MRI	63–83	78–80
Computed tomography	67	87

Adapted from Durkan JA. A new diagnostic test for carpal tunnel syndrome. J Bone Joint Surg Am 1991;73(4):536; with permission.

following cortisone injection,[15] whereas in a later survey 90% indicated that they used EDS before recommending surgery.[16] A more recent survey of 134 physicians in Michigan, however, found that 57% required a diagnostic test before recommending surgery for CTS (most often EDS).[17] EDS, although most commonly used, add little to the diagnosis of CTS.[18] The AAOS CPG notes limited evidence that a hand-held nerve conduction study may be helpful in the diagnosis of CTS. With a sensitivity of 49% to 84% and specificity of 95% to 99%, EDS are no more sensitive or specific than physical examination testing. The CPG also reports moderate/limited evidence that supports not using MRI or ultrasound for diagnosis. These adjunctive tests are expensive, and the benefit/cost ratio should be carefully considered before using them.

TREATMENT
Nonoperative Treatment
Many patients with mild or moderate CTS respond to nonoperative treatment, and generally an initial trial of conservative treatment is recommended. Cha and colleagues,[19] however, found that outcomes were not as good in patients who initially had nonoperative treatment and delayed surgery for an average of 6 months compared with those who had surgery as their initial treatment.

Nonoperative modalities with the strongest evidence of benefit are bracing/splinting[20,21] and steroid injections.[22,23] Both wrist splints and soft wrist braces have been shown to obtain improvement in symptoms and function when compared with wrists with no treatment.[20,21,24] Corticosteroid injections have been reported to be successful in relieving symptoms, at least at short-term; longer-term outcomes are variable. Blazar and colleagues[23] reported that a single corticosteroid injection obtained symptom relief in 79% of 52 wrists at 6 weeks; at 6 months and 12 months only 53% and 31%, respectively, were symptom-free. Others have described early symptom relief in up to 80% of patients,[25–27] but with steadily decreasing success at longer-term follow-up and surgical treatment required in 15% to 94% of patients at 12 to 18 months.[25–28]

The use of multiple injections remains in question. Berger and colleagues[29] reported that 30 of 120 patients had good outcomes with a single injection, 11 required a second injection, and five needed a third injection to reach a good outcome; 28 (52%) had good outcomes at 1 year. At 6 weeks, 79% of patients reported by Blazar and colleagues[23] had symptom relief with a single injection.

Identified predictors for failure of conservative treatment include diabetes,[23,27] age more than 50 years,[30] and severity of symptoms.[28]

Operative Treatment
Several high-quality studies have demonstrated the superior effectiveness of operative treatment compared with nonoperative treatment,[25,31–36] and strong evidence supports the operative treatment of CTS.[1]

Inpatient versus outpatient
Although CTR has historically been done in an operating room with general anesthesia, currently most CTR procedures are done in a surgery center or clinic procedure room. A 2015 survey of ASSH members found that 65% performed most of their CTR surgery in an outpatient surgery center.[16] CTR procedures done in an operating room are four times more expensive than those done in an ambulatory surgery center or clinic procedure room and are much less efficient.[37–39] Nguyen and colleagues[39] determined that using an ambulatory center could lower charges for CTR surgery approximately 30%, and Rhee and colleagues[40] calculated that, in their military medical center, performing CTR surgery in the clinic with wide-awake local anesthesia would result in an 85% cost savings.

Simultaneous or staged bilateral surgery
Bilateral CTS is reported to occur in from 22% to 87% of patients.[41] Park and colleagues[42] showed that bilateral simultaneous CTR had lower total costs and higher total effectiveness than bilateral staged surgeries; however, patients with bilateral simultaneous releases have more severe functional impairment during the first few postoperative days, but after 2 or 3 days limitations are similar to those with unilateral release.[43] Patients with simultaneous releases seem to return to work in a much shorter time (2.5 weeks) than those with the second surgery 1 to 3 weeks later (8.5 weeks) or more than 3 weeks later (6 weeks).[44] Herisson and colleagues[41] reported that 93% of their 25 patients were satisfied with simultaneous release and would choose the same technique again. Bilateral simultaneous CTR is well-tolerated by patients and is associated with lower total costs compared with staged release.[41,43–45]

Prophylactic antibiotics
Whether prophylactic antibiotics are indicated for CTR remains an area of controversy, especially in the current medicolegal environment. In a survey of ASSH members, the percentages of those who routinely gave antibiotics for CTR and those who did not were comparable (33% and 39%, respectively).[46] Two studies showed no statistically significant difference between those with perioperative antibiotics and those without.[47,48] The current AAOS CPG states that "limited evidence supports that there is no benefit for routine use of prophylactic antibiotics prior to CTR because there is not a demonstrated reduction in postoperative surgical site infection with the use of antibiotics."[1] Overall the deep infection rate for CTR is less than 1%.[46,47,49] Certain comorbidities and patient factors that may increase the risk of infection include a history of previous infection, diabetes, rheumatoid arthritis, and surgery time longer than 4 hours.[46–49] Several adverse possibilities should be considered before the routine use of prophylactic antibiotics: higher financial cost, anaphylaxis, and development of antibiotics resistance.[48] Szabo[46] suggested that, considering the low frequency of infection and no proven clear benefit of prophylactic antibiotics, concerns about emerging drug-resistant organisms probably should outweigh routine use of antibiotics in CTR.

Anesthesia
Anesthesia choices for CTR include local anesthesia (with or without sedation), intravenous regional, or general anesthesia. The WALANT (wide-awake, local anesthesia, no tourniquet) technique has become a popular option because it reduces postoperative nausea and vomiting, decreases cost, increases procedural efficiency, and produces high patient satisfaction.[50,51] In a prospective cohort study comparing CTR done with local anesthetic in the clinic (100 patients) with surgery with sedation in the operating room (100 patients), Davison and colleagues[52] found that patients were equally satisfied with their procedures and would have the same type of anesthesia again; however, those with sedation had more preoperative anxiety, required more preoperative testing, used more postoperative opioids (67% vs 5%), had more nausea and vomiting, and spent more time in the hospital (4 hours vs 2.6 hours). Better pain control with local anesthesia also may result in less frequent use of postoperative opioids and shorter hospital stays.[53]

Operative technique
Regardless of the technique chosen, operative treatment of CTS generally is a successful procedure, with excellent long-term results. Louie and colleagues[54] reported an 88% satisfaction

rate 13 years after open release in 113 patients, and Means and colleagues[55] reported low recurrence rates and good function scores 8 to 10 years after 115 endoscopic releases. Studies comparing techniques have had varying conclusions. Larsen and colleagues[56] compared standard incision, short incision, and endoscopic techniques and found no significant differences at 24 weeks. Better early satisfaction rates with mini-incision and endoscopic techniques compared with standard open technique were reported by Aslani and colleagues[57]; outcomes were similar after 4 months. Zuo and colleagues,[58] in a meta-analysis, concluded that endoscopic release and open release have similar benefits and complication rates, despite earlier studies that showed more major complications with endoscopic technique. Even with similar outcomes, Kang and colleagues[59] found that 34 (65%) of 52 patients with bilateral releases (one endoscopic, one mini-open) preferred the endoscopic technique. Endoscopic release also has been noted to have fewer complications, lower recurrence rates, and quicker return to work than open techniques.[60–63] In their meta-analysis, Sayegh and Strauch[62] noted that high-level evidence from randomized controlled trials indicates that endoscopic release allows earlier return to work and improved strength during the early postoperative period. Results at 6 months or later are similar except that patients undergoing endoscopic release are at greater risk of nerve injury and lower risk of scar tenderness compared with open release.

POSTOPERATIVE MANAGEMENT
Pain Management
The overuse of opioids currently is an area of much concern. Chapman and colleagues,[64] in a prospective study of 277 patients, recorded an average consumption of 4.3 pills per patient even though 21 pills were prescribed. Opioid consumption was more influenced by age and gender than by anesthesia, insurance, or opioid type.

Splinting/Dressing
At least three high-level studies have shown that postoperative wrist splinting is not necessary after CTR.[65–67] Immobilization does not decrease scar pain or improve pinch strength and may delay functional recovery.[68]

Ritting and colleagues[69] reviewed 94 consecutive patients with mini-open releases who had their bulky postoperative dressings removed at 48 to 72 hours or at their 2-week follow-up. There were no wound complications in either group and no differences in function or symptom relief. Williams and colleagues[70] prospectively randomized 100 patients to wear a bulky postoperative dressing for 24 hours or 2 weeks and found no differences in postsurgical pain or wound healing.

COMPLICATIONS

Complications are infrequent after CTR, reported to occur in from 1% to 25% of patients, and most are minor and transient.[71] A study based on the National Survey of Ambulatory Surgery database (400,000 patients) found a perioperative or postoperative "problem" in 10%.[72] Risk factors for a complication included male gender and age greater than or equal to 45 years. A recent systematic review compared complications associated with endoscopic and open CTR and determined that endoscopic procedures had a higher rate of transient nerve lesions, but there was no difference in permanent injury rates.[73]

The development of a trigger finger after CTR has been reported in 5% to 32% of patients, with the thumb and ring finger most commonly involved.[74,75] In a nationwide, population-based retrospective cohort study, Lin and colleagues[75] found that the overall risk of trigger digits was nearly four times greater in those with CTR. Most trigger digits developed within the first 6 months after surgery. In three large case series involving 2315 patients,[76–78] trigger digits developed in 9%. The frequency of concomitant and subsequent trigger digits in patients with CTS suggests a common pathophysiologic process,[75,79,80] but this has not been proven.

SUMMARY

CTS is one of the most common musculoskeletal disorders of the upper extremity. Comorbidities associated with the development of CTS include diabetes and obesity. Although a high rate of repetitive hand/wrist motions is a risk factor, there is insufficient evidence to implicate computer use in the development of CTS. Initial treatment generally is nonoperative, with the strongest evidence supporting bracing/splinting. Strong evidence supports operative treatment, regardless of technique, as superior to nonoperative treatment. Complications are infrequent and most are minor and transient.

REFERENCES

1. American Academy of Orthopaedic Surgeons. Management of carpal tunnel syndrome.

Evidence-based clinical practice guideline. 2016. Available at: https://www.aaos.org/uploadedFiles/PreProduction/Quality/Guidelines_and_Reviews/guidelines/CTS%20CPG_2.29.16.pdf. Accessed July 25, 2017.

2. Centers for Disease Control and Prevention. Morbidity and Mortality Weekly Report, 2011. Available at: https://www.cdc.gov/mmwr/preview/mmwrhtml/mm6049a4.htm?s_cid=mm6049a4_w. Accessed November 21, 2017.

3. Dale AM, Harris-Adamson C, Rempel D, et al. Prevalence and incidence of carpal tunnel syndrome in US working populations: pooled analysis of six prospective studies. Scand J Work Environ Health 2013;39:495–505.

4. United States Department of Labor, Bureau of Labor Statistics. Nonfatal occupational injuries and illnesses requiring days away from work. 2015. Available at: https://www.bls.gov/news.release/osh2.nr0.htm. Accessed July 25, 2017.

5. Zyluk A, Puchalski P. A comparison of outcomes of carpal tunnel release in diabetic and non-diabetic patients. J Hand Surg Eur Vol 2013;38:485–8.

6. Ricco M, Cattani S, Signorelli C. Personal risk factors for carpal tunnel syndrome in female visual display unit workers. Int J Occup Med Environ Health 2016;29:927–36.

7. Toosi KK, Hogaboom NS, Oyster ML, et al. Computer keyboarding biomechanics and acute changes in median nerve indicative of carpal tunnel syndrome. Clin Biomech (Bristol, Avon) 2015;30:546–50.

8. Kozak A, Schedlbauer G, Wirth T, et al. Associated between work-related biomechanical risk factors and the occurrence of carpal tunnel syndrome: an overview of systematic reviews and a meta-analysis of current research. BMC Musculoskelet Disord 2015,16:231.

9. Mattioil S, Violante FS, Bonfiglioli R. Upper extremity and neck disorders associated with keyboard and mouse use. Handb Clin Neurol 2015;131:427–33.

10. Mediouni Z, Bodin J, Dale AM, et al. Carpal tunnel syndrome and computer exposure at work in two large complementary cohorts. BMJ Open 2015;5(9):e008156.

11. Pourmemari MH, Shiri R. Diabetes as a risk factor for carpal tunnel syndrome: a systematic review and meta-analysis. Diabet Med 2016;33:10–6.

12. Shiri R, Pourmemari MH, Falah-Hassani K, et al. The effect of excess body mass on the risk of carpal tunnel syndrome: a meta-analysis of 58 studies. Obes Rev 2015;16:1094–104.

13. Durkan JA. A new diagnostic test for carpal tunnel syndrome. J Bone Joint Surg Am 1991;73:535–8.

14. Graham B, Regehr G, Wright JG. Delphi as a method to establish consensus for diagnostic criteria. J Clin Epidemiol 2003;56:1150–6.

15. Lane LB, Starecki M, Olson A, et al. Carpal tunnel syndrome diagnosis and treatment: a survey of members of the American Society for Surgery of the Hand. J Hand Surg Am 2014;39:2181–7.

16. Munns JJ, Awan HM. Trends in carpal tunnel surgery: an online survey of members of the American Society for Surgery of the Hand. J Hand Surg Am 2015;40:767–71.

17. Sears ED, Lu YU, Wood SM, et al. Diagnostic testing requested before surgical evaluation for carpal tunnel syndrome. J Hand Surg Am 2017;42(8):623–9.e1.

18. Graham B. The value added by electrodiagnostic testing the diagnosis of carpal tunnel syndrome. J Bone Joint Surg Am 2008;90:2587–93.

19. Cha SM, Shin HD, Ahn JS, et al. Differences in the postoperative outcomes according to the primary treatment options chosen by patients with carpal tunnel syndrome: conservative versus operative treatment. Ann Plast Surg 2016;77:80–4.

20. Hall B, Lee HC, Fitzgerald H, et al. Investigating the effectiveness of full-time wrist splinting and education in the treatment of carpal tunnel syndrome: a randomized controlled trial. Am J Occup Ther 2013;67:448–59.

21. Manente G, Torrieri F, De Blasio F, et al. An innovative hand brace for carpal tunnel syndrome: a randomized controlled trial. Muscle Nerve 2001;24:1020–5.

22. Atroshi I, Flondell M, Hofer M, et al. Methylprednisolone injections for the carpal tunnel syndrome: a randomized, placebo-controlled trial. Ann Intern Med 2013;159:309–17.

23. Blazar PE, Floyd WE 4th, Han CH, et al. Prognostic indicators for recurrent symptoms after a single corticosteroid injection for carpal tunnel syndrome. J Bone Joint Surg Am 2015;97:1563–70.

24. De Angelis MV, Pierfelice F, Di Giovanni P, et al. Efficacy of a soft hand brace and a wrist splint for carpal tunnel syndrome: a randomized controlled study. Acta Neurol Scand 2009;119:68–74.

25. Andreu JL, Ly-Pen D, Millán I, et al. Local injection versus surgery in carpal tunnel syndrome: neurophysiologic outcomes of a randomized clinical trial. Clin Neurophysiol 2014;125:1479–84.

26. Dammers JW, Veering MM, Vermeulen M. Injection with methylprednisolone proximal to the carpal tunnel: randomised double bind trial. BMJ 1999;319:884–6.

27. Jenkins PJ, Duckworth AD, Watts AC, et al. Corticosteroid injection for carpal tunnel syndrome: a 5-year survivorship analysis. Hand (N Y) 2012;7:151–6.

28. Meys V, Thissen S, Roseman S, et al. Prognostic factors in carpal tunnel syndrome treated with a corticosteroid injection. Muscle Nerve 2011;44:763–8.

29. Berger M, Vermeulen M, Koelman JH, et al. The long-term follow-up of treatment with corticosteroid injections in patients with carpal tunnel

syndrome. When are multiple injections indicated? J Hand Surg Eur Vol 2013;38:634–9.

30. Kaplan SJ, Glickel SZ, Eaton RG. Predictive factors in the non-surgical treatment of carpal tunnel syndrome. J Hand Surg Br 1990;15:106–8.

31. Gerritsen AA, de Vet HC, Scholten RJ, et al. Splinting vs surgery in the treatment of carpal tunnel syndrome: a randomized controlled trial. JAMA 2002; 288:1245–51.

32. Hui AC, Wong S, Leung CH, et al. A randomized controlled trial of surgery vs steroid injection for carpal tunnel syndrome. Neurology 2005;64: 2074–8.

33. Ismatullah J. Local steroid injection or carpal tunnel release for carpal tunnel syndrome—which is more effective? J Postgrad Med Instit 2013. Available at: http://www.jpmi.org.pk/index.php/jpmi/article/view/1497. Accessed November 21, 2017.

34. Jarvik JG, Comstock BA, Kilot M, et al. Surgery versus non-surgical therapy for carpal tunnel syndrome: a randomised parallel-group trial. Lancet 2009;374:1074–81.

35. Ly-Pen D, Andréu JL. Treatment of carpal tunnel syndrome. Med Clin 2005;125:585–9.

36. Ly-Pen D, Andréu JL, Millan I, et al. Comparison of surgical decompression and local steroid injection in the treatment of carpal tunnel syndrome: 2-year clinical results from a randomized trial. Rheumatology (Oxford) 2012;51:1447–54.

37. Chatterjee A, McCarthy JE, Montagne SA, et al. A cost, profit, and efficiency analysis of performing carpal tunnel surgery in the operating room versus the clinic setting in the United States. Ann Plast Surg 2011;66:245–8.

38. Leblanc MR, Lalonde J, Lalonde DH. A detailed cost and efficiency analysis of performing carpal tunnel surgery in the main operating room versus the ambulatory setting in Canada. Hand (N Y) 2007;2:173–8.

39. Nguyen C, Milstein A, Hernandez-Boussard T, et al. The effect of moving carpal tunnel releases out of hospitals on reducing United States health care charges. J Hand Surg Am 2015;40:1657–62.

40. Rhee PC, Fischer MM, Rhee LS, et al. Cost savings and patient experience of a clinic-based, wide-awake hand surgery program at a military medical center: a critical analysis of the first 100 procedures. J Hand Surg Am 2017;42:e139–47.

41. Herisson O, Dury M, Rapp E, et al. Bilateral carpal tunnel surgery in one operation: retrospective study. Hand Surg Rehabil 2016;35:199–202.

42. Park KW, Boyer MI, Gelberman RH, et al. Simultaneous bilateral versus staged bilateral carpal tunnel release: a cost-effectiveness analysis. J Am Acad Orthop Surg 2016;24:796–804.

43. Osei DA, Calfee RP, Stepan JG, et al. Simultaneous bilateral or unilateral carpal tunnel release? A prospective cohort study of early outcomes and limitations. J Bone Joint Surg Am 2014;96:889–96.

44. Nesbitt KS, Innis PC, Dubin NH, et al. Staged versus simultaneous bilateral endoscopic carpal tunnel release: an outcome study. Plast Reconstr Surg 2006;118:139–45.

45. Fehringer EV, Tiedeman JJ, Dobler K, et al. Bilateral endoscopic carpal tunnel releases: simultaneous versus staged operative intervention. Arthroscopy 2002;18:316–21.

46. Szabo RM. Perioperative antibiotics for carpal tunnel surgery. J Hand Surg Am 2010;35:122–4.

47. Harness NG, Inacio MC, Pfeil FF, et al. Rate of infection after carpal tunnel release surgery and effect of antibiotic prophylaxis. J Hand Surg Am 2010;35:189–96.

48. Tosti R, Fowler J, Dwyer J, et al. Is antibiotric prophylaxis necessary in elective sort tissue hand surgery? Orthopedics 2012;35:e829–33.

49. Hanssen AD, Amadio PC, DeSilva SP. Deep postoperative wound infection after carpal tunnel release. J Hand Surg 1989;14:869–73.

50. Lalonde DH. "Hole-in-one" local anesthesia for wide-awake carpal tunnel surgery. Plast Reconstr Surg 2010;126:1642–4.

51. Lalonde D, Martin A. Tumescent local anesthesia for hand surgery: improved results, cost effectiveness, and wide-awake patient satisfaction. Arch Plast Surg 2014;41:312–6.

52. Davison PG, Cobb T, Lalonde DH. The patient's perspective on carpal tunnel surgery related to the type of anesthesia: a prospective cohort study. Hand (N Y) 2013;8:47–53.

53. Sørensen AM, Dalsgaard J, Hansen TB. Local anaesthesia versus intravenous regional anaesthesia in endoscopic carpal tunnel release: a randomized controlled trial. J Hand Surg Eur Vol 2013;38:481–4.

54. Louie DL, Earp BE, Collins JE, et al. Outcomes of open carpal tunnel release at a minimum of ten years. J Bone Joint Surg Am 2013;95:1067–73.

55. Means KR Jr, Dubin NH, Patel KM, et al. Long-term outcomes following single-portal endoscopic carpal tunnel release. Hand (N Y) 2014;9:384–8.

56. Larsen MB, Sørensen AI, Crone KL, et al. Carpal tunnel release: a randomized comparison of three surgical methods. J Hand Surg Eur Vol 2013;38: 646–50.

57. Aslani HR, Alizadeh K, Eajazi A, et al. Comparison of carpal tunnel release with three different techniques. Clin Neurol Neurosurg 2012;114:965–8.

58. Zuo D, Zhou Z, Wang H, et al. Endoscopic versus open carpal tunnel release for idiopathic carpal tunnel syndrome: a meta-analysis of randomized controlled trials. J Orthop Surg Res 2015;10:12.

59. Kang HJ, Koh IH, Lee TJ, et al. Endoscopic carpal tunnel release is preferred over mini-open despite

similar outcome: a randomized trial. Clin Orthop Relat Res 2013;471:1548–54.

60. Calotta NA, Lopez J, Deune EG. Improved surgical outcomes with endoscopic carpal tunnel release in patients with severe median neuropathy. Hand (N Y) 2017;12:252–7.

61. Gümüştas SA, Ekmekci B, Tosun HB, et al. Similar effectiveness of the open versus endoscopic technique for carpal tunnel syndrome: a prospective randomized trial. Eur J Orthop Surg Traumatol 2015;25:1253–60.

62. Sayegh ET, Strauch RJ. Open versus endoscopic carpal tunnel release: a meta-analysis of randomized controlled trials. Clin Orthop Relat Res 2015; 473:1120–32.

63. Vasiliadis HS, Georgoulas P, Shrier I, et al. Endoscopic release for carpal tunnel syndrome. Cochrane Database Syst Rev 2014;(1):CD008265.

64. Chapman T, Kim N, Maltenfort M, et al. Prospective evaluation of opioid consumption following carpal tunnel release surgery. Hand (N Y) 2017;12:39–42.

65. Bury TF, Akelman E, Weiss AP. Prospective, randomized trial of splinting after carpal tunnel release. Ann Plast Surg 1995;35:19–22.

66. Cook AC, Szabo RM, Birkholz SW, et al. Early mobilization following carpal tunnel release. A prospective randomized study. J Hand Surg Br 1995;20: 228–30.

67. Finsen V, Andersen K, Russwurm H. No advantage from splinting the wrist after open carpal tunnel release. A randomized study of 82 wrists. Acta Orthop Scand 1999;70:288–92.

68. Hermiz SJ, Kalliainen LK. Evidence-based medicine: current evidence in the diagnosis and management of carpal tunnel syndrome. Plast Reconstr Surg 2017;140:120e–9e.

69. Ritting AW, Leger R, O'Malley MP, et al. Duration of postoperative dressing after mini-open carpal tunnel release: a prospective, randomized trial. J Hand Surg Am 2012;37:3–8.

70. Williams AM, Baker PA, Platt AJ. The impact of dressings on recovery from carpal tunnel decompression. J Plast Reconstr Aesthet Surg 2008;61:1493–5.

71. Neuhaus V, Christoforou D, Cheriyan T, et al. Evaluation and treatment of failed carpal tunnel release. Orthop Clin North Am 2012;43:439–47.

72. Rozanski M, Neuhaus V, Thornton E, et al. Symptoms during or shortly after isolated carpal tunnel release and problems within 24 hours after surgery. J Hand Microsurg 2015;7:30–5.

73. Faucher GK, Daruwalla JH, Seiler JG 3rd. Complications of surgical release of carpal tunnel syndrome: a systematic review. J Surg Orthop Adv 2017;26:18–24.

74. Lin FY, Wu CI, Cheng HT. Coincidence or complication? A systematic review of trigger digit after carpal tunnel release. J Plast Surg Hand Surg 2017;7:1–7.

75. Lin FY, Manrique OJ, Lin CL, et al. Incidence of trigger digits following carpal tunnel release: a nationwide population-based retrospective cohort study. Medicine (Baltimore) 2017;96:e7355.

76. Kim JH, Gong HS, Lee HJ, et al. Pre- and postoperative comorbidities in idiopathic carpal tunnel syndrome: cervical arthritis, basal joint arthritis of the thumb, and trigger digit. J Hand Surg Eur Vol 2013;38:50–6.

77. King BA, Stern PJ, Kiefhaber TR. The incidence of trigger finger or de Quervain's tendinitis after carpal tunnel release. J Hand Surg Eur Vol 2013;38:82–3.

78. Lee SK, Bae KW, Choy WS. The relationship of trigger finger and flexor tendod volar migration after carpal tunnel release. J Hand Surg Eur Vol 2014; 39:694–8.

79. Kumar P, Chakrabarti I. Idiopathic carpal tunnel syndrome and trigger finger: is there an association? J Hand Surg Eur Vol 2009;34:58–9.

80. Rottgers SA, Lewis D, Wollstein RA. Concomitant presentation of carpal tunnel syndrome and trigger finger. J Brachial Plex Peripher Nerve Inj 2009;4:13.

Shoulder and Elbow

Injection Therapies for Rotator Cuff Disease

Kenneth M. Lin, MD, Dean Wang, MD*, Joshua S. Dines, MD

KEYWORDS

- Injection • Therapy • Rotator cuff • Calcific tendinitis • Corticosteroid • Prolotherapy
- Platelet-rich plasma • Stem cell

KEY POINTS

- Numerous injection therapies have been used for the treatment of rotator cuff disease, including corticosteroid, prolotherapy, platelet-rich plasma, stem cells, and ultrasound-guided barbotage for calcific tendinitis.
- Although the cornerstone of injection therapy consists of administration of corticosteroids, its efficacy remains debatable in terms of pain relief, improvement in range of motion, and return of shoulder function.
- Existing evidence on prolotherapy, platelet-rich plasma, and stem cell injection therapies for the treatment of rotator cuff disease remains limited.
- Ultimately, improved understanding of the underlying structural and compositional deficiencies of the injured rotator cuff tissue is needed to identify the biological needs that can potentially be targeted with injection therapies.

INTRODUCTION

Shoulder pain is common among the general population, with a reported prevalence of 6.9% to 34.0%,[1] and comprises the third leading musculoskeletal complaint behind back and neck complaints as reasons for physician consultation.[2] Rotator cuff disease accounts for a large proportion of shoulder complaints, especially with increasing age.[3–5] Depending on the patients' precise pathologic conditions, age, activity level, symptoms, level of dysfunction, and findings on physical examination and imaging, a wide variety of treatment modalities have been described for rotator cuff disease. Nonoperative modalities include activity modification, nonsteroidal antiinflammatory drugs (NSAIDs), physical therapy, and various injection therapies. Operative management is generally reserved for select patients or when nonoperative modalities have been exhausted.

Historically, the injection therapy of choice was corticosteroids; however, more recently numerous other injectable therapies have been used for rotator cuff disease, including platelet-rich plasma (PRP), stem cells, and prolotherapy. The purpose of this review is to summarize the current evidence for each type of injection therapy reported in the relevant literature. Although injection therapies are also frequently used in other shoulder conditions, such as adhesive capsulitis (frozen shoulder) and osteoarthritis, these conditions are not discussed in this review.

INDICATIONS

Injections can be used for both diagnostic and therapeutic purposes in rotator cuff disease. For patients presenting with shoulder pain, history and physical examination alone is frequently diagnostic. However, when patients present with shoulder weakness and are unable to participate in a thorough examination because of pain, a subacromial injection consisting of local anesthetic with or without corticosteroids will aid in differentiating between weakness caused by impingement (with improvement in strength

Disclosure Statement: The authors have nothing to disclose.
Sports Medicine and Shoulder Service, Hospital for Special Surgery, 535 East 70th Street, New York, NY, USA
* Corresponding author.
E-mail address: wangde@hss.edu

after injection) or true rotator cuff tear (no change in strength after injection). From a therapeutic standpoint, injections for symptom relief are generally offered for patients with significant symptoms unrelieved by a trial of NSAIDs. The diagnoses in which injection therapies are frequently used are subacromial impingement, degenerative rotator cuff tendinopathy, and calcific tendinitis.

Subacromial impingement is a common diagnosis that represents a spectrum of severity from bursitis to rotator cuff tendinopathy to full-thickness tears, which comprise the 3 Neer stages of the impingement process.[6] The subacromial space refers to the area between the coracoacromial arch and the humeral head where the supraspinatus tendon and biceps lie.[3] The pathology in subacromial impingement originates from compression of the rotator cuff against the lateral acromion most prominently during the arc of shoulder abduction leading to bursitis and cuff inflammation.[7] Predisposing structural factors to subacromial impingement include a type III or hooked acromion,[8,9] acromial spurs as a result of ossification of the coracoacromial ligament insertion,[10] and acromioclavicular joint arthritis.[11] When symptoms are consistent with subacromial impingement and there is absence of acute injury or radiographic findings, patients may be indicated for a subacromial injection.[3] Alternatively, intrinsic rotator cuff tendinopathy leading to thickening of the rotator cuff is also thought to contribute to subacromial impingement and can itself be a cause of shoulder pain. Intrinsic causes of rotator cuff tendinopathy include diminished vascular supply, age-related degeneration, and tensile forces leading to mechanical failure.[6]

Calcific tendinitis is another common rotator cuff condition that should be discussed as a separate entity from subacromial impingement and degenerative rotator cuff tendinopathy. The term *calcific tendinitis* refers to calcium deposition, predominately in the form of hydroxyapatite in the rotator cuff tendons, most frequently the supraspinatus.[12,13] Calcific tendinitis is reported to occur in 2.5% to 7.5% of healthy shoulders, preferentially affecting women and patients in the fifth decade of life.[14] Symptomatically, patients may have a range of presentations from subacute to acute shoulder pain depending on the stage of the disease and the body's immune response to the calcific deposits and, rarely, fevers due to rupture of calcifications into local tissue. Calcific tendinitis is thought to be a self-limited disease that is generally managed with physical therapy and NSAIDs; however, for severe cases, pain

and dysfunction can become significant, warranting more invasive treatment modalities, such as ultrasound-guided barbotage.[15]

CORTICOSTEROIDS

Corticosteroid injections are widely used in orthopedics and general practice and traditionally have been the cornerstone injection therapy in a variety of shoulder conditions.[16] A survey showed that 96% of practitioners, including primary care physicians and physiatrists, think that subacromial corticosteroid injections are efficacious in managing rotator cuff tendinitis.[17] Frequently used corticosteroids in the literature are methylprednisolone and triamcinolone, which are thought to have equivalent potency, followed by betamethasone and dexamethasone, which are proportionally more potent than both methylprednisolone and triamcinolone and, thus, are administered in smaller doses.[16,18,19] Most of the literature on injection therapies for rotator cuff disease focuses on corticosteroids; however, although some studies have reported efficacy in reducing pain and improving function, there is little reproducible evidence.

Historical studies from the 1980s and 1990s reported conflicting results regarding the efficacy of subacromial steroid injection over NSAIDs with respect to improvement in pain, function, or range of motion (ROM), as reported in a 2003 Cochrane systematic review.[19] Although several studies report a benefit of subacromial steroid injection over placebo at short-term time points (4–6 weeks), there was significant heterogeneity among populations and methodologies, precluding pooled analysis across various studies. Of note, a 1990 double-blinded randomized controlled trial (RCT) by Adebajo and colleagues[20] reported an improvement in visual analog scale (VAS) pain score of 3.6 points and an improvement active abduction of 45° versus control at the final follow-up in patients receiving triamcinolone versus placebo injection, both of which were statistically and clinically significant. A similar study by Petri and colleagues[21] reported statistically significant improvements in pain scores as well as an improvement in active shoulder abduction of 28°. A 1996 double-blind RCT by Blair and colleagues[22] corroborated this trend, reporting a 14° improvement in forward elevation compared with controls at 28 weeks. However, numerous other studies have reported no statistical differences in pain scores, ROM, or functional scores compared with placebo.[23–26] A Cochrane systematic review comparing steroid injections and concomitant oral NSAIDs to NSAIDs alone yielded no difference in pain, function, and abduction ROM at various time points.[19]

Similar to the Cochrane review, a more recent systematic review by Koester and colleagues[16] in 2007 concluded that although there are existing data to suggest that subacromial corticosteroid injections relieve pain, increase ROM, and improve function in patients with rotator cuff disease, most studies are limited by methodological flaws leading to little reproducible evidence. Importantly, the investigators noted that when interpreting results from randomized studies, a distinction must be made between clinical and statistical significance. All but one randomized study reported statistically significant differences in pain scores on the magnitude of 0.5 to 1.0 points (centimeters) on the VAS scale, which were deemed clinically insignificant.[16,20–27] Only 2 of 8 studies included that reported on ROM yielded results that reached a minimal clinically important difference (MCID)[20,21] as indicated by a difference in VAS pain score by greater than 0.9 to 1.3 cm.[16,28,29] For ROM, a concrete cutoff for clinical relevance has not established; however, it must be noted ROM assessments have poor interobserver and intraobserver reliability leading to variations up to 10° to 15°.[16,30,31]

A more recent RCT studying the effectiveness of corticosteroid injections versus hyaluronic acid versus placebo in patients with subacromial impingement showed that at the 3-, 6-, and 12-week follow-up, patients receiving corticosteroids had improved pain and functional scores compared with those receiving hyaluronic acid but similar results to the placebo group.[32] Specifically, at 12 weeks, there was a reduction in VAS score of 7% in the hyaluronic acid group, 28% in the corticosteroid group, and 23% in the placebo group; by 26 weeks, there was no difference among any of the groups.

A 2016 meta-analysis of subacromial corticosteroid injections for pain due to rotator cuff tendinosis pooled 726 patients from 11 studies and found no significant reduction in pain compared with placebo at 3 months.[33] However, they did note a statistically significant relief in pain at a magnitude of a standardized mean difference VAS score of 0.52 (corrected for variability in pooling) in corticosteroid injection compared with placebo between 4 and 8 weeks, which they classify as minimally to mildly clinically relevant. Furthermore, they found that multiple injections in succession do not provide an added benefit over a single injection at any time point.

Finally, regarding subacromial corticosteroid injections, the accuracy of injection must be taken into account. Several studies have assessed injection accuracy and its impact on clinical outcomes (Table 1). A Japanese study using arthrographic evaluation concluded that injections using a lateral approach reached the subacromial space 70% of the time. Unintentionally, 21% were in the deltoid, 4% in the glenohumeral joint, and 5% subcutaneously.[34] A recent prospective study similarly reported an injection accuracy of 70%, although, among all injections, there was no difference in terms of pain, function, or patient satisfaction in patients who received accurate and inaccurate injections at 3 months.[35]

PROLOTHERAPY

Another injection therapy that has been described for the treatment of chronic painful rotator cuff tendinopathy is prolotherapy or hypertonic dextrose injection.[37] Although the exact mechanism of this type of treatment remains unclear, it is thought that injection of an irritant solution at painful ligament and tendon insertions stimulates local healing through proliferation of scar tissue.[38] Most of the literature on prolotherapy is limited to the treatment of knee osteoarthritis, and the literature on prolotherapy in the shoulder is limited to small retrospective series outside of North America. Lee and colleagues[39] conducted a retrospective case-control study among a heterogeneous Korean population with rotator cuff disease showing that prolotherapy injection led to improvement in VAS score, Shoulder Pain and Disability Index (SPADI) score, isometric strength, and active ROM compared with continued conservative management without injection. A similar study conducted in a Turkish population by Seven and colleagues[40] showed similar results with improvement in VAS, SPADI, and Western Ontario Rotatory Cuff Index at up to 1 year in patients treated with prolotherapy versus no injection. To the authors' knowledge, there are no comparative studies of prolotherapy with other injection therapies and no RCTs investigating prolotherapy in the literature. Further clinical data as well as an improved understanding of the exact mechanism of action of prolotherapy are needed.

PLATELET-RICH PLASMA

PRP injections locally deliver high concentrations of biological factors essential to the healing process to augment musculoskeletal tissue repair. As a result, the use of PRP for the treatment of

Table 1
Outcomes from recent level I studies of subacromial corticosteroid injection

Study (Type), Year	Location	N	Average Age (y)	Intervention and Control	Follow-up	Outcome Measures	Final Effect Size (Intervention-Control)	Other Notable Findings
McInerney et al,[24] (RCT), 2003	United Kingdom	98	49	Methylprednisolone vs bupivicaine[a]	3, 6, 12 wk	VAS Abduction	0 cm (P = .99) 1.4° (P = .8)	—
Akgun et al,[27] (RCT), 2004	Turkey	32	49	Methylprednisolone vs lignocaine[a]	1, 3 mo	VAS Constant score	0.1 (P>.05) 0 (P>.05)	Difference in VAS of 1.1 at 1 mo (P<.001)
Alvarez et al,[23] (RCT), 2005	Canada	58	55	Betamethasone vs xylocaine[a]	3, 6 mo	WORC ASES DASH	-8.0 (P = .38) -1.9 (P = .89) 0.3 (P = .86)	—
Hong et al,[36] (RCT), 2011	South Korea	54	50	Triamcinolone vs lidocaine[a]	2, 4, 8 wk	VAS Forward flexion Abduction	-2.7 cm (P<.05) 7° (P = .21) 23.5° (P<.05)	—
Penning et al,[32] (RCT), 2012	Netherlands	106	53	Triamcinolone vs lidocaine[a]	3, 6, 12, 26 wk	VAS Constant score	-0.1 cm (P>.05) -1.9 (P>.05)	Difference in VAS of 1.2 at 6 wk (P<.001)
Mohamadi et al,[33] (meta-analysis), 2017	Multicenter	726 (pooled)		Results: minimal to mild statistically and clinically significant improvement in pain at 4–8 wk, adjusted standardized mean difference VAS score 0.52, NNT = 5				

Abbreviations: ASES, American Shoulder and Elbow Surgeons standardized form; DASH, disabilities of the arm, shoulder, and hand; NNT, number needed to treat; WORC, Western Ontario Rotator Cuff Index.
[a] Intervention injection also contained local anesthetic.

rotator cuff disease has been extensively studied through multiple RCTs and meta-analyses. However, it is important to note that there remains substantial variability in the methods of PRP production among commercial systems.[41–43] Furthermore, within a given separation technique, there is a high degree of intersubject and intrasubject variability in the composition of PRP produced.[44] This variability, along with the heterogeneity among studies regarding the means of administration, tear size, and repair technique (single or double row), make it difficult to draw any definitive conclusions on the efficacy of PRP treatment of rotator cuff disease.

Present level I studies report no difference in clinical outcomes in patients who received PRP injection for rotator cuff tendinopathy compared with controls.[45,46] In an RCT of patients with chronic rotator cuff tendinopathy randomized to arthroscopic acromioplasty alone or in combination with a PRP injection, reduced vascularity and cellularity and increased levels of apoptosis were noted in tissue biopsy specimens taken from PRP-treated patients.[45] Additionally, most level I and II studies report no differences in pain and functional scores in patients who received PRP injection as an augment to rotator cuff repair compared with controls.[47–51] In a meta-analysis, Warth and colleagues[47] showed a significantly decreased improvement in the constant score when PRP was injected over the surface of the repaired tendon as opposed to application at the tendon-bone interface; however, this difference was not greater than the threshold for an MCID. The effect of PRP treatment on retear rates after rotator cuff repair remains debatable. Of the studies that assessed the repair site integrity at least 6 months postoperatively, most demonstrated no difference in retear rates.[47,50–53] Nevertheless, some studies have shown that PRP applied at the tendon-bone interface resulted in significantly lower retear rates after the repair of medium to large tears.[47,54,55]

MESENCHYMAL STEM CELLS

Mesenchymal stem cells (MSCs) derived from bone marrow (Fig. 1) and adipose (Fig. 2) have garnered the most attention for use in rotator cuff healing because of their multipotent potential and ability to exert paracrine effects, such as modulating and controlling inflammation, stimulating endogenous cell repair and proliferation, inhibiting apoptosis, and improving blood flow.[56,57] Like PRP augmentation therapy, continued research is needed to identify the optimal cell source and the ideal treatment protocol needed to drive cell differentiation and create an optimal healing environment that directs regeneration of the native fibrocartilaginous enthesis. Currently, only a few studies have examined the effect of augmentative MSC therapy on rotator cuff repair in humans, with early results suggesting a possible improvement in repair site healing.[58–60] In a level III study, Kim and colleagues[58] reported no difference in pain and functional scores in patients who received an injection of adipose-derived

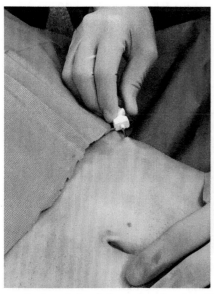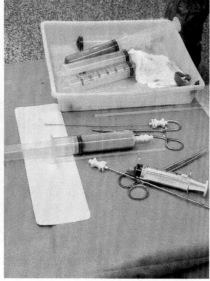

Fig. 1. Lipo-aspiration of the abdominal midsection. The lipo-aspirate is then processed to form an injectable solution containing MSCs.

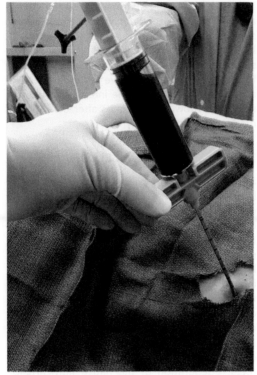

Fig. 2. Bone marrow aspirate is taken from the iliac crest with the use of a needle. The bone marrow aspirate is then processed and concentrated to form an injection solution containing MSCs.

MSCs as an augment to rotator cuff repair compared with controls. However, MRI obtained at a minimum of 1 year indicated a significantly lower retear rate (14.3%) in patients treated with MSCs compared with controls (28.5%).

ULTRASOUND-GUIDED NEEDLE THERAPIES FOR CALCIFIC TENDINITIS

Severe cases of calcific tendinitis that require invasive treatment modalities have traditionally been treated with subacromial corticosteroid injections; however, more recently, barbotage has become increasingly popular (Fig. 3).[15] Barbotage was first introduced in 1937[61] and involves image-guided insertion of a needle directly into a calcific deposit, followed by lavage (usually with normal saline) to dissolve the deposit.[15,62] The increasing use of ultrasound as an imaging alternative has made this technique radiation free and more accessible.[61]

A 2013 systematic review assessing the efficacy of ultrasound-guided needle treatments for calcific tendinitis included 11 articles and concluded that all studies in the literature were of low quality and that there was no difference in pain relief between needle lavage and other interventions.[63] A recent RCT in the Netherlands compared barbotage with subacromial corticosteroid injection and found that clinical and radiographic outcomes at 1 year were superior in the barbotage group.[15] Specifically, at 1 year they reported a 12.1-point improvement in the mean constant score, 6.5-mm improvement in calcification size decrease, and a greater proportion of total resorption in the barbotage group compared with the corticosteroid group. These results corroborate those from a previously reported prospective nonrandomized trial of ultrasound-guided barbotage versus control in Italy showing a 13.3-point improvement in the constant score and a 1.8-point improvement in the VAS score at 1 year.[62] In this study, significant improvements in the constant score and the VAS score were seen as early as 1 month and maintained beyond 1 year but were no longer present at the follow-up at 5 and 10 years.

Interestingly, some investigators think that some of the observed therapeutic effects of barbotage may be attributed to fenestration of the tendon causing a natural healing response.[64] A recent small randomized study in China

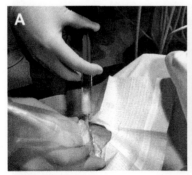
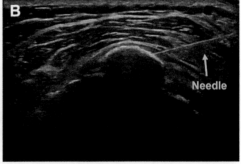

Fig. 3. (A) Ultrasound-guided barbotage of calcific tendinitis in the supraspinatus. (B) Ultrasound image demonstrating insertion of a needle directly into a calcific deposit, followed by lavage (usually with normal saline) to dissolve the deposit.

showed that patients undergoing ultrasound-guided barbotage versus ultrasound-guided fenestration experienced a similar degree of pain relief from 1 to 36 weeks.[65]

Although limited evidence does exist to support the use of ultrasound-guided needle therapies in calcific tendinitis of the shoulder, at least in the short-term, further high-quality studies are required to more definitively determine its efficacy and understand its mechanism of action. Apart from improved study quality, further studies should also aim to clarify whether certain patient populations (based on number and size of calcifications) may benefit more than others.[63]

SUMMARY

Rotator cuff disease affects a large proportion of the overall population and encompasses a wide spectrum of pathologies, including subacromial impingement, rotator cuff tendinopathy or tear, and calcific tendinitis. Various injection therapies have been used for the treatment of rotator cuff disease. Although the cornerstone of traditional injection therapy involves the administration of corticosteroids, the evidence on its efficacy remains debatable in terms of pain relief, improvement in ROM, and return of shoulder function. Several newer injection therapies have gained popularity, including prolotherapy, PRP, stem cells, and ultrasound-guided barbotage for calcific tendinitis. However, the existing evidence for each type of therapy is currently limited. Ultimately, improved understanding of the underlying structural and compositional deficiencies of the injured rotator cuff tissue is needed to identify the biological needs that can potentially be targeted with injection therapies.

REFERENCES

1. Chard MD, Hazleman R, Hazleman BL, et al. Shoulder disorders in the elderly: a community survey. Arthritis Rheum 1991;34(6):766–9.

2. Rekola KE, Keinanen-Kiukaanniemi S, Takala J. Use of primary health services in sparsely populated country districts by patients with musculoskeletal symptoms: consultations with a physician. J Epidemiol Community Health 1993;47(2):153–7.

3. Gruson KI, Ruchelsman DE, Zuckerman JD. Subacromial corticosteroid injections. J Shoulder Elbow Surg 2008;17(1):118S–30S.

4. Varkey DT, Patterson BM, Creighton RA, et al. Initial medical management of rotator cuff tears: a demographic analysis of surgical and nonsurgical treatment in the United States Medicare population. J Shoulder Elbow Surg 2016;25(12):e378–85.

5. Schmidt CC, Jarrett CD, Brown BT. Management of rotator cuff tears. J Hand Surg Am 2015;40(2):399–408.

6. Harrison AK, Flatow EL. Subacromial impingement syndrome. J Am Acad Orthop Surg 2011;19(11):701–8.

7. Watson-Jones R. Fractures and other bone and joint injuries. Baltimore (MD): Williams & Wilkins; 1940.

8. Epstein RE, Schweitzer ME, Frieman BG, et al. Hooked acromion: prevalence on MR images of painful shoulders. Radiology 1993;187(2):479–81.

9. Toivonen DA, Tuite MJ, Orwin JF. Acromial structure and tears of the rotator cuff. J Shoulder Elbow Surg 1995;4(5):376–83.

10. Neer CS 2nd. Anterior acromioplasty for the chronic impingement syndrome in the shoulder: a preliminary report. J Bone Joint Surg Am 1972;54(1):41–50.

11. Chen AL, Rokito AS, Zuckerman JD. The role of the acromioclavicular joint in impingement syndrome. Clin Sports Med 2003;22(2):343–57.

12. Bosworth B. Calcium deposits in the shoulder and subacromial bursitis: a survey of 12,122 shoulders. J Am Med Assoc 1941;116(22):2477–82.

13. Mole D, Gonzalvez M, Roche O, et al. Introduction to calcifying tendinitis. In: Gazielly D, Gleyze P, Thomas T, editors. The cuff. Paris: Elsevier; 1997. p. 141–3.

14. Speed CA, Hazleman BL. Calcific tendinitis of the shoulder. N Engl J Med 1999;340(20):1582–4.

15. de Witte PB, Selten JW, Navas A, et al. Calcific tendinitis of the rotator cuff: a randomized controlled trial of ultrasound-guided needling and lavage versus subacromial corticosteroids. Am J Sports Med 2013;41(7):1665–73.

16. Koester MC, Dunn WR, Kuhn JE, et al. The efficacy of subacromial corticosteroid injection in the treatment of rotator cuff disease: a systematic review. J Am Acad Orthop Surg 2007;15(1):3–11.

17. Johansson K, Oberg B, Adolfsson L, et al. A combination of systematic review and clinicians' beliefs in interventions for subacromial pain. Br J Gen Pract 2002;52(475):145–52.

18. Schimmer BP, Parker KL. Adrenocorticotropic hormone, adrenocortical steroids and their synthetic analogs; inhibitors of the synthesis and actions of adrenocortical hormones. In: Hardman JG, Limbird LE, editors. Goodman and Gillman's the parmacological basis of therapeutics. 10th edition. New York: McGraw-Hill; 2001. p. 1649–78.

19. Buchbinder R, Green S, Youd JM. Corticosteroid injections for shoulder pain. Cochrane Database Syst Rev 2003;(1):CD004016.

20. Adebajo AO, Nash P, Hazleman BL. A prospective double blind dummy placebo controlled study comparing triamcinolone hexacetonide injection with oral diclofenac 50 mg TDS in patients with rotator cuff tendinitis. J Rheumatol 1990;17(9):1207–10.

21. Petri M, Dobrow R, Neiman R, et al. Randomized, double-blind, placebo-controlled study of the treatment of the painful shoulder. Arthritis Rheum 1987;30(9):1040–5.

22. Blair B, Rokito AS, Cuomo F, et al. Efficacy of injections of corticosteroids for subacromial impingement syndrome. J Bone Joint Surg Am 1996;78(11): 1685–9.

23. Alvarez CM, Litchfield R, Jackowski D, et al. A prospective, double-blind, randomized clinical trial comparing subacromial injection of betamethasone and xylocaine to xylocaine alone in chronic rotator cuff tendinosis. Am J Sports Med 2005; 33(2):255–62.

24. McInerney JJ, Dias J, Durham S, et al. Randomised controlled trial of single, subacromial injection of methylprednisolone in patients with persistent, post-traumatic impingement of the shoulder. Emerg Med J 2003;20(3):218–21.

25. Vecchio PC, Hazleman BL, King RH. A double-blind trial comparing subacromial methylprednisolone and lignocaine in acute rotator cuff tendinitis. Br J Rheumatol 1993;32(8):743–5.

26. Withrington RH, Girgis FL, Seifert MH. A placebo-controlled trial of steroid injections in the treatment of supraspinatus tendonitis. Scand J Rheumatol 1985;14(1):76–8.

27. Akgun K, Birtane M, Akarirmak U. Is local subacromial corticosteroid injection beneficial in subacromial impingement syndrome? Clin Rheumatol 2004;23(6):496–500.

28. Kelly A. The minimum clinically significant difference in visual analogue scale pain score does not differ with severity of pain. Emerg Med J 2001; 18(3):205–7.

29. Todd KH. Clinical versus statistical significance in the assessment of pain relief. Ann Emerg Med 1996;27(4):439–41.

30. Hoving J, Buchbinder R, Green S, et al. How reliably do rheumatologists measure shoulder movement? Ann Rheum Dis 2002;61(7):612–6.

31. Mallon WJ, Herring CL, Sallay PI, et al. Use of vertebral levels to measure presumed internal rotation at the shoulder: a radiographic analysis. J Shoulder Elbow Surg 1996;5(4):299–306.

32. Penning LI, de Bie RA, Walenkamp GH. The effectiveness of injections of hyaluronic acid or corticosteroid in patients with subacromial impingement: a three-arm randomised controlled trial. J Bone Joint Surg Br 2012;94(9):1246–52.

33. Mohamadi A, Chan JJ, Claessen FM, et al. Corticosteroid injections give small and transient pain relief in rotator cuff tendinosis: a meta-analysis. Clin Orthop Relat Res 2017;475(1):232–43.

34. Yamakado K. The targeting accuracy of subacromial injection to the shoulder: an arthrographic evaluation. Arthroscopy 2002;18(8):887–91.

35. Kang MN, Rizio L, Prybicien M, et al. The accuracy of subacromial corticosteroid injections: a comparison of multiple methods. J Shoulder Elbow Surg 2008;17(1 Suppl):61s–6s.

36. Hong JY, Yoon S-H, Moon DJ, et al. Comparison of high- and low-dose corticosteroid in subacromial injection for periarticular shoulder disorder: a randomized, triple-blind, placebo-controlled trial. Arch Phys Med Rehabil 2011; 92(12):1951–60.

37. Bertrand H, Reeves KD, Bennett CJ, et al. Dextrose prolotherapy versus control injections in painful rotator cuff tendinopathy. Arch Phys Med Rehabil 2016;97(1):17–25.

38. Rabago D, Patterson JJ, Mundt M, et al. Dextrose prolotherapy for knee osteoarthritis: a randomized controlled trial. Ann Fam Med 2013;11(3):229–37.

39. Lee DH, Kwack KS, Rah UW, et al. Prolotherapy for refractory rotator cuff disease: retrospective case-control study of 1-year follow-up. Arch Phys Med Rehabil 2015;96(11):2027–32.

40. Seven MM, Ersen O, Akpancar S, et al. Effectiveness of prolotherapy in the treatment of chronic rotator cuff lesions. Orthop Traumatol Surg Res 2017; 103(3):427–33.

41. Castillo TN, Pouliot MA, Kim HJ, et al. Comparison of growth factor and platelet concentration from commercial platelet-rich plasma separation systems. Am J Sports Med 2011;39(2):266–71.

42. Oh JH, Kim W, Park KU, et al. Comparison of the cellular composition and cytokine-release kinetics of various platelet-rich plasma preparations. Am J Sports Med 2015;43(12):3062–70.

43. Degen RM, Bernard JA, Oliver KS, et al. Commercial separation systems designed for preparation of platelet-rich plasma yield differences in cellular composition. HSS J 2017;13(1):75–80.

44. Mazzocca AD, McCarthy MB, Chowaniec DM, et al. Platelet-rich plasma differs according to preparation method and human variability. J Bone Joint Surg Am 2012;94(4):308–16.

45. Carr AJ, Murphy R, Dakin SG, et al. Platelet-rich plasma injection with arthroscopic acromioplasty for chronic rotator cuff tendinopathy: a randomized controlled trial. Am J Sports Med 2015; 43(12):2891–7.

46. Kesikburun S, Tan AK, Yilmaz B, et al. Platelet-rich plasma injections in the treatment of chronic rotator cuff tendinopathy: a randomized controlled trial with 1-year follow-up. Am J Sports Med 2013; 41(11):2609–16.

47. Warth RJ, Dornan GJ, James EW, et al. Clinical and structural outcomes after arthroscopic repair of full-thickness rotator cuff tears with and without platelet-rich product supplementation: a meta-analysis and meta-regression. Arthroscopy 2015; 31(2):306–20.

48. Flury M, Rickenbacher D, Schwyzer HK, et al. Does pure platelet-rich plasma affect postoperative clinical outcomes after arthroscopic rotator cuff repair? A randomized controlled trial. Am J Sports Med 2016;44(8):2136–46.

49. Castricini R, Longo UG, De Benedetto M, et al. Platelet-rich plasma augmentation for arthroscopic rotator cuff repair: a randomized controlled trial. Am J Sports Med 2011;39(2):258–65.

50. Malavolta EA, Gracitelli ME, Ferreira Neto AA, et al. Platelet-rich plasma in rotator cuff repair: a prospective randomized study. Am J Sports Med 2014;42(10):2446–54.

51. Wang A, McCann P, Colliver J, et al. Do postoperative platelet-rich plasma injections accelerate early tendon healing and functional recovery after arthroscopic supraspinatus repair? A randomized controlled trial. Am J Sports Med 2015;43(6):1430–7.

52. Randelli P, Arrigoni P, Ragone V, et al. Platelet rich plasma in arthroscopic rotator cuff repair: a prospective RCT study, 2-year follow-up. J Shoulder Elbow Surg 2011;20(4):518–28.

53. Ruiz-Moneo P, Molano-Munoz J, Prieto E, et al. Plasma rich in growth factors in arthroscopic rotator cuff repair: a randomized, double-blind, controlled clinical trial. Arthroscopy 2013;29(1):2–9.

54. Pandey V, Bandi A, Madi S, et al. Does application of moderately concentrated platelet-rich plasma improve clinical and structural outcome after arthroscopic repair of medium-sized to large rotator cuff tear? A randomized controlled trial. J Shoulder Elbow Surg 2016;25(8):1312–22.

55. Jo CH, Shin JS, Shin WH, et al. Platelet-rich plasma for arthroscopic repair of medium to large rotator cuff tears: a randomized controlled trial. Am J Sports Med 2015;43(9):2102–10.

56. Caplan AI. Review: mesenchymal stem cells: cell-based reconstructive therapy in orthopedics. Tissue Eng 2005;11(7–8):1198–211.

57. Veronesi F, Giavaresi G, Tschon M, et al. Clinical use of bone marrow, bone marrow concentrate, and expanded bone marrow mesenchymal stem cells in cartilage disease. Stem Cell Dev 2013;22(2):181–92.

58. Kim YS, Sung CH, Chung SH, et al. Does an injection of adipose-derived mesenchymal stem cells loaded in fibrin glue influence rotator cuff repair outcomes? A clinical and magnetic resonance imaging study. Am J Sports Med 2017;45(9):2010–8.

59. Hernigou P, Flouzat Lachaniette CH, Delambre J, et al. Biologic augmentation of rotator cuff repair with mesenchymal stem cells during arthroscopy improves healing and prevents further tears: a case-controlled study. Int Orthop 2014;38(9):1811–8.

60. Ellera Gomes JL, da Silva RC, Silla LM, et al. Conventional rotator cuff repair complemented by the aid of mononuclear autologous stem cells. Knee Surg Sports Traumatol Arthrosc 2012;20(2):373–7.

61. Comfort TH, Arafiles RP. Barbotage of the shoulder with image-intensified fluoroscopic control of needle placement for calcific tendinitis. Clin Orthop Relat Res 1978;(135):171–8.

62. Serafini G, Sconfienza LM, Lacelli F, et al. Rotator cuff calcific tendonitis: short-term and 10-year outcomes after two-needle us-guided percutaneous treatment–nonrandomized controlled trial. Radiology 2009;252(1):157–64.

63. Vignesh KN, McDowall A, Simunovic N, et al. Efficacy of ultrasound-guided percutaneous needle treatment of calcific tendinitis. AJR Am J Roentgenol 2015;204(1):148–52.

64. Chiavaras MM, Jacobson JA. Ultrasound-guided tendon fenestration. Semin Musculoskelet Radiol 2013;17(1):85–90.

65. Zhu J, Jiang Y, Hu Y, et al. Evaluating the long-term effect of ultrasound-guided needle puncture without aspiration on calcifying supraspinatus tendinitis. Adv Ther 2008;25(11):1229–34.

Antibiotic Prophylaxis and Prevention of Surgical Site Infection in Shoulder and Elbow Surgery

K. Keely Boyle, MD*, Thomas R. Duquin, MD

KEYWORDS

- Antibiotic prophylaxis • Surgical site infection • Infection prevention • Shoulder surgery
- Elbow surgery • Shoulder arthroplasty

KEY POINTS

- The Centers for Disease Control and Prevention and the Musculoskeletal Infection Society current recommendations for prevention of surgical site infection incorporate the following: risk mitigation by host optimization, appropriate selection of perioperative antibiotics, preoperative skin preparation, operative environment, and wound management.
- Antibiotic prophylaxis in the shoulder and elbow should be carefully considered when assessing the unique susceptibility patterns of the common bacteria within this microbiome, especially *Propionibacterium acnes*.
- Standard surgical site sterilization protocols have been unable to eliminate bacterial contamination. Residual bacterial contamination, specifically *P acnes*, has been identified in superficial and deep tissues during clean procedures. Further research is needed to determine the significance of this contamination and the role of additional techniques for surgical site preparation.
- The potential mechanical advantage of irrigation before closure for reduction of bacterial burden is recognized, but the abundance of conflicting evidence precludes consensus on recommending any agent versus another.
- A summary of the author's current practice is included, although additional research is needed to help guide treatment protocols that allow for the highest level of prevention while avoiding unnecessary or potentially detrimental interventions.

INTRODUCTION

Infection after orthopedic procedures is a devastating and serious complication associated with significant clinical and financial challenges to the health care system and the unfortunate suffering patient. Surgical site infections (SSIs) are associated with extensive therapeutic regimens, technically difficult revision surgeries, poor patient outcomes, and substantially increased costs to the health care system. There has been an increase in the number of orthopedic procedures performed in the United States, especially upper extremity arthroplasty procedures.[1,2] The growth rates of upper extremity arthroplasty procedures are noted to be between 7% to 13% annually and have been shown to be comparable to growth rates for total hip and knee procedures. Between 1993 and 2007, primary total shoulder and total elbow arthroplasty

Disclosure Statement: Neither author has any commercial or financial disclosures that are relevant to the creation of this article. There was no external funding provided for the development of this article.
Department of Orthopaedics, State University of New York at Buffalo, Erie County Medical Center, 462 Grider Street, Buffalo, NY 14215, USA
* Corresponding author.
E-mail address: kkboyle@buffalo.edu

procedures increased by 369% and 248%, respectively.[3] Total shoulder arthroplasty rates are projected to increase by more than 150% by the year 2020.[1] A similar trend has been noted in recent years, in which a significant increase has been witnessed in the incidence of arthroscopic and open procedures treating shoulder and elbow injuries.[4–11] This includes a notable 600% increase in the number of arthroscopic rotator cuff repairs witnessed between 1996 and 2006.[5]

Periprosthetic joint infection (PJI) accounts for a substantial percentage of shoulder arthroplasty procedure complications, with failure rates reported as high as 15.4%.[12–15] The prevalence of SSI for all orthopedic procedures is reported to be between 0.6% and 2.55%.[16,17] There is growing concern surrounding the current and predicted economic burden of PJI and SSI due to the rapid increase in the number of arthroplasty and other orthopedic procedures being performed, and the increasing rate of infection.[18] Most cost analysis data and fiscal implications for treating infection stems from total knee arthroplasty (TKA) and total hip arthroplasty (THA) procedures and can be used as a framework for assessing the financial impact associated with revisions for infection of shoulder and elbow procedures. The direct medical cost for treating a case of infected THA is 2.8 times higher than for other causes of revision and 4.8 times higher than primary THA.[19] Early literature reported costs per case averaging $100,000, resulting in financial losses for hospitals between $15,000 and $30,000 per patient, with inpatient costs expected to double by 2020.[18–22] This cost disparity is largely driven by the characteristics associated with revision procedures for infection: longer operative times with a higher number of total surgical procedures, longer length of stay, subsequent hospitalizations with higher inpatient charges, higher complication rates, administration of long-term antibiotics, and more outpatient visits.[23] The time and resource-intensive nature of treating infection after orthopedic procedures has turned attention toward enhancing preventative efforts and establishing quality improvement measures. Infection prevention strategies include risk mitigation, host optimization, reducing bacterial burden, and wound management throughout all phases of the perioperative period.

PREVENTION OF SURGICAL SITE INFECTION AND PERIPROSTHETIC JOINT INFECTION

In 2002, the Centers for Disease Control and Prevention (CDC) and Centers for Medicare and Medicaid Services (CMS) instituted the Surgical Infection Prevention project, which later became the Surgical Care Improvement Program (SCIP). The expansion to SCIP included enhanced antimicrobial prophylaxis recommendations, patient hair removal at the surgical site, glycemic control, and normothermia process measures.[24,25] In 2009, the US Department of Health and Human Services set a 5-year target goal of a 25% reduction in SSI detected on admission and readmission through the implementation of the *National Action Plan to Prevent Health Care-Associated Infections: Road Map to Elimination*. The CMS Hospital Inpatient Quality Reporting Program has required hospitals to report SSI outcome data since 2012; through the Deficit Reduction Act of 2005, payments are adjusted downward for health care–associated infections.[26] In May of 2017, the CDC released guidelines for prevention of SSI that are generalizable across surgical procedures and recommended integration of these guidelines to improve patient safety.[25] The first two aspects of prevention discussed are parenteral and nonparenteral antimicrobial prophylaxis. A summary of the relevant recommendations is found in Table 1.

Despite technological advances, scientific discoveries, and improved care pathways, infection continues to provide a very complex and difficult problem for the treating surgeon. The Musculoskeletal Infection Society (MSIS) and the European Bone and Joint Infection Society, along with numerous other societies, developed an interdisciplinary team of more than 400 experts from orthopedic surgery, infectious disease, musculoskeletal disease, microbiology, dermatology, rheumatology, musculoskeletal radiology, pharmaceutics, and scientists to critically evaluate the current evidence and reach a consensus on recommendations. The consensus statements on current practices for preventing SSI and PJI were presented at the most recent International Consensus Meeting on Surgical Site and Periprosthetic Joint Infection in 2013.[23] The recommendations included risk mitigation, perioperative antibiotics, preoperative skin preparation, operative environment, and wound management.

RISK MITIGATION AND HOST OPTIMIZATION

Host optimization incorporates various defined categories termed modifiable risk factors that have the potential to be changed or optimized in the perioperative period to help reduce the

Table 1
Centers for Disease Control and Prevention 2017 guidelines for prevention of surgical site infection

Core Section	Relevant Recommendations	Recommendation Category
Parenteral Antimicrobial Prophylaxis	Administer preoperative antimicrobial agents only when indicated, timed such that serum or tissue bactericidal concentration is established before incision	Category IB
	Weight-adjusted dosing No literature to support effects on risk of SSI	No recommendation
	Do not administer additional antibiotics after surgical incision is closed for clean or clean-contaminated procedures	Category IA
Nonparenteral Antimicrobial Prophylaxis	Do not apply antimicrobial agents to surgical incision	Category IB
	Application autologous platelet-rich plasma not necessary	Category II
	Antimicrobial dressings applied to surgical incision after primary closure	No recommendation
Glycemic Control	Implement perioperative glycemic control, blood glucose target <200 mg/dL	Category IA
	Optimal HbA1C target	No recommendation
Normothermia	Maintain perioperative normothermia	Category IA
Oxygenation	Administer increased fraction of inspired oxygen during surgery and immediate postoperative period to optimize tissue oxygen delivery, maintain perioperative normothermia and adequate volume replacement (normal pulmonary function)	Category IA
Antiseptic Prophylaxis	Advise patients to shower or bathe with soap or antiseptic agent on at least the night before operative day	Category IB
	Application microbial sealant after intraoperative skin preparation not necessary	Category II
	Consider intraoperative irrigation of deep or subcutaneous tissues with aqueous iodophor solution	Category II
Blood Transfusion	Do not withhold transfusion of necessary blood products from surgical patients as a means to prevent SSI	Category IB
Systemic Immunosuppressive Therapy	Available evidence suggests uncertain tradeoffs between benefits and harms of systemic corticosteroid or immunosuppressive therapies on risk of SSI	No recommendation or unresolved issue
Intraarticular Corticosteroid Injection	Available evidence suggests uncertain tradeoffs between benefits and harms of use and timing of perioperative intraarticular corticosteroid infection on SSI	No recommendation or unresolved issue
Anticoagulation	Available evidence suggests uncertain tradeoffs between benefits and harms of venous thromboembolism prophylaxis on incidence of SSI	No recommendation or unresolved issue
Orthopedic Surgical Space Suit	Available evidence suggests uncertain tradeoffs between benefits and harms of orthopedic space suits or the health care personnel who should wear them	No recommendation or unresolved issue

(continued on next page)

Core Section	Relevant Recommendations	Recommendation Category
Drain Use	Do not administer additional antibiotics after surgical incision is closed in presence of a drain	Category IA
Biofilm	Prosthesis modifications or use of biofilm control agents, dispersants quorum-sensing inhibitors novel antimicrobial agents for prevention of biofilm formation or SSI	No recommendation or unresolved issue

Category IA, a strong recommendation supported by high to moderate-quality evidence suggesting net clinical benefits or harms; Category IB, a strong recommendation supported by low-quality evidence suggesting net clinical benefits or harms or an accepted practice supported by low to very low-quality evidence; Category IC, a strong recommendation required by state or federal regulation; Category II, a weak recommendation supported by any quality evidence suggesting a trade-off between clinical benefits and harms; No recommendation or unresolved issue, An issue for which there is low to very low-quality evidence with uncertain tradeoffs between the benefits and harms or no published evidence on outcomes.
 Abbreviation: HbA1C, hemoglobin A1C.
 Data from Berrios-Torres SI, Umscheid CA, Bratzler DW, et al. Centers for Disease Control and Prevention Guideline for the Prevention of Surgical Site Infection, 2017. JAMA Surg 2017;152(8):784–91.

associated risk of SSI and PJI. The MSIS assessed and reached a consensus on the areas in which risk mitigation and host optimization would be most influential in preventing SSI or PJI after arthroplasty procedures (Table 2).[23,25,27]

UNIQUE ISSUES RELATED TO THE SHOULDER
Offending Organisms
Understanding the most common offending organisms of the shoulder and their hypothesized mechanism of infection is crucial to selecting appropriate preventative measures. The most common organism isolated from SSIs from orthopedic procedures of the shoulder and elbow are Propionibacterium acnes, Staphylococcus aureus, and coagulase-negative staphylococci (CONS).[28] The microbiome of the shoulder demonstrates distinctive qualities compared with other orthopedic surgical sites, including the presence of sebaceous and apocrine glands.[29] The skin surrounding the shoulder is colonized by a diverse milieu of microorganisms, most of which are harmless or can be beneficial to their host. Several factors influence colonization, including the skin surface topography, endogenous host factors, and exogenous environmental factors.[30] The axilla harbors high concentrations of sebaceous glands that are connected to a hair follicle, forming a pilosebaceous unit that secretes a lipid-rich substance called sebum, which protects and lubricates the skin providing antibacterial qualities. The growth of P acnes, a facultative anaerobe, is supported by this lipid-rich environment.[31] This common commensal bacterium encodes many genes for lipases that degrade sebum and produce free fatty acids, which contribute to the acidic pH of the axilla.[32] Subsequently, common pathogens, such as S aureus, are inhibited by this acidic pH, which then favors the growth of CONS and cornyebacteria.[33] Interestingly, skin occlusion results in an increased pH, which in turn the favors the growth of S aureus.[34]

Propionibacterium acnes
The prevalence of P acnes in periprosthetic shoulder infections has been shown to equal or exceed that of other common offending organisms.[35] A recent study of 48 subjects who underwent revision shoulder arthroplasty with positive intraoperative cultures noted that 38% were infected with P acnes, 35% with CONS, and 13% with S aureus.[36] The high prevalence of P acnes is unique to the shoulder and other groups have noted a similar trend and distribution of offending organisms in patients determined to have a definite periprosthetic shoulder infection.[37] P acnes was previously thought to be a culture contaminant, mainly because of the presumed indolent nature of the bacterium, as well as identification on normal skin flora and maintenance of the microbiome. P acnes is now recognized and accepted in the orthopedic community as a pathogenic organism. Genomic studies have isolated distinct phylotypes (IA, IB, II, III) that are associated with orthopedic implants. Type IB is the most commonly isolated phylotype from infected prostheses.[38] These phylotypes have varying adaptive virulence properties that may influence pathogenic potential, including the ability to degrade and invade

Table 2
Risk mitigation and host optimization in prevention of surgical site infection and periprosthetic joint infection

Potential Risk Factors		Modifiable Risk Factors	
		Risk Factor	Recommended Target
Morbid obesity	BMI >40 kg/m^2	Obesity	<40 kg/m^2
Poorly controlled diabetes	Glucose >200 mg/L or HbA1C >7%	Diabetes	Fasting glucose <180 mg/dL; HbA1C <7%
Malnutrition	—	Rheumatoid arthritis	—
Chronic renal disease	ESRD on hemodialysis	Depression	—
Active liver disease	Asymptomatic hepatitis and cirrhosis	Immunosuppressive medications	—
Excessive smoking	>1 pack per day	Nicotine use	Tobacco-free 4 wk before surgery
History of previous surgery on affected joint	Appropriate infection workup before revision surgery; ESR, CRP, CBC, aspiration if elevated inflammatory markers	Malnutrition[a] (serum levels)	Albumin 3.5–5.0 g/dL, prealbumin 15–35 mg/dL, transferrin 204–360 mg/dL, total lymphocyte count 800–2000 mm^3
Excessive alcohol consumption	>40 units per week	Anemia of chronic disease	—
IV drug abuse	—	Alcohol abuse	Cessation 4 wk before surgery
Recent hospitalization	Within 6 mo	IV drug abuse	Complete cessation before offering elective procedure
Extended stay in rehabilitation facility	—	Human immunodeficiency virus	CD4 count >400 cells/mL, undetectable viral load
Male gender	—	Operating time	<115 min
Diagnosis of posttraumatic arthritis	—	Operative normothermia	—
Diagnosis of inflammatory arthropathy	—	Allogeneic blood transfusion	—
Severe immunodeficiency	Human immunodeficiency virus	S aureus colonization	—

Abbreviations: BMI, body mass index (kg/m^2); CBC, complete blood count; CRP, C-reactive protein; ESR, erythrocyte sedimentation rate; ESRD, end-stage renal disease; IV, intravenous.

[a] Although optimal method of malnutrition correction is unknown, current suggestions include high-protein supplements, vitamin and mineral supplementation, appropriate calorie intake, appropriate weight loss, nutrition counseling, early mobilization, and physiotherapy.

host cells, produce an enhanced host inflammatory response, form biofilms on orthopedic implants, and demonstrate antibiotic resistance.[39–41] Beta-hemolytic activity has been noted in certain strains of P acnes and may be directly correlated with the bacteria's pathogenicity (Fig. 1).[42] The cohemolytic Christie-Atkins-Munch-Peterson (CAMP) factor is found in the P acnes genome and functions as a toxin to host cells, which may be responsible for this observed beta-hemolytic activity.[40,43]

Interestingly, a recent study by Levy and colleagues[44] discovered a high prevalence of P acnes in primary shoulder arthroplasty in subjects

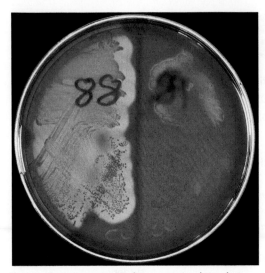

Fig. 1. *P acnes* strain 88 demonstrating hemolysis on *Brucella* blood agar medium.

presenting with glenohumeral arthritis. This generated a novel hypothesis about a possible relationship between *P acnes* and osteoarthritis with a potential role in the development of glenohumeral arthropathy. *P acnes* is currently recognized as a pathogenic organism, along with other common offending organisms, such as CONS and *S aureus*, with the capability of causing infection in upper extremity orthopedic procedures. *P acnes* is unique in that it presents a constellation of subjective and objective diagnostic challenges for the treating surgeon.

Diagnosing infection with *P acnes* is challenging due to the indolent clinical presentation and unreliable nature of classic inflammatory markers, as well as synovial fluid aspirations.[40,45] There has been an enhanced effort placed on infection prevention strategies because of these diagnostic challenges associated with upper extremity procedures and the known devastating complications, associated patient morbidity, and increased burden on the health care system. Recent investigations have focused on reduction of bacterial load through appropriate antibiotic prophylaxis, decolonization methods, surgical preparation solutions, various intraoperative irrigation agents, and topical antimicrobial protection.

ANTIBIOTIC PROPHYLAXIS

The most recent CDC guidelines outline a strong recommendation and suggested acceptance into clinical practice for the administration of appropriate preoperative antimicrobial agents timed such that bactericidal concentration is established in the serum and tissues when the incision is made.[25] The appropriateness of prophylactic antibiotics is imperative to successful prevention of upper extremity SSI. The CDC identified that 20% to 50% of all antibiotics prescribed in United States acute care hospitals are either unnecessary or inappropriate, leading to resistance and inability to effectively prevent and treat the ever-increasing range of infections according the World Health Organization.[46] The Joint Commission on Accreditation of Healthcare Organizations (JCAHO) recently developed the antimicrobial standard after participating in the White House Forum for Antibiotic Stewardship for hospitals, critical access hospitals, nursing care centers, ambulatory care organizations, and office-based surgery practices. Included in the performance measures as determined by JCAHO and CMS for hospitals is the development of a protocol for the proper use of prophylactic antibiotics based on scientific literature.

Perioperative Antibiotics

Most SSIs are acquired at the time of surgery, with the patient's skin being the most common cause, as well as airborne organisms from operating room personnel and traffic.[28] Antibiotic prophylaxis effectiveness in orthopedic surgery was confirmed by Lidwell and colleagues[47] in a study from 1984, which showed a 3-fold reduction in PJI using antibiotic prophylaxis following THA and TKA. The American Academy of Orthopedic Surgeons (AAOS) recommended the use of cefazolin or cefuroxime for arthroplasty patients in 2008, with most institutions in the United States using cefazolin as their antibiotic of choice for prophylaxis.[48] Studies have shown similar success rates for SSI prevention with the use of cefazolin and cefuroxime in the primary arthroplasty literature.[49] Cefazolin is a water soluble, first-generation cephalosporin that exhibits bactericidal action by inhibiting cell wall biosynthesis, causing bacteria to lyse. Cefazolin provides coverage against most *S aureus* and some gram-negative organisms, but it does not provide adequate coverage for CONS. Cephalosporins are not effective against methicillin-resistant *S aureus* (MRSA). Cefazolin has been shown to have good penetration in bone, synovium, and muscle with a long half-life of 1.8 hours following intravenous (IV) administration and an acceptable safety profile.[50] In synovial fluid, the concentration of cefazolin becomes comparable to that in the serum about 4 hours after IV administration. Standard recommended dosing for cefazolin is as follows: 1 g for patients less than 60 kg, 2 g for patients less than 120 kg, and 3 g for patients greater than 120 kg. There is a prospective randomized study currently being conducted assessing the pharmacokinetics of cefazolin in morbidly obese (body mass index >40 kg/m^2) patients after administration of a standard recommended 2 to 3 g dose versus a weight-based dosing (30 mg/kg).

Antibiotic susceptibility to *P acnes* should be carefully considered when deciding on prophylactic management for all patients undergoing orthopedic shoulder procedures because this bacterium is now recognized as the most common offending pathogen in shoulder infections. There remains a paucity of data on *P acnes* antibiotic susceptibility patterns in this subset of patients.[51–53] Prior work from the authors' institution has shown a high percentage of clindamycin-resistant strains from patients who have undergone an orthopedic shoulder procedure.[53,54] Antibiotics with the lowest minimum inhibitory concentration (MIC) values against *P acnes*, signifying susceptibility, included penicillin G and the first-generation cephalosporins. Current research from the authors' group has found similar resistance patterns to clindamycin of 31%, which is a nearly 3 times higher rate of resistance than reported in the literature.[42,53] One of the strains that was resistant to clindamycin was also resistant to vancomycin and ciprofloxacin. Our findings concerning clindamycin resistance were confirmed in a recent *P acnes* animal implant infection model in which clindamycin was found to have the highest minimal bactericidal concentration and minimal biofilm eradication concentration.[55] Clindamycin provides coverage for gram-positive and anaerobic bacteria but does not usually have adequate activity against aerobic gram-negative bacteria. The AAOS has recommended the use of clindamycin for patients with a beta-lactam allergy, although cautionary use of this antibiotic is advised based on the resistance profile seen with *P acnes*.[48]

CONS are gram-positive, catalase-positive organisms that occur in irregular clusters and encompass many *Staphylococcus* species, including *S epidermidis*, *S lugdunensis*, and *S haemolyticus*. Resistance to methicillin has been detected in 67.5% to 80% of isolates and resistance to penicillin approaches 95%.[56] Many strains demonstrated enhanced resistance patterns to erythromycin, clindamycin, tetracycline, gentamicin, trimethoprim-sulfamethoxazole, and ciprofloxacin, but all strains were susceptible to vancomycin.[57] Vancomycin is a heat stable glycopeptide antibiotic produced by the *Actinobacteria* species that inhibits cell wall synthesis in gram-positive bacteria, including CONS, MRSA, and methicillin-susceptible *S aureus* (MSSA). The routine use of systemic vancomycin as a prophylactic agent is not indicated due to the increasing emergence of vancomycin-resistant enterococci.[58] The CDC Hospital Infection Control Practices Advisory Committee has restricted the use of the vancomycin to a certain number of specific indications. Included in those indications is the use of vancomycin in surgical prophylaxis for major procedures involving implantation of a prostheses in institutions with a high rate of MRSA or MRSE (Methicillin-resistant Staphylococcus Epidermidis), as well as for patients with anaphylactic reactions to beta-lactam antibiotics.[58] For this subset of patients who are MRSA carriers or have a severe beta-lactam allergy, weight-based dosing of vancomycin is recommended, using 15 mg/kg with a maximal dose of 2 g. One dose is recommended preoperatively within 2 hours of surgical incision.[23]

The current suggested protocols for antibiotic prophylaxis in orthopedic procedures, especially arthroplasty, recommend against dual antibiotic administration.[23] Antibiotic prophylaxis in the shoulder and elbow should be carefully considered when assessing the unique susceptibility patterns of the common bacteria within this microbiome.

Optimal Timing and Duration

The goal of preoperative administration of antibiotics is to allow for adequate tissue concentrations to develop as measured by exceeding the MIC for the organisms likely to be encountered before incision. Previous literature has suggested that the first 2 hours after incision are the most crucial for maintaining this concentration of antibiotic.[59] The current recommendation for optimal timing of antibiotic prophylaxis is within 1 hour before the surgical procedure based on recommendations from the AAOS, CDC, and SCIP guidelines, which may be extended to 2 hours for the use of vancomycin and fluoroquinolones because of their extended infusion times.[23] European guidelines recommend a single preoperative dose of antibiotics within 30 minutes before incision.[60] Multiple studies have demonstrated an increased rate of SSI when prophylactic antibiotics were administrated more than 60 minutes before incision.[48,60–64] A recent pharmacokinetic study in the bariatric literature determined that a single 2 g dose of cefazolin given as an IV bolus 3 to 5 minutes before skin incision provided protective levels of the antibiotics (>MIC of MSSA) in the adipose tissue for 4.8 hours.[65] Perioperative redosing is recommended every 4 hours for cefazolin.

Discontinuation of antibiotic prophylaxis is recommended within 24 hours after cessation of the operation based on the US advisory statement and the AAOS. The AAOS advises against the continuation of antibiotic prophylaxis past 24 hours postoperatively irrespective of drains or catheters.[59] For clean and clean-contaminated procedures, the CDC recommends against administration of additional prophylactic antimicrobial agent dosing after the surgical incision is closed in the operating room, even in the presence of a drain.[25] Prior studies in the hip and knee arthroplasty literature have found no difference in the rate of SSI in patients who received antibiotic prophylaxis for 1 day compared with those who received a 3 or 7 day course.[66] There are multiple metaanalyses and systematic reviews demonstrating supportive evidence for the use of single-dose antibiotic prophylaxis based on both elective orthopedic and trauma surgical procedures, although this is not often reflected in current practice.[49,67,68] This hesitation to change common protocol is multifactorial but is most likely due to an underlying fear of infection and the known associated complications, morbidity, and excessive health care costs.

DECOLONIZATION METHODS
Methicillin-Resistant *Staphylococcus aureus* and Methicillin-Susceptible *Staphylococcus aureus* Preoperative Screening and Decolonization
The rate of SSI and incidence of staphylococcal and nonstaphylococcal infections has been shown to decrease with preoperative screening for *S aureus* (MSSA and MRSA) and decolonization protocols.[69–72] The carriage of *S aureus* in the anterior nares has demonstrated to be an important reservoir for bacteria and the colonization rates have been studied extensively in patients and hospital employees.[70,73] The current accepted method of decolonization for MRSA and MSSA is the short-term nasal application of mupirocin, according to the MSIS.[71] Controversy exists for universal screening and decolonization protocols, although a recent prospective study suggested no identifiable advantage in screening and decolonizing carriers before total joint arthroplasty. A recent prospective study suggested no identifiable advantage in screening and decolonizing carriers before total joint arthroplasty.[74] The development of bacterial resistance is a concern with long-term use of this agent.

Patient compliance has been identified as an issue with perioperative decolonization protocols. Intranasal antimicrobial photodisinfection therapy combined with chlorhexidine gluconate body wipes significantly reduced the SSI rate, with an excellent compliance record.[75] Unfortunately, this unique method is not currently approved by the US Food and Drug Administration and is not available in the United States. Based on the most recent consensus meeting in 2013, the MSIS does not recommend the universal screening and decolonization of all patients; although future research is warranted to further define this area of infection prevention.[23]

Perioperative Skin Preparation
Various methods of preadmission and preoperative skin decolonization protocols have been proposed in the orthopedic literature, including total body chlorhexidine gluconate showers and wipes, chlorhexidine gluconate combined with isopropyl alcohol, iodine-based solutions, and benzoyl peroxide. There is conflicting literature regarding the effectiveness of showering with chlorhexidine gluconate or using chlorhexidine gluconate wipes before surgery. In a recent prospective randomized series of subjects undergoing THA and TKA procedures, subjects who used chlorhexidine gluconate wipes 1 day preoperatively and the morning of surgery were found to have a lower incidence of SSI than those who did not comply with the protocol.[69,76]

The most commonly isolated native organisms from the shoulder before skin preparation are *P acnes* and CONS. Chlorhexidine gluconate combined with isopropyl alcohol (ChloraPrep; Care Fusion Corp, San Diego, CA, USA) has been recognized as an effective agent for surgical site skin preparation as measured by reduction of bacterial load.[77] Saltzman and colleagues[77] determined that ChloraPrep was more effective than povidone-iodine and iodine povacrylex-isopropyl alcohol (DuraPrep; 3M Healthcare, St Paul, MN, USA) at eliminating CONS from the shoulder, with an overall 7% positive culture rate compared with 31% and 19% with the other preparation solutions, respectively. There was no significant difference noted between the agents evaluated in their ability to eliminate *P acnes* from the surgical site. Concern remains surrounding the residual bacteria that reside on the skin immediately after skin preparation as *P acnes* has been found to persist 7% to 29% of the time.[77,78] Interestingly, *P acnes* has been identified by dermal biopsy in 70% of subjects after surgical site preparation.[79] A recent study by Sabetta and colleagues[80] showed a reduction in the rate at which residual *P acnes* is identified when topical benzoyl peroxide was used 48 hours before surgery for a total of 5 applications, in addition to ChloraPrep use at time of surgery, for surgical site preparation.

OPERATIVE ENVIRONMENT

Traditional methods to reduce the bacterial load in the operating room setting include implementation of laminar flow ventilation, ultraviolet light, decreasing operating room traffic, orthopaedic body space suits, and sterile draping. Charnley[81] and Lidwell and colleagues[82] conducted studies in the 1970s and 1980s that supported the use of laminar flow ventilation, whereas more recent studies provide conflicting results.[83,84] Hooper and colleagues[85] revealed an increased early infection rate with laminar flow use independent of patient characteristics, operative time, surgeon, or institution, based on the New Zealand joint registry. Salvati and colleagues[86] found that horizontal laminar flow increased the risk of PJI in TKA, whereas other studies have found no significant differences. Further investigation is recommended because of the variation in study results and the complex nature of this technology with associated institutional maintenance requirements.[87]

Ultraviolet light has previously been shown to significantly reduce the bacterial count in the operating room, but it is harmful to personnel and the patient due to the increased risk of corneal injuries and skin cancer. The CDC guidelines recommend against the use of ultraviolet lights in the operating room setting as a method to prevent SSIs.[24,88,89] To further decrease the risk of contamination, foot pedals to control operating room lights have been proposed instead of reaching overhead. One study found a 14.5% rate of contamination of light handles during arthroplasty cases.[90] The MSIS recommends minimal handling of overhead operating room lights with the notion that there is a need for future development of ways to minimize this source of contamination. The utilization of orthopedic body space suits is a controversial topic and, currently, there is no conclusive evidence to suggest routine use in arthroplasty procedures.[85,91]

Other techniques to reduce the risk of SSI have been evaluated, including application of sticky U-drapes before and after skin preparation to seal the operative field from the nonprepped area, iodine-impregnated occlusive drapes, changing the knife blade after skin incision for the deeper tissues, changing suction tips regularly, various gown materials, and frequent glove changes.[90,92–95] Although the results of these techniques may vary or may be insufficient to draw conclusion, increased surgical time is a factor that has been shown to clearly correlate with increased incidence of SSI and PJI.[96]

WOUND MANAGEMENT
Intraoperative Irrigation
Irrigation is commonly used to dilute contamination by removing particulate matter and bacteria, as well as remove nonviable tissue from the wound. In a study by Niki and colleagues,[97] the diluting capacity and ability to eliminate particulate matter plateaued when pulse lavage was used with 4 L of sterile saline. There is conflicting evidence evaluating pulsatile lavage (high or low) and bulb-syringe lavage. In vitro models have shown that pulsatile lavage results in greater bacterial seeding in bone and can spread contamination to nearby tissues.[98,99] In contrast, a prospective randomized controlled trial compared pulsatile lavage to bulb-syringe lavage and found a lower incidence of PJI with use of pulsatile lavage during cemented hemiarthroplasty for hip fracture.[100]

There are several types of commercial irrigation solutions available for sterilization of the wound before closure, including detergents, antibiotic laden lavage, and antiseptics agents. Detergents or surface agents inhibit the bacteria's ability to adhere to soft tissue and bone by disrupting their hydrophobic and electrostatic forces. Numerous detergents have been studied in musculoskeletal wounds in vitro, including benzalkonium chloride and castile soap, demonstrating their superiority compared with saline or antibiotic solution for bacterial removal.[101] Recently, a wound lavage system with active ingredients of ethanol (solvent), acetic acid (pH modifier), sodium acetate (buffer), benzalkonium chloride (surface agent), and water (Bactirsure; Zimmer Biomet, Warsaw, IN, USA) has been proposed to remove debris, microorganisms, and structurally resistant forms of bacteria, including biofilms. This agent is currently undergoing a prospective, multicenter, single-arm study to quantitatively and qualitatively assess synovial fluid in TKA for presence of bacteria before and after lavage using quantitative real-time polymerase chain reaction assay.

Antibiotics instilled through irrigation at the end of the procedure should have broad coverage, have low systemic absorption, and preserve host tissues. The most commonly used topical antibiotics for irrigation include cephalosporins, neomycin, glycopeptides, chloramphenicol, polymyxin, and bacitracin. The addition of antibiotics to lavage for prophylaxis is controversial. Earlier reports provided evidence that topical administration of antibiotics is more efficacious than normal saline, although similar reproducible results are limited.[102] There is evidence to support that topical antibiotics decrease bacterial inoculum in clean wounds, but this method has not been shown to be advantageous compared with IV prophylactic antibiotics with regard to decreasing the incidence of SSI.[103,104] Antibiotic irrigation solutions have been associated with a higher rate of wound complications, dermatitis, and hypersensitivity reactions.[105,106]

Wound irrigation with antiseptic agents has been shown to be effective for prevention of SSI by reducing bacterial load without creating resistance.[107,108] One of the major concerns about these agents is their inherent cytotoxicity, which potentially could impair wound healing, lead to development of necrotic tissue, and potentiate infection.[109,110] A recent study by van Meurs and colleagues,[111] evaluated the performance of 5 antiseptic agents to determine the optimal dilution that resulted in minimal cytotoxicity against human fibroblasts and stromal progenitor cells while retaining a bacterial load reduction of at least 99.9%. All agents tested, except polyhexanide, were bactericidal and cytotoxic at commercially available concentrations against *S aureus* and *S epidermidis*. When diluted, only povidone-iodine was bactericidal at concentrations in which some cells remained viable when diluted to 1.3 g/L. Before wound closure, irrigation with dilute povidone-iodine solution (0.35%) has been shown to decrease the risk of SSI and PJI in arthroplasty and spine procedures, with no reported adverse effects on wound healing, bone union, or clinical outcome.[107,112] Although these studies have shown promising results, the shoulder is unique due to the overwhelming presence of *P acnes* and, based on prior studies, the ability of *P acnes* to persist after preparation with povidone-iodine solution.[77]

There has been a developing interest in using a jet lavage containing low-dose chlorhexidine gluconate 0.05% in sterile water (Irrisept; IrriMax Corp, Lawrenceville, GA, USA) for intraoperative irrigation before wound closure because this agent has been designed to mechanically remove bacteria and debris without harming underlying tissues. Dilute hydrogen peroxide has been used in multiple areas of orthopedic surgery to decrease infection rates because it has

been shown to be synergistic with chlorhexidine and dilute povidone-iodine, especially against *Streptococcus* and *Staphylococcus* species.[113,114] Basic science studies have shown articular cartilage cytotoxic effects of hydrogen peroxide by inhibiting normal chondrocyte metabolic function, depletion of adenosine triphosphate in cells, and reduction of proteoglycan and hyaluronic acid synthesis.[115,116] Another serious potential complication that has been reported is air embolism from the formation of copious amounts of oxygen gas during breakdown of hydrogen peroxide.[117,118] Multiple studies, including a recent review of hydrogen peroxide use for wound irrigation in orthopedic surgery, recommend against the use of hydrogen peroxide for medullary canal irrigation, as well as immediate application before wound closure.[119]

The MSIS recognizes the mechanical advantage of irrigation before closure for reduction of bacterial burden, but the abundance of conflicting evidence precludes a consensus on recommending any agent versus another.[23] Further research is recommended for an optimal irrigation solution for orthopedic shoulder and elbow procedures.

Local Intrawound Powdered Antibiotics

Lyophilized powder applied just before wound closure is an additional modality for local delivery of antibiotics. This technique was first described before the evolution of efficacious systemic antibiotic prophylaxis for prevention of infection in abdominal surgery.[120] *P acnes* has been discovered by culture at the end of surgical procedures 41% to 63% of the time.[80] This raises concern for patients undergoing technically challenging or revision procedures in which the surgical time will be longer. This has prompted surgeons to use alternative methods such as intrawound topical powdered antibiotics just before closure. A potential concern is that administration of topical antibiotics can potentiate bacterial selection effects and subsequently create resistance.[121] There is a paucity of data supporting the use of this technique, with most stemming from spine literature. A single prospective randomized controlled trial evaluated the addition of topical powdered vancomycin in the muscle, fascia, and subcutaneous tissue to systemic antibiotic prophylaxis with cefuroxime for 24 hours and found no difference in the rate of SSI between the control and treatment groups.[122] A recent retrospective study of 272 patients undergoing open release of posttraumatic elbow stiffness found a statistically lower rate of SSI in patients who had 1 g of topical vancomycin compared with IV cefazolin alone.[123] For many surgeons, administration of local antibiotics in conjunction with systemic antibiotics is an attractive option when attempting to reduce the rate of SSI. However, high-quality evidence is lacking in orthopedic surgery, especially shoulder and elbow.[124] The role of local intrawound powdered antibiotics needs to be further defined through future research.

SUMMARY OF AUTHORS' RECOMMENDATIONS

The authors' current practice is as follows: in the preoperative holding area, the surgical site is cleaned with a single-use chlorhexidine wipe and hair is removed from the surgical site, if necessary (Table 3). In the operating room, the surgical site is prepped with a betadine soap solution, followed by ChloraPrep before and after application of a sticky impervious drape to isolate the surgical site. The skin is covered

Table 3
Summary of authors' current practice

Preoperative Holding	• Surgical site cleaned with single-use chlorhexidine wipe • Hair removal from operative site using clippers
Intraoperative Surgical Site Skin Preparation	• Betadine soap solution, then ChloraPrep before and after application of sticky impervious drapes • Skin is covered with an iodine-impregnated isolation drape
Intraoperative Irrigation	• During the procedure, and before closure, irrigation with normal saline is preformed using a pulsatile lavage system
Orthopedic Body Space Suits	• Currently not used during arthroplasty or nonarthroplasty procedures
Outpatient Procedures	• No additional measures performed or antibiotics prescribed beyond the standard prophylaxis given before incision
Revision or Contaminated Procedures or Suspected Infection	• Multiple sterile cultures obtained: synovial fluid via aspiration with 18-gauge needle before violation of capsule, capsular tissue, tissue surrounding implants • Cultures held in aerobic and anaerobic conditions for 21 d • Cultures are evaluated for the presence of hemolysis if P acnes is present • Irrigation with dilute betadine solution after debridement and cultures • Vancomycin powder placed in wound at time of closure

Antibiotic Protocol	Prophylaxis	Revisions
No beta-lactam allergy	Cefazolin 2g or 3g IV 30–60 min before skin incision, then cefazolin 2g or 3g IV every 8 h for 24 h	Cefazolin 2g or 3g IV every 8 h until discharge, then amoxicillin 500 mg po every 8 h until cultures finalized
Beta-lactam allergy	Vancomycin IV (15 mg/kg)[a] and clindamycin 600 mg IV 60–90 min before skin incision, then vancomycin every 12 h and clindamycin 600 mg IV every 6 h for 24 h	Vancomycin (15 mg/kg) IV q12 h and clindamycin 600 mg IV every 6 h until discharge, then ciprofloxacin 500 mg po every 12 h or doxycycline 100 mg po every 12 h until cultures finalized

Abbreviation: po, by mouth.
[a] Maximal dose of vancomycin when using weight-based dosing is 2 g.

with an iodine-impregnated isolation drape (Ioban; 3M, St Paul, MN, USA). Our routine for antibiotic prophylaxis includes the use of cefazolin 30 to 60 minutes before skin incision or, in beta-lactam allergic patients, the use of weight-based dosing of vancomycin at least 60 minutes before surgery. Antibiotics are continued for 24 hours after the procedure for all joint replacement procedures. For outpatient procedures, no additional antibiotics are prescribed beyond the standard prophylaxis given before incision as previously listed. During the procedure, and before closure, irrigation with normal saline is preformed using a pulsatile lavage system.

In revision procedures or cases in which infection or contamination is suspected, multiple cultures are sent and held in aerobic and anaerobic conditions for 21 days. If new implants are inserted, vancomycin powder is placed in the wound before closure and the patient is continued on antibiotics until culture results are final (see Table 3).

One of the greatest challenges faced by orthopedic surgeons is successfully treating SSI and PJI. The authors' bias is to do everything conceivable that could heighten our ability to prevent infection. This bias often leads surgeons away from evidence-based practices and can result in harm to patients or contribute to the development of antibiotic-resistant strains of bacteria. Additional research is needed to help guide treatment protocols that allow for the highest level of prevention while avoiding unnecessary or potentially detrimental interventions.

REFERENCES

1. Kim SH, Wise BL, Zhang Y, et al. Increasing incidence of shoulder arthroplasty in the United States. J Bone Joint Surg Am 2011;93(24):2249–54.
2. Kurtz S, Ong K, Lau E, et al. Projections of primary and revision hip and knee arthroplasty in the United States from 2005 to 2030. J Bone Joint Surg Am 2007;89(4):780–5.
3. Day JS, Lau E, Ong KL, et al. Prevalence and projections of total shoulder and elbow arthroplasty in the United States to 2015. J Shoulder Elbow Surg 2010;19(8):1115–20.
4. Leong NL, Cohen JR, Lord E, et al. Demographic trends and complication rates in arthroscopic elbow surgery. Arthroscopy 2015;31(10):1928–32.
5. Colvin AC, Egorova N, Harrison AK, et al. National trends in rotator cuff repair. J Bone Joint Surg Am 2012;94(3):227–33.
6. Owens BD, Harrast JJ, Hurwitz SR, et al. Surgical trends in Bankart repair: an analysis of data from the American Board of Orthopaedic Surgery certification examination. Am J Sports Med 2011;39(9):1865–9.
7. Vellios EE, Nazemi AK, Yeranosian MG, et al. Demographic trends in arthroscopic and open biceps tenodesis across the United States. J Shoulder Elbow Surg 2015;24(10):e279–285.
8. Hasty EK, Jernigan EW 3rd, Soo A, et al. Trends in surgical management and costs for operative treatment of proximal humerus fractures in the elderly. Orthopedics 2017;40(4):e641–7.
9. Motisi M, Kurowicki J, Berglund DD, et al. Trends in management of radial head and olecranon fractures. Open Orthop J 2017;11:239–47.
10. Schoch BS, Padegimas EM, Maltenfort M, et al. Humeral shaft fractures: national trends in management. J Orthop Trauma 2017;18(3):259–63.
11. Popovic D, King GJ. Fragility fractures of the distal humerus: what is the optimal treatment? J Bone Joint Surg Br 2012;94(1):16–22.
12. Delanois RE, Mistry JB, Gwam CU, et al. Current epidemiology of revision total knee arthroplasty in the United States. J Arthroplasty 2017;32(9):2663–8.
13. Gwam CU, Mistry JB, Mohamed NS, et al. Current epidemiology of revision total hip arthroplasty in the United States: National Inpatient Sample 2009 to 2013. J Arthroplasty 2017;32(7):2088–92.
14. Nelson GN, Davis DE, Namdari S. Outcomes in the treatment of periprosthetic joint infection after shoulder arthroplasty: a systematic review. J Shoulder Elbow Surg 2016;25(8):1337–45.
15. Sperling JW, Kozak TK, Hanssen AD, et al. Infection after shoulder arthroplasty. Clin Orthop Relat Res 2001;(382):206–16.
16. Al-Mulhim FA, Baragbah MA, Sadat-Ali M, et al. Prevalence of surgical site infection in orthopedic surgery: a 5-year analysis. Int Surg 2014;99(3):264–8.
17. de Lissovoy G, Fraeman K, Hutchins V, et al. Surgical site infection: incidence and impact on hospital utilization and treatment costs. Am J Infect Control 2009;37(5):387–97.
18. Kurtz SM, Lau E, Watson H, et al. Economic burden of periprosthetic joint infection in the United States. J Arthroplasty 2012;27(8 Suppl):61–5.e1.
19. Bozic KJ, Ries MD. The impact of infection after total hip arthroplasty on hospital and surgeon resource utilization. J Bone Joint Surg Am 2005;87(8):1746–51.
20. Kurtz SM, Ong KL, Lau E, et al. Prosthetic joint infection risk after TKA in the Medicare population. Clin Orthop Relat Res 2010;468(1):52–6.
21. Ong KL, Kurtz SM, Lau E, et al. Prosthetic joint infection risk after total hip arthroplasty in the Medicare population. J Arthroplasty 2009;24(6 Suppl):105–9.

22. Parvizi J, Pawasarat IM, Azzam KA, et al. Periprosthetic joint infection: the economic impact of methicillin-resistant infections. J Arthroplasty 2010;25(6 Suppl):103–7.

23. Parvizi J, Gehrke T, Chen AF. Proceedings of the International Consensus on Periprosthetic Joint Infection. Bone Joint J 2013;95-B(11):1450–2.

24. Mangram AJ, Horan TC, Pearson ML, et al. Guideline for prevention of surgical site infection, 1999. Centers for Disease Control and Prevention (CDC) Hospital Infection Control Practices Advisory Committee. Am J Infect Control 1999;27(2):97–132 [quiz: 133–4]; [discussion: 196].

25. Berrios-Torres SI, Umscheid CA, Bratzler DW, et al. Centers for Disease Control and Prevention guideline for the prevention of surgical site infection, 2017. JAMA Surg 2017;152(8):784–91.

26. McKibben L, Horan T, Tokars JI, et al. Guidance on public reporting of healthcare-associated infections: recommendations of the Healthcare Infection Control Practices Advisory Committee. Am J Infect Control 2005;33(4):217–26.

27. Perry KI, Hanssen AD. Orthopaedic infection: prevention and diagnosis. J Am Acad Orthop Surg 2017;25(Suppl 1):S4–6.

28. Fletcher N, Sofianos D, Berkes MB, et al. Prevention of perioperative infection. J Bone Joint Surg Am 2007;89(7):1605–18.

29. Leeming JP, Holland KT, Cunliffe WJ. The microbial ecology of pilosebaceous units isolated from human skin. J Gen Microbiol 1984;130(4):803–7.

30. Grice EA, Segre JA. The skin microbiome. Nat Rev Microbiol 2011;9(4):244–53.

31. Hentges DJ. The anaerobic microflora of the human body. Clin Infect Dis 1993;16(Suppl 4):S175–80.

32. Bruggemann H, Henne A, Hoster F, et al. The complete genome sequence of Propionibacterium acnes, a commensal of human skin. Science 2004;305(5684):671–3.

33. Korting HC, Hubner K, Greiner K, et al. Differences in the skin surface pH and bacterial microflora due to the long-term application of synthetic detergent preparations of pH 5.5 and pH 7.0. Results of a crossover trial in healthy volunteers. Acta Derm Venereol 1990;70(5):429–31.

34. Aly R, Shirley C, Cunico B, et al. Effect of prolonged occlusion on the microbial flora, pH, carbon dioxide and transepidermal water loss on human skin. J Invest Dermatol 1978;71(6):378–81.

35. Singh JA, Sperling JW, Schleck C, et al. Periprosthetic infections after total shoulder arthroplasty: a 33-year perspective. J Shoulder Elbow Surg 2012;21(11):1534–41.

36. Grosso MJ, Sabesan VJ, Ho JC, et al. Reinfection rates after 1-stage revision shoulder arthroplasty for patients with unexpected positive intraoperative cultures. J Shoulder Elbow Surg 2012;21(6):754–8.

37. Piper KE, Jacobson MJ, Cofield RH, et al. Microbiologic diagnosis of prosthetic shoulder infection by use of implant sonication. J Clin Microbiol 2009;47(6):1878–84.

38. Sampedro MF, Piper KE, McDowell A, et al. Species of Propionibacterium and Propionibacterium acnes phylotypes associated with orthopedic implants. Diagn Microbiol Infect Dis 2009;64(2):138–45.

39. Nakatsuji T, Tang DC, Zhang L, et al. Propionibacterium acnes CAMP factor and host acid sphingomyelinase contribute to bacterial virulence: potential targets for inflammatory acne treatment. PLoS One 2011;6(4):e14797.

40. Achermann Y, Goldstein EJ, Coenye T, et al. Propionibacterium acnes: from commensal to opportunistic biofilm-associated implant pathogen. Clin Microbiol Rev 2014;27(3):419–40.

41. Gristina AG, Naylor P, Myrvik Q. Infections from biomaterials and implants: a race for the surface. Med Prog Technol 1988;14(3–4):205–24.

42. Nodzo SR, Hohman DW, Crane JK, et al. Hemolysis as a clinical marker for Propionibacterium acnes orthopedic infection. Am J Orthop (Belle Mead NJ) 2014;43(5):E93–7.

43. McDowell A, Valanne S, Ramage G, et al. Propionibacterium acnes types I and II represent phylogenetically distinct groups. J Clin Microbiol 2005;43(1):326–34.

44. Levy O, Iyer S, Atoun E, et al. Propionibacterium acnes: an underestimated etiology in the pathogenesis of osteoarthritis? J Shoulder Elbow Surg 2013;22(4):505–11.

45. Piper KE, Fernandez-Sampedro M, Steckelberg KE, et al. C-reactive protein, erythrocyte sedimentation rate and orthopedic implant infection. PLoS One 2010;5(2):e9358.

46. Joint Commission on Hospital Accreditation. APPROVED: New Antimicrobial Stewardship Standard. Jt Comm Perspect 2016;36(7):1, 3–4, 8.

47. Lidwell OM, Lowbury EJ, Whyte W, et al. Infection and sepsis after operations for total hip or knee-joint replacement: influence of ultraclean air, prophylactic antibiotics and other factors. J Hyg (Lond) 1984;93(3):505–29.

48. Prokuski L. Prophylactic antibiotics in orthopaedic surgery. J Am Acad Orthop Surg 2008;16(5):283–93.

49. Tang WM, Chiu KY, Ng TP, et al. Efficacy of a single dose of cefazolin as a prophylactic antibiotic in primary arthroplasty. J Arthroplasty 2003;18(6):714–8.

50. Neu HC. Cephalosporin antibiotics as applied in surgery of bones and joints. Clin Orthop Relat Res 1984;(190):50–64.

51. Kurokawa I, Nishijima S, Kawabata S. Antimicrobial susceptibility of *Propionibacterium acnes* isolated from acne vulgaris. Eur J Dermatol 1999;9(1):25–8.

52. Nishijima S, Kurokawa I, Katoh N, et al. The bacteriology of acne vulgaris and antimicrobial susceptibility of *Propionibacterium acnes* and *Staphylococcus epidermidis* isolated from acne lesions. J Dermatol 2000;27(5):318–23.

53. Crane JK, Hohman DW, Nodzo SR, et al. Antimicrobial susceptibility of *Propionibacterium acnes* isolates from shoulder surgery. Antimicrob Agents Chemother 2013;57(7):3424–6.

54. Wright TE, Boyle KK, Duquin TR, et al. *Propionibacterium acnes* susceptibility and correlation with hemolytic phenotype. Infect Dis (Auckl) 2016;9:39–44.

55. Furustrand Tafin U, Corvec S, Betrisey B, et al. Role of rifampin against *Propionibacterium acnes* biofilm in vitro and in an experimental foreign-body infection model. Antimicrob Agents Chemother 2012;56(4):1885–91.

56. Diekema DJ, Pfaller MA, Schmitz FJ, et al. Survey of infections due to *Staphylococcus* species: frequency of occurrence and antimicrobial susceptibility of isolates collected in the United States, Canada, Latin America, Europe, and the Western Pacific region for the SENTRY Antimicrobial Surveillance Program, 1997-1999. Clin Infect Dis 2001;32(Suppl 2):S114–32.

57. Koksal F, Yasar H, Samasti M. Antibiotic resistance patterns of coagulase-negative staphylococcus strains isolated from blood cultures of septicemic patients in Turkey. Microbiol Res 2009;164(4):404–10.

58. Hospital Infection Control Practices Advisory Committee (HICPAC). Recommendations for preventing the spread of vancomycin resistance. Infect Control Hosp Epidemiol 1995;16(2):105–13.

59. Meehan J, Jamali AA, Nguyen H. Prophylactic antibiotics in hip and knee arthroplasty. J Bone Joint Surg Am 2009;91(10):2480–90.

60. Bratzler DW, Houck PM, Surgical Infection Prevention Guideline Writers Workgroup. Antimicrobial prophylaxis for surgery: an advisory statement from the National Surgical Infection Prevention Project. Am J Surg 2005;189(4):395–404.

61. van Kasteren ME, Mannien J, Ott A, et al. Antibiotic prophylaxis and the risk of surgical site infections following total hip arthroplasty: timely administration is the most important factor. Clin Infect Dis 2007;44(7):921–7.

62. Galandiuk S, Polk HC Jr, Jagelman DG, et al. Re-emphasis of priorities in surgical antibiotic prophylaxis. Surg Gynecol Obstet 1989;169(3):219–22.

63. Hawn MT, Richman JS, Vick CC, et al. Timing of surgical antibiotic prophylaxis and the risk of surgical site infection. JAMA Surg 2013;148(7):649–57.

64. de Jonge SW, Gans SL, Atema JJ, et al. Timing of preoperative antibiotic prophylaxis in 54,552 patients and the risk of surgical site infection: a systematic review and meta-analysis. Medicine (Baltimore) 2017;96(29):e6903.

65. Chen X, Brathwaite CE, Barkan A, et al. Optimal cefazolin prophylactic dosing for bariatric surgery: no need for higher doses or intraoperative redosing. Obes Surg 2017;27(3):626–9.

66. Williams DN, Gustilo RB. The use of preventive antibiotics in orthopaedic surgery. Clin Orthop Relat Res 1984;(190):83–8.

67. Southwell-Keely JP, Russo RR, March L, et al. Antibiotic prophylaxis in hip fracture surgery: a meta-analysis. Clin Orthop Relat Res 2004;(419):179–84.

68. Bryson DJ, Morris DL, Shivji FS, et al. Antibiotic prophylaxis in orthopaedic surgery: difficult decisions in an era of evolving antibiotic resistance. Bone Joint J 2016;98-B(8):1014–9.

69. Johnson AJ, Daley JA, Zywiel MG, et al. Preoperative chlorhexidine preparation and the incidence of surgical site infections after hip arthroplasty. J Arthroplasty 2010;25(6 Suppl):98–102.

70. Perl TM, Golub JE. New approaches to reduce *S aureus* nosocomial infection rates: treating *S. aureus* nasal carriage. Ann Pharmacother 1998;32(1):S7–16.

71. Kallen AJ, Wilson CT, Larson RJ. Perioperative intranasal mupirocin for the prevention of surgical-site infections: systematic review of the literature and meta-analysis. Infect Control Hosp Epidemiol 2005;26(12):916–22.

72. van Rijen MM, Bonten M, Wenzel RP, et al. Intranasal mupirocin for reduction of *Staphylococcus aureus* infections in surgical patients with nasal carriage: a systematic review. J Antimicrob Chemother 2008;61(2):254–61.

73. Kalmeijer MD, van Nieuwland-Bollen E, Bogaers-Hofman D, et al. Nasal carriage of *Staphylococcus aureus* is a major risk factor for surgical-site infections in orthopedic surgery. Infect Control Hosp Epidemiol 2000;21(5):319–23.

74. Sousa RJ, Barreira PM, Leite PT, et al. Preoperative *Staphylococcus aureus* screening/decolonization protocol before total joint arthroplasty-results of a small prospective randomized trial. J Arthroplasty 2016;31(1):234–9.

75. Bryce E, Wong T, Forrester L, et al. Nasal photodisinfection and chlorhexidine wipes decrease surgical site infections: a historical control study and propensity analysis. J Hosp Infect 2014;88(2):89–95.

76. Zywiel MG, Daley JA, Delanois RE, et al. Advance pre-operative chlorhexidine reduces the incidence of surgical site infections in knee arthroplasty. Int Orthop 2011;35(7):1001–6.

77. Saltzman MD, Nuber GW, Gryzlo SM, et al. Efficacy of surgical preparation solutions in shoulder surgery. J Bone Joint Surg Am 2009;91(8):1949–53.

78. Hudek R, Sommer F, Kerwat M, et al. *Propionibacterium acnes* in shoulder surgery: true infection, contamination, or commensal of the deep tissue? J Shoulder Elbow Surg 2014;23(12):1763–71.

79. Lee MJ, Pottinger PS, Butler-Wu S, et al. *Propionibacterium* persists in the skin despite standard surgical preparation. J Bone Joint Surg Am 2014;96(17):1447–50.

80. Sethi PM, Sabetta JR, Stuek SJ, et al. Presence of *Propionibacterium acnes* in primary shoulder arthroscopy: results of aspiration and tissue cultures. J Shoulder Elbow Surg 2015;24(5):796–803.

81. Charnley J. Postoperative infection after total hip replacement with special reference to air contamination in the operating room. Clin Orthop Relat Res 1972;87:167–87.

82. Lidwell OM, Lowbury EJ, Whyte W, et al. Effect of ultraclean air in operating rooms on deep sepsis in the joint after total hip or knee replacement: a randomised study. Br Med J (Clin Res Ed) 1982; 285(6334):10–4.

83. Breier AC, Brandt C, Sohr D, et al. Laminar airflow ceiling size: no impact on infection rates following hip and knee prosthesis. Infect Control Hosp Epidemiol 2011;32(11):1097–102.

84. Gastmeier P, Breier AC, Brandt C. Influence of laminar airflow on prosthetic joint infections: a systematic review. J Hosp Infect 2012;81(2): 73–8.

85. Hooper GJ, Rothwell AG, Frampton C, et al. Does the use of laminar flow and space suits reduce early deep infection after total hip and knee replacement?: the ten-year results of the New Zealand Joint Registry. J Bone Joint Surg Br 2011;93(1).85–90.

86. Salvati EA, Robinson RP, Zeno SM, et al. Infection rates after 3175 total hip and total knee replacements performed with and without a horizontal unidirectional filtered air-flow system. J Bone Joint Surg Am 1982;64(4):525–35.

87. Brandt C, Hott U, Sohr D, et al. Operating room ventilation with laminar airflow shows no protective effect on the surgical site infection rate in orthopedic and abdominal surgery. Ann Surg 2008; 248(5):695–700.

88. Berg M, Bergman BR, Hoborn J. Ultraviolet radiation compared to an ultra-clean air enclosure. Comparison of air bacteria counts in operating rooms. J Bone Joint Surg Br 1991;73(5):811–5.

89. Taylor GJ, Bannister GC, Leeming JP. Wound disinfection with ultraviolet radiation. J Hosp Infect 1995;30(2):85–93.

90. Davis N, Curry A, Gambhir AK, et al. Intraoperative bacterial contamination in operations for joint replacement. J Bone Joint Surg Br 1999;81(5): 886–9.

91. Miner AL, Losina E, Katz JN, et al. Deep infection after total knee replacement: impact of laminar airflow systems and body exhaust suits in the modern operating room. Infect Control Hosp Epidemiol 2007;28(2):222–6.

92. Lewis DA, Leaper DJ, Speller DC. Prevention of bacterial colonization of wounds at operation: comparison of iodine-impregnated ('Ioban') drapes with conventional methods. J Hosp Infect 1984;5(4):431–7.

93. Johnston DH, Fairclough JA, Brown EM, et al. Rate of bacterial recolonization of the skin after preparation: four methods compared. Br J Surg 1987;74(1):64.

94. Greenough CG. An investigation into contamination of operative suction. J Bone Joint Surg Br 1986;68(1):151–3.

95. Schindler OS, Spencer RF, Smith MD. Should we use a separate knife for the skin? J Bone Joint Surg Br 2006;88(3):382–5.

96. Maoz G, Phillips M, Bosco J, et al. The Otto Aufranc Award: Modifiable versus nonmodifiable risk factors for infection after hip arthroplasty. Clin Orthop Relat Res 2015;473(2):453–9.

97. Niki Y, Matsumoto H, Otani T, et al. How much sterile saline should be used for efficient lavage during total knee arthroplasty? Effects of pulse lavage irrigation on removal of bone and cement debris. J Arthroplasty 2007;22(1):95–9.

98. Bhandari M, Schemitsch EH, Adili A, et al. High and low pressure pulsatile lavage of contaminated tibial fractures: an in vitro study of bacterial adherence and bone damage. J Orthop Trauma 1999; 13(8):526–33.

99. Kalteis T, Lehn N, Schroder HJ, et al. Contaminant seeding in bone by different irrigation methods: an experimental study. J Orthop Trauma 2005; 19(9):591–6.

100. Hargrove R, Ridgeway S, Russell R, et al. Does pulse lavage reduce hip hemiarthroplasty infection rates? J Hosp Infect 2006;62(4):446–9.

101. Anglen JO, Gainor BJ, Simpson WA, et al. The use of detergent irrigation for musculoskeletal wounds. Int Orthop 2003;27(1):40–6.

102. Rambo WM. Irrigation of the peritoneal cavity with cephalothin. Am J Surg 1972;123(2):192–5.

103. McHugh SM, Collins CJ, Corrigan MA, et al. The role of topical antibiotics used as prophylaxis in surgical site infection prevention. J Antimicrob Chemother 2011;66(4):693–701.

104. Greig J, Morran C, Gunn R, et al. Wound sepsis after colorectal surgery: the effect of cefotetan lavage. Chemioterapia 1987;6(2 Suppl):595–6.

105. Dirschl DR, Wilson FC. Topical antibiotic irrigation in the prophylaxis of operative wound infections in

orthopedic surgery. Orthop Clin North Am 1991; 22(3):419–26.

106. Anglen JO. Comparison of soap and antibiotic solutions for irrigation of lower-limb open fracture wounds. A prospective, randomized study. J Bone Joint Surg Am 2005;87(7):1415–22.

107. Brown NM, Cipriano CA, Moric M, et al. Dilute betadine lavage before closure for the prevention of acute postoperative deep periprosthetic joint infection. J Arthroplasty 2012;27(1):27–30.

108. Russell AD. Antibiotic and biocide resistance in bacteria: introduction. Symp Ser Soc Appl Microbiol 2002;(31):1S–3S.

109. Muller G, Kramer A. Biocompatibility index of antiseptic agents by parallel assessment of antimicrobial activity and cellular cytotoxicity. J Antimicrob Chemother 2008;61(6):1281–7.

110. Thomas GW, Rael LT, Bar-Or R, et al. Mechanisms of delayed wound healing by commonly used antiseptics. J Trauma 2009;66(1):82–90 [discussion: 90-81].

111. van Meurs SJ, Gawlitta D, Heemstra KA, et al. Selection of an optimal antiseptic solution for intraoperative irrigation: an in vitro study. J Bone Joint Surg Am 2014;96(4):285–91.

112. Cheng MT, Chang MC, Wang ST, et al. Efficacy of dilute betadine solution irrigation in the prevention of postoperative infection of spinal surgery. Spine (Phila Pa 1976) 2005;30(15):1689–93.

113. Steinberg D, Heling I, Daniel I, et al. Antibacterial synergistic effect of chlorhexidine and hydrogen peroxide against Streptococcus sobrinus, Streptococcus faecalis and Staphylococcus aureus. J Oral Rehabil 1999;26(2):151–6.

114. Zubko EI, Zubko MK. Co-operative inhibitory effects of hydrogen peroxide and iodine against bacterial and yeast species. BMC Res Notes 2013;6:272.

115. Asada S, Fukuda K, Oh M, et al. Effect of hydrogen peroxide on the metabolism of articular chondrocytes. Inflamm Res 1999;48(7):399–403.

116. Asada S, Fukuda K, Nishisaka F, et al. Hydrogen peroxide induces apoptosis of chondrocytes; involvement of calcium ion and extracellular signal-regulated protein kinase. Inflamm Res 2001;50(1):19–23.

117. Timperley AJ, Bracey DJ. Cardiac arrest following the use of hydrogen peroxide during arthroplasty. J Arthroplasty 1989;4(4):369–70.

118. Henley N, Carlson DA, Kaehr DM, et al. Air embolism associated with irrigation of external fixator pin sites with hydrogen peroxide. A report of two cases. J Bone Joint Surg Am 2004;86-A(4): 821–2.

119. Lu M, Hansen EN. Hydrogen peroxide wound irrigation in orthopaedic surgery. J Bone Jt Infect 2017;2(1):3–9.

120. Huiras P, Logan JK, Papadopoulos S, et al. Local antimicrobial administration for prophylaxis of surgical site infections. Pharmacotherapy 2012;32(11): 1006–19.

121. Harkaway KS, McGinley KJ, Foglia AN, et al. Antibiotic resistance patterns in coagulase-negative staphylococci after treatment with topical erythromycin, benzoyl peroxide, and combination therapy. Br J Dermatol 1992;126(6):586–90.

122. Tubaki VR, Rajasekaran S, Shetty AP. Effects of using intravenous antibiotic only versus local intrawound vancomycin antibiotic powder application in addition to intravenous antibiotics on postoperative infection in spine surgery in 907 patients. Spine (Phila Pa 1976) 2013;38(25): 2149–55.

123. Yan H, He J, Chen S, et al. Intrawound application of vancomycin reduces wound infection after open release of post-traumatic stiff elbows: a retrospective comparative study. J Shoulder Elbow Surg 2014;23(5):686–92.

124. Fleischman AN, Austin MS. Local intra-wound administration of powdered antibiotics in orthopaedic surgery. J Bone Jt Infect 2017;2(1): 23–8.

Venous Thromboembolism Prophylaxis in Shoulder Surgery

William R. Aibinder, MD,
Joaquin Sanchez-Sotelo, MD, PhD*

KEYWORDS

- Deep vein thrombosis • Pulmonary embolism • Thromboembolism prophylaxis
- Shoulder surgery • Shoulder arthroplasty • Arthroscopy

KEY POINTS

- A venous thromboembolic event (VTE) is rare after shoulder surgery.
- VTE is more common after shoulder surgery for fracture and shoulder arthroplasty, compared with shoulder arthroscopy.
- The main risk factors for VTE are malignancy, other procoagulopathic conditions or treatments, dehydration, obesity, and advanced age.
- Mechanical prophylaxis could be universally considered given its risk-benefit profile.
- Chemical prophylaxis should be considered in patients with risk factors for VTE but weighed against the risk of bleeding complications.

INTRODUCTION

Venous thrombosis is thought to be causally related to 3 factors that comprise Virchow triad: hypercoagulability, stasis, and endothelial injury.[1] Venous thromboembolic events (VTEs) after elective orthopedic surgery can have devastating complications and be costly and potentially fatal.[2–4] Prevention of VTE is key to minimizing risk to patients and the associated increased economic burden.

VTE has been extensively studied as a complication of lower extremity orthopedic surgery.[5–9] Without prophylaxis, the rate of a deep vein thrombosis (DVT) after lower extremity arthroplasty or fracture has been reported between 40% and 60%.[5] As a result, some sort of VTE prophylaxis is routinely recommended after hip arthroplasty and knee arthroplasty.[10]

Historically, rates of VTE after upper extremity surgery were largely unknown but anecdotally considered less than that after lower extremity surgery. The early descriptions of VTE after shoulder surgery were in the form of case reports.[11–18] Subsequently, several larger series have shown that the rate of DVT after shoulder surgery is not insignificant and may be as high as 13%.[19–21] Unlike lower extremity arthroplasty, there is a paucity of evidence regarding thromboembolic prophylaxis after upper extremity surgery; thus, the American Academy of Orthopaedic Surgeons does not make strong recommendations.[22,23]

The first case report of a symptomatic DVT after shoulder surgery was described by Burkhart[11] in 1990 and was attributed to an underlying undiagnosed previously asymptomatic Hodgkin lymphoma. Arcand and colleagues[16] reported 1 case of axillary DVT with a resultant nonfatal pulmonary embolism (PE) in a 32-year-old man after shoulder arthroplasty. The investigators surmised that traction on the arm during the procedure may have caused an endothelial injury leading to thrombus formation.[1] Scott[12] reported a nonfatal PE in a 24-year-old man after arthroscopic glenohumeral débridement. Saleem and

---

Department of Orthopedic Surgery, Mayo Clinic, 200 First Street Southwest, Rochester, MN 55905, USA
* Corresponding author.
E-mail address: Sanchezsotelo.Joaquin@mayo.edu

Orthop Clin N Am 49 (2018) 257–263
https://doi.org/10.1016/j.ocl.2017.11.012
0030-5898/18/© 2017 Elsevier Inc. All rights reserved.

Markel[14] reported a fatal PE in a 68-year-old man after shoulder arthroplasty; death occurred on postoperative day 1. The investigators speculated the event was related to the patient's long drive prior to surgery. Creighton and Cole[18] reported a symptomatic brachial DVT and subsequent symptomatic PE in a 43-year-old man undergoing an arthroscopic labral repair. Due to the absence of obvious risk factors, the authors attributed the thrombus to the beach chair position. Amarasekera and colleagues[17] reported a symptomatic subclavian DVT with subsequent symptomatic PE after an arthroscopic rotator cuff repair. Madhusudhan and colleagues[15] reported a fatal PE in a 73-year-old woman after shoulder arthroplasty originating from a symptomatic lower extremity DVT. The only risk factors the authors noted was a body mass index (BMI) of 34 kg/m^2. Several other case reports exist in the literature.[13] Consistent throughout these singular cases, however, is the variability in patient age, procedure, and symptoms.

To some extent, these limitations in the literature are related to the overall low occurrence of VTEs. Additionally, studies vary in regard to study population and end points. This article attempts to delineate the reported rates of symptomatic versus asymptomatic DVTs as well as fatal versus nonfatal PE. This article also attempts to differentiate the rates after shoulder arthroplasty, arthroscopy, and trauma. Lastly, literature is reviewed in regard to recommendations for venous thromboembolism prophylaxis after shoulder surgery.

INCIDENCE

The true incidence of VTE after shoulder surgery is difficult to extrapolate from the literature due to variations in diagnostic criteria, endpoints, and procedures analyzed. Ojike and colleagues[24] performed a systematic review on 8 separate studies in an effort to determine the incidence, risk factors, and diagnosis of VTE after shoulder surgery. Seven of the studies included were considered level II evidence, whereas 1 study was level IV. The study collected information on a total of 40,537 patients. Of these, 7314 had undergone an anatomic total shoulder arthroplasty, 9432 a hemiarthroplasty, and the remaining 23,791 an arthroscopic procedure. The overall reported rate of DVT in these studies ranged from 0.02% to 13%. The overall rate of VTE across all patients was 0.35%, with 0.24% of these having a DVT and 0.11% having a PE. VTE was more common for arthroplasty procedure with a rate of 0.7%, compared with 0.08% for arthroscopic procedures (Fig. 1).

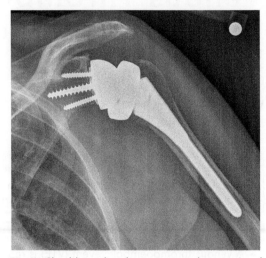

Fig. 1. Shoulder arthroplasty seems to be associated with a higher risk of VTE than shoulder arthroscopy.

Three recent prospective studies have attempted to delineate the incidence of VTE after shoulder arthroplasty,[19] arthroscopy,[20] and trauma[21] (Table 1). Willis and colleagues[19] prospectively studied 100 consecutive patients undergoing shoulder arthroplasty (73 anatomic total shoulder arthroplasties and 27 hemiarthroplasties). All patients underwent 4-limb surveillance Doppler ultrasounds 2 days after surgery. Additionally, 50 patients underwent a repeat ultrasound at 12 weeks postoperatively. The investigators documented 13 (13%) DVTs in 12 patients, 10 of which had occurred by day 2, whereas 3 were diagnosed at week 12. The location of the DVTs varied, with 6 in the ipsilateral upper extremity, 5 in the ipsilateral lower extremity, and 2 in the contralateral lower extremity. None of these patients seemed symptomatic. In this cohort, there were 2 (2%) symptomatic nonfatal PEs and 1 (1%) fatal PE at 7 weeks postoperatively.

Takahashi and colleagues[20] prospectively studied 175 consecutive patients undergoing shoulder arthroscopy. Similarly, all patients underwent 4-limb Doppler ultrasound. Unlike the study by Willis and colleagues,[19] these investigators performed preprocedural baseline ultrasound scans, scans at 1 to 2 days postoperatively, and scans 3 weeks to 3 months postoperatively. Ultrasound detected 10 (5.7%) DVTs in this cohort, with only 1 occurring in the upper extremity and only 1 occurring in the subacute (3 weeks to 3 months) phase. Additionally, 1 patient was noted to have an asymptomatic PE in the subacute phase. The same institution performed surveillance scans in

Table 1					
Summary of prospective studies evaluating the incidence of venous thromboembolic events after shoulder surgery					
Study	**Surgery**	**Sample Size**	**Prophylactic Measures**	**Diagnostic Method**	**Incidence**
Willis et al,[19] 2009	Arthroplasty	100	• Enteric-coasted aspirin • Pneumatic compression devices • Early mobilization	4-limb surveillance Doppler ultrasound at: • 2 d postoperatively • 12 wk postoperatively	DVT: 13% PE: 3%
Takahashi et al,[20] 2014	Arthroscopy	175	• Elastic stockings • Pneumatic compression devices • Early mobilization	4-limb surveillance Doppler ultrasound at: • Preoperatively • 1–2 d postoperatively • 3–12 wk postoperatively	DVT: 5.7% PE: 0.6%
Widmer et al,[21] 2011	Trauma	50	• Enteric-coated aspirin • Pneumatic compression devices • Early mobilization	3-limb surveillance Doppler ultrasound at: • 7–21 d operatively	DVT: 0% PE: 0%

patients undergoing total knee arthroplasty, and they observed a 33% incidence of asymptomatic DVT.

Widmer and colleagues[21] prospectively studied 50 patients treated for a proximal humerus with open reduction internal fixation or hemiarthroplasty. Patients underwent Doppler ultrasounds of the operative extremity and the bilateral lower extremities at a single time point, between 7 days and 21 days postoperatively. No patient had evidence of DVT or PE.

These studies highlight the challenges in defining the true incidence of VTE after shoulder surgery. First, the sample size in each study is low, given the known low number of absolute events. Second, prophylactic measures varied in each study (see Table 1). Third, surveillance ultrasounds capture subclinical events, which may not be useful for altering treatment management or instituting prevention modalities. Lastly, surveillance was performed at various time points. Without a preoperative scan, it is uncertain whether the large number of DVTs identified by Willis and colleagues[19] were present prior to surgery.

Several retrospective reviews have analyzed the incidence of VTE after shoulder surgery (Table 2). The rates in these studies tend to be lower than those reported in the aforementioned prospective studies, because only symptomatic, clinically significant events are captured. A recent database study from the United Kingdom analyzing 2341 patients noted an overall incidence of symptomatic VTE of 0.43%.[25] The rate for arthroplasty procedures

was 1.42% compared with 0.31% for arthroscopic procedures. Lyman and colleagues[26] reported on 13,759 shoulder arthroplasties performed in New York State and noted the overall incidence of symptomatic DVT was 0.5% and for symptomatic PE was 0.23%. Navarro and colleagues[27] performed a similar database study in the United States reviewing 2574 patients undergoing shoulder arthroplasty and noted a VTE rate of 1.01%. There was a slight trend toward increased risk of VTE in patients undergoing arthroplasty for trauma rather than on elective basis for nontraumatic etiology. A larger nationwide database study from the United Kingdom showed a similar increase in VTE risk in patients undergoing shoulder surgery for trauma (Fig. 2).[28] One study reported a high 5.1% rate of symptomatic nonfatal PE after treatment of a proximal humerus fracture.[29] The same group reported a symptomatic nonfatal PE rate of 0.17% in patients undergoing shoulder arthroplasty.[30] Most other studies have also noted that the rate of VTE after arthroscopic shoulder surgery is generally lower than that after arthroplasty or trauma-related procedures.[24,25,28,31–33]

Few studies clearly separate whether the DVT observed occurred in the upper extremity or the lower extremity. In their systematic review, based on 5 of the 8 studies included, Ojike and colleagues[24] reported that 58% of DVTs occurred in the upper extremity. Several studies have shown that upper extremity DVT carries a significant risk of PE and has a higher rate of mortality relative to lower extremity DVT.[34]

Table 2
Summary of retrospective studies evaluating the incidence of VTE after shoulder surgery

Study	Surgery	Sample Size	Venous Thromboembolic Event (%)	Incidence Deep Vein Thrombosis (%)	Pulmonary Embolism (%)
Lyman et al,[26] 2006	Arthroplasty	13,759	—	0.5	0.23
Sperling and Cofield,[30] 2002	Arthroplasty	2885	—	—	0.17
Navarro et al,[27] 2013	Arthroplasty	2574	1.01	0.51	0.54
Wronka et al,[25] 2014	Arthroplasty	352	1.42	0.56	0.85
	Arthroscopy	1281	0.31	0.23	0.08
Jameson et al,[28] 2011	Arthroplasty	10,229	0.15	0.06	0.11
	Arthroscopy	65,302	0.01	0.004	0.008
	Trauma	4696	0.51	0.19	0.40
Hoxie et al,[29] 2007	Trauma	137	—	—	5.1
Kuremsky et al,[31] 2011	Arthroscopy	1908	0.47	0.26	0.21
Randelli et al,[32] 2010	Arthroscopy	9385	0.06	0.05	0.01
Bongiovanni et al,[33] 2009	Arthroscopy	1082	—	0.27	—
Day et al,[36] 2015	Arthroplasty	130,258	0.53	—	—

RISK FACTORS

The limitations of the studies, outlined previously regarding VTE after shoulder surgery, make it difficult to identify specific risk factors. Nonetheless, it is clear that there is a VTE risk

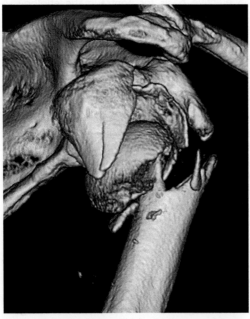

Fig. 2. Shoulder surgery for trauma seems associated with an increased risking of VTE.

associated with shoulder surgery where a fatal PE may occur.[14,15,19]

The United Kingdom National Institute for Health and Clinical Excellence has described a set of risk factors for VTE.[35] These include age older than 60 years, dehydration, admission to critical care, active malignancy or active cancer treatment, obesity, known thrombophilia, prior VTE, history of a first-degree family member with a VTE, estrogen-containing contraception, hormone replacement therapy, and pregnancy or recent childbirth. Willis and colleagues,[19] in their prospective surveillance study, noted that increasing age, BMI, prolonged operative time, and prior history of VTE all trended toward an increased risk of VTE. Lyman and colleagues[26] suggested that increasing age, traumatic etiology, and active malignancy were risk factors for VTE.

More recently, Day and colleagues[36] reviewed the national Medicare data to determine the incidence of symptomatic VTE as well as the patient-specific risk factors. This study focused specifically on arthroplasty procedures. The overall incidence of VTE was 0.53%. The investigators did not demonstrate that increasing age was a risk factor for VTE. The risk of VTE was significantly increased in patients treated for a diagnosis of fracture and those with a prior history of VTE as well as in the presence of a metastatic tumor, coagulopathy, cardiac arrhythmia, congestive heart failure, alcohol abuse, or obesity. In particular, the PE risk was increased 5-fold for patients undergoing anatomic total shoulder arthroplasty and 3-fold for patients undergoing hemiarthroplasty.

Dattani and colleagues[22] performed a systematic review of 14 studies. The VTE rate after arthroscopic surgery was 0.038%, after arthroplasty procedures was 0.45%, and after surgery for shoulder trauma was 0.82%. Risk factors identified by these investigators included diabetes mellitus, rheumatoid arthritis, and ischemic heart disease. The investigators also mentioned that the lateral decubitus position may be a risk factor for VTE (the first described case of VTE after arthroscopic shoulder surgery by Burkhart[11] occurred in the lateral position). As discussed previously, some investigators have theorized that traction on the arm may cause injury and incite the Virchow triad. In most case reports of VTE after arthroscopic surgery in the lateral decubitus position, however, other intrinsic risk factors are identified, such as a compressive mass.[11] The beach chair position with the lower extremity in a dependent position may itself be a risk factor for VTE. Yet, case reports have usually identified other potential risk factors, such as age, estrogen use, and obesity.[37]

PREVENTION

As discussed previously, chemical prophylaxis is commonly used for lower extremity arthroplasty. There are few data in regard to chemical or mechanical prophylaxis as preventative for VTE in upper extremity surgery. In a survey of 99 American Shoulder and Elbow Surgeons members, only 37 reported using chemical prophylaxis routinely after shoulder arthroplasty.[36] A small proportion of surgeons routinely used mechanical measures, whereas a majority used no form of VTE prophylaxis.

Several studies have discussed the use of aspirin as a form of chemoprophylaxis, but it has not been shown to decrease the risk of VTE after shoulder surgery.[19,21,36] Based on the available literature, understanding of minimizing the risk of VTE after shoulder surgery should be based largely on understanding of the Virchow triad. Patients who are considered hypercoagulable should be given consideration for chemical and mechanical prophylactic measures. These include those on estrogen therapy, who have had recent trauma, with a history of active malignancy, with recent sedentary travel, or with history of a coagulopathy or prior VTE. Additional measures may be considered to limit venous stasis, such as the application of pneumatic compression devices in the operating room, particularly in patients in the beach chair position with dependent lower extremities. Lastly, endothelial injury should be limited by minimizing traction on the arm for arthroscopic procedures in the lateral decubitus position, avoiding excessive retraction during shoulder arthroplasty, and minimizing operative time.

The authors believe that utilization of pneumatic compression devices in the operating room and during admission for those undergoing inpatient surgeries should be considered due to relative low cost and absence of complications. Early patient mobilization after surgery should be encouraged as well. Patients with substantial risk factors or on pharmacologic prophylaxis previously generally receive some form of chemical prophylaxis, which is weighed against the risk of bleeding complications for their respective procedures.

SUMMARY

VTE after shoulder surgery is a rare but potentially fatal event. DVTs can occur in the operative upper extremity as well as in the lower extremity. Due to the low overall incidence of symptomatic VTE, it is difficult to clearly identify potential risk factors. Risk factors that likely place patients at risk for VTE complicating shoulder surgery may include a prolonged operative time in the lateral decubitus or beach chair position, history of trauma (in particular surgery for shoulder fracture), prior history of VTE, obesity, increasing age, and estrogen use. A high index of suspicion is required to diagnosis a DVT or PE after shoulder surgery. Doppler ultrasound of the upper and lower extremities should be considered for DVT, and a CT angiography of the chest should be ordered to evaluate for PE (Fig. 3). Treatment should be prompt to avoid potential complications. There is little evidence to guide VTE prophylaxis for shoulder surgery. Mechanical prophylaxis, such as the use of pneumatic compression devices, represents a reasonable, safe, and cost-effective option for most patients. Chemical prophylaxis should be considered for patients with intrinsic risk factors and weighed against the potential risks of postoperative hematoma and wound problems. Evidence-based medicine is difficult to apply to VTE complicating shoulder surgery for all the reasons discussed previously. Undoubtedly, further larger prospective

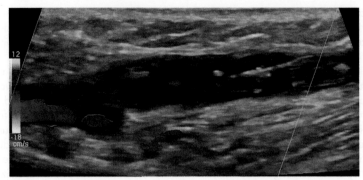

Fig. 3. Doppler ultrasound of an 80-year-old woman demonstrating evidence of a DVT in the lower extremity with no flow on color Doppler and thrombus present. The patient underwent a reverse total shoulder arthroplasty 7 weeks prior to DVT symptoms. The patient was taking enteric-coated aspirin prior to surgery and continued after surgery. Risk factors included advanced age and history of lung adenocarcinoma. Surgery was performed in the beach chair position and operative time was 102 minutes. The patient was started on apixaban.

multicenter studies and better consensus reports should be pursued to provide better guidance for patients and surgeons.

REFERENCES

1. Bagot CN, Arya R. Virchow and his triad: a question of attribution. Br J Haematol 2008;143(2):180–90.
2. Oster G, Ollendorf DA, Vera-Llonch M, et al. Economic consequences of venous thromboembolism following major orthopedic surgery. Ann Pharmacother 2004;38(3):377–82.
3. MacDougall DA, Feliu AL, Boccuzzi SJ, et al. Economic burden of deep-vein thrombosis, pulmonary embolism, and post-thrombotic syndrome. Am J Health Syst Pharm 2006;63(20 Suppl 6):S5–15.
4. Haake DA, Berkman SA. Venous thromboembolic disease after hip surgery. Risk factors, prophylaxis, and diagnosis. Clin Orthop Relat Res 1989;(242):212–31.
5. Geerts WH, Bergqvist D, Pineo GF, et al. Prevention of venous thromboembolism: American College of Chest Physicians Evidence-Based Clinical Practice Guidelines (8th Edition). Chest 2008;133(6 Suppl):381S–453S.
6. Freedman KB, Brookenthal KR, Fitzgerald RH Jr, et al. A meta-analysis of thromboembolic prophylaxis following elective total hip arthroplasty. J Bone Joint Surg Am 2000;82-A(7):929–38.
7. Clarke MT, Green JS, Harper WM, et al. Screening for deep-venous thrombosis after hip and knee replacement without prophylaxis. J Bone Joint Surg Br 1997;79(5):787–91.
8. Stulberg BN, Insall JN, Williams GW, et al. Deep-vein thrombosis following total knee replacement. An analysis of six hundred and thirty-eight arthroplasties. J Bone Joint Surg Am 1984;66(2):194–201.
9. Warwick D, Williams MH, Bannister GC. Death and thromboembolic disease after total hip replacement. A series of 1162 cases with no routine chemical prophylaxis. J Bone Joint Surg Br 1995;77(1):6–10.
10. American Academy of Orthopaedic Surgeons. Preventing venous thromboembolic disease in patients undergoing elective hip and knee arthroplasty: evidence-based guideline and evidence report. 2011. Available at: https://www.aaos.org/uploadedFiles/PreProduction/Quality/Guidelines_and_Reviews/VTE_full_guideline_10.31.16.pdf. Accessed June 12, 2017.
11. Burkhart SS. Deep venous thrombosis after shoulder arthroscopy. Arthroscopy 1990;6(1):61–3.
12. Scott DL. Pulmonary embolism after elective glenohumeral joint debridement. Orthopedics 2001;24(5):495–7.
13. Rockwood CA Jr, Wirth MA, Blair S. Warning: pulmonary embolism can occur after elective shoulder surgery-report of two cases and survey of the members of the American Shoulder and Elbow Surgeons. J Shoulder Elbow Surg 2003;12(6):628–30.
14. Saleem A, Markel DC. Fatal pulmonary embolus after shoulder arthroplasty. J Arthroplasty 2001;16(3):400–3.
15. Madhusudhan TR, Shetty SK, Madhusudhan S, et al. Fatal pulmonary embolism following shoulder arthroplasty: a case report. J Med Case Rep 2009;3:8708.
16. Arcand M, Burkhead WZ Jr, Zeman C. Pulmonary embolism caused by thrombosis of the axillary vein after shoulder arthroplasty. J Shoulder Elbow Surg 1997;6(5):486–90.
17. Amarasekera SS, van Dalen J, Thompson TJ, et al. Pulmonary embolism after acromioplasty and rotator cuff repair. J Shoulder Elbow Surg 2008;17(5):e13–4.

18. Creighton RA, Cole BJ. Upper extremity deep venous thrombosis after shoulder arthroscopy: a case report. J Shoulder Elbow Surg 2007;16(1): e20–2.

19. Willis AA, Warren RF, Craig EV, et al. Deep vein thrombosis after reconstructive shoulder arthroplasty: a prospective observational study. J Shoulder Elbow Surg 2009;18(1):100–6.

20. Takahashi H, Yamamoto N, Nagamoto H, et al. Venous thromboembolism after elective shoulder surgery: a prospective cohort study of 175 patients. J Shoulder Elbow Surg 2014;23(5):605–12.

21. Widmer BJ, Bassora R, Warrender WJ, et al. Thromboembolic events are uncommon after open treatment of proximal humerus fractures using aspirin and compression devices. Clin Orthop Relat Res 2011;469(12):3332–6.

22. Dattani R, Smith CD, Patel VR. The venous thromboembolic complications of shoulder and elbow surgery: a systematic review. Bone Joint J 2013; 95-B(1):70–4.

23. American Academy of Orthopaedic Surgeons. The treatment of glenohumeral joint osteoarthritis: guideline and evidence report. 2009. Available at: https://www.aaos.org/research/guidelines/gloguideline.pdf. Accessed June 12, 2017.

24. Ojike NI, Bhadra AK, Giannoudis PV, et al. Venous thromboembolism in shoulder surgery: a systematic review. Acta Orthop Belg 2011;77(3):281–9.

25. Wronka KS, Pritchard M, Sinha A. Incidence of symptomatic venous thrombo-embolism following shoulder surgery. Int Orthop 2014;38(7):1415–8.

26. Lyman S, Sherman S, Carter TI, et al. Prevalence and risk factors for symptomatic thromboembolic events after shoulder arthroplasty. Clin Orthop Relat Res 2006;448:152–6.

27. Navarro RA, Inacio MC, Burke MF, et al. Risk of thromboembolism in shoulder arthroplasty: effect of implant type and traumatic indication. Clin Orthop Relat Res 2013;471(5):1576–81.

28. Jameson SS, James P, Howcroft DW, et al. Venous thromboembolic events are rare after shoulder surgery: analysis of a national database. J Shoulder Elbow Surg 2011;20(5):764–70.

29. Hoxie SC, Sperling JW, Cofield RH. Pulmonary embolism after operative treatment of proximal humeral fractures. J Shoulder Elbow Surg 2007;16(6): 782–3.

30. Sperling JW, Cofield RH. Pulmonary embolism following shoulder arthroplasty. J Bone Joint Surg Am 2002;84-A(11):1939–41.

31. Kuremsky MA, Cain EL Jr, Fleischli JE. Thromboembolic phenomena after arthroscopic shoulder surgery. Arthroscopy 2011;27(12):1614–9.

32. Randelli P, Castagna A, Cabitza F, et al. Infectious and thromboembolic complications of arthroscopic shoulder surgery. J Shoulder Elbow Surg 2010; 19(1):97–101.

33. Bongiovanni SL, Ranalletta M, Guala A, et al. Case reports: heritable thrombophilia associated with deep venous thrombosis after shoulder arthroscopy. Clin Orthop Relat Res 2009;467(8):2196–9.

34. Hingorani A, Ascher E, Lorenson E, et al. Upper extremity deep venous thrombosis and its impact on morbidity and mortality rates in a hospital-based population. J Vasc Surg 1997; 26(5):853–60.

35. Anakwe RE, Middleton SD, Beresford-Cleary N, et al. Preventing venous thromboembolism in elective upper limb surgery. J Shoulder Elbow Surg 2013;22(3):432–8.

36. Day JS, Ramsey ML, Lau E, et al. Risk of venous thromboembolism after shoulder arthroplasty in the Medicare population. J Shoulder Elbow Surg 2015;24(1):98–105.

37. Cortes ZE, Hammerman SM, Gartsman GM. Pulmonary embolism after shoulder arthroscopy: could patient positioning and traction make a difference? J Shoulder Elbow Surg 2007;16(2): e16–7.

Foot and Ankle

Venous Thromboembolism Disease Prophylaxis in Foot and Ankle Surgery

Bonnie Y. Chien, MD[a,*], Tonya Dixon, MD, MPH[b],
Daniel Guss, MD, MBA[b,c], Christopher DiGiovanni, MD[b,c]

KEYWORDS

- VTED prophylaxis • Foot and ankle • Mechanical • Chemical prophylaxis

---

KEY POINTS

- Indications for venous thromboembolism disease (VTED) prophylaxis in foot and ankle surgery remain unclear, with available evidence frequently of low quality and often contradictory in its conclusions.
- Consider all potential individual risk factors for VTED when making any decision to pursue chemical prophylaxis after foot and ankle surgery.
- The need for perioperative chemical prophylaxis in foot and ankle surgery is most clear for patients who have a known history of VTED, hereditary predisposition, or a positive family history.
- Certain subpopulations of patients may be at higher risk, such as ankle fracture in those older than 50, acute Achilles tendon injury, or preexisting inflammatory connective tissue disorders. The need for VTED prophylaxis, the type of prophylaxis recommended, as well as its efficacy in preventing VTED remains controversial.
- Higher-powered level I data will be necessary to definitively answer these VTED questions and develop consensus for the foot and ankle population.

INTRODUCTION

The fundamental reason for preventing postoperative deep vein thrombosis (DVT) is to avoid clinically significant chronic venous stasis, phlebitis, and, most importantly, potentially fatal pulmonary embolism (PE). Accordingly, numerous specialty society guidelines underscore the importance of postoperative venous thromboembolism disease (VTED) prophylaxis after hip or knee arthroplasty or in the setting of hip fracture, for which there is robust literature supporting the use of such preventive measures. In contrast, few data exist to guide patients or providers alike regarding the use of VTED prophylaxis after foot and ankle surgery. Current recommendations are often inconsistent and are generally based on weak or insufficient evidence (Table 1). Therefore, the recommendations currently in use after hip and knee arthroplasty may not be safely extrapolated to foot and ankle surgery patients, especially in light of the wide variability in procedure type and severity, as well as differences in postoperative immobilization protocols. These shortcomings continue to render safe and effective VTED care of the foot and ankle patient somewhat challenging.

Published surveys of foot and ankle surgeons have repeatedly demonstrated that providers use a wide variety of prophylactic regimens

---

Disclosure Statement: None.
[a] Harvard Combined Orthopaedic Residency Program, Harvard University, 55 Fruit Street, Boston, MA 02114, USA; [b] Department Foot and Ankle Center, Massachusetts General Hospital Orthopaedics, 55 Fruit Street, Yawkey Building, Suite 3F, Boston, MA 02114, USA; [c] Foot and Ankle Center, Newton-Wellesley Hospital, 2014 Washington Street, Newton, MA 02462, USA
* Corresponding author.
E-mail address: bchien@partners.org

Orthop Clin N Am 49 (2018) 265–276
https://doi.org/10.1016/j.ocl.2017.11.013
0030-5898/18/Published by Elsevier Inc.

Table 1	
Recommendations for venous thromboembolism disease prophylaxis from different committees	
Committee	**Recommendation**
American College of Chest Physicians (ACCP) 2012[1]	Use chemical prophylaxis or an intermittent pneumatic compression device for patients undergoing major orthopedic surgery (total hip arthroplasty, total knee arthroplasty, or hip fracture surgery). *No chemical prophylaxis is needed for patients with a lower extremity (distal to knee) injury that requires immobilization-weak recommendation based on low quality evidence*
American Academy of Orthopedic Surgeons (AAOS) 2012[2]	Use pharmacologic or mechanical prophylaxis for venous thromboembolism disease in patients undergoing elective hip or knee arthroplasty without risk factors. *No specific recommendation regarding foot and ankle surgery*
American Orthopedic Foot & Ankle Society (AOFAS) 2013[3]	*Insufficient evidence* to make recommendation for or against use of venous thromboembolism disease prophylaxis

without clear patterns of use, including aspirin, low molecular weight heparin (LMWH), sequential compression devices, and other forms of prophylaxis. This ongoing confusion is highlighted by the inconsistent guidelines published to date, and demonstrates the lack of consensus necessary to properly care for this patient population. One survey found that even though fewer than 50% of surgeons used prophylaxis, 70% believed it was sometimes necessary, with great variation in use.[4–6] Although some surgeons have argued that prophylaxis is not uniformly necessary for the foot and ankle population based on an overall lower incidence of VTED as compared with the hip and knee population, most acknowledge that not all the foot and ankle population is risk free. Unfortunately, an assumption that VTED prophylaxis is unnecessary at the population level does not predicate an ability to perform a risk-benefit analysis at the individual patient level.

INCIDENCE

Foot and ankle surgery encompasses a disparate array of procedures, making it challenging to project heterogeneous procedure data at the population level onto a single individual. The incidence of VTED events in foot and ankle surgery as described in the literature is therefore often marked by enormous variability. Many of the largest studies to date depend on large-scale state or national databases, and thereby insert their own confounders. A large-scale study that retrospectively examined a California statewide database found a very low incidence of DVT, and recommended no need for prophylaxis.[7] This study, however, relied on hospital

readmissions to capture DVTs, likely underestimating the incidence of such events. Another retrospective population study conducted within a single, large-scale California health system also found a low rate of DVT, but the overwhelming majority of these procedures were located in the forefoot, which may also underestimate VTED rates by virtue of being low-risk procedures.[8] Meanwhile, another prospective study exploring VTED after acute Achilles injuries found DVTs in more than a third of patients, suggesting a markedly high risk.[9] This study, however, performed routine ultrasound screening of all patients, including asymptomatic ones, arguably overestimating the incidence of clinically significant events. Meanwhile, there are studies published in well-regarded journals concluding that the simple act of below-knee cast immobilization requires DVT prophylaxis, colored by other studies that suggest DVT prophylaxis may not work in preventing VTED events.[10–12] Ultimately, providers and patients alike find themselves mired in uncertainty.

At the population level, the overall risk of VTED for patients without risk factors undergoing foot and ankle surgery is approximately 3:1000, compared with the overall population rate of 1:1000.[13] The risk of VTED increases to more than 4% in the presence of previous VTED history and 2 or more of the following risk factors: obesity with a body mass index (BMI) greater than 30 kg/m^2, age older than 40, medical comorbidities, use of a contraceptive pill, and immobilization.[14] Felcher and colleagues[15] found that history of VTED conferred a 23 times greater risk (multivariate odds ratio 23, 95% confidence interval 9–58) of subsequent VTED event among 7264 patients who underwent foot surgery. Saragas and colleagues[16] also found that active or previous malignancy was present in 27.3% of those who developed VTED after foot or ankle surgery compared with only 11.7% of their non-VTED patients. Another retrospective study of 602 patients with a 4% incidence of symptomatic VTED suggested that inflammatory connective tissue conditions, such as rheumatoid arthritis, were significant risk factors ($P = .04$).[17]

A generalized, overall incidence remains difficult to determine given the wide range of host factors and foot and ankle disorders and procedures that exist for this particular population. Some of these values are summarized in Table 2. One major confounding factor in attempting to determine actual risk stratification for this group of patients is the fact that:

1. Most published studies involve only level 4 evidence,
2. Few accurately record whether or not patients received prophylaxis, what kind, or for how long, and
3. None have ever been sufficiently powered to study this problem in a statistically responsible manner.

As alluded to previously, one retrospective study of readmission rates from VTED in 57,183 patients undergoing surgery for ankle fractures in California demonstrated readmission rates of 0.05% for DVT and 0.34% for PE.[7] In another study of 4481 patients undergoing calcaneal fracture repair, VTED readmission was 0.25%.[20] Although these numbers are globally lower than that for the hip and knee population, they likely underestimate the VTED incidence by including only patients with severe enough VTED events to warrant admission, which likely fails to capture most patients with VTED who are generally treated on an outpatient basis. Similarly, the English National Health Service found low rates, including DVT 0.12%, PE 0.17% among 45,949 ankle fracture surgeries; DVT 0.01%, PE 0.02% among 33,626 first metatarsal osteotomies; and DVT 0.03%, PE 0.11% among 7033 hindfoot fusions. This study is limited in its dependence on diagnostic codes for diagnosis and its inability to ascertain whether VTED prophylaxis was actually used.[18] A large prospective multicenter study found that the incidence of PE was 0.15% across a broad spectrum of foot and ankle surgeries, consistent with the rates reported previously.[6]

Despite the approximations in Table 2, the true incidence of VTED events for both standard and high-risk patients remains elusive as a result of the differing reports that confound symptomatic versus asymptomatic events, which may not be of equivalent clinical importance. In reviewing

Table 2
Reported venous thromboembolism disease incidence according to different foot and ankle surgeries/injuries

Type of Surgery/Injury	Reported Incidence of VTED
First ray surgery	0.01% (symptomatic DVT), 0.02%[18] (PE) *Did not state if patients had received prophylaxis or not*
Metatarsal fracture	0.2%[8] (PE); no DVT rate reported *Did not state if patients had received prophylaxis or not*
Hindfoot fusion	0.03% (symptomatic DVT), 0.11%[18] (PE) *Did not state if patients had received prophylaxis or not*
Total ankle arthroplasty	3.9% (symptomatic VTED)[19]; *all received LMWH* 0.06% (PE)[18]; *unclear if patients had received prophylaxis or not*
Ankle trauma	0.05%–28%[14] (VTED), 5% symptomatic *Mixed in whether received prophylaxis*
Achilles tendon	5%–36%[14] (VTED) *Unclear if symptomatic and mixed in whether received prophylaxis, although higher end of range was observed in those who did not receive chemical prophylaxis*
Lower extremity cast and brace immobilization	4.3%–40% in no prophylaxis group, 0%–37% in LMWH group[10]; *not stated whether symptomatic or not* 2.5% in no prophylaxis group, 0.3% in LMWH group had symptomatic VTED[10]

Abbreviations: DVT, deep vein thrombosis; LMWH, low molecular weight heparin; PE, pulmonary embolism; VTED, venous thromboembolism disease.

the literature, it is crucial to separate incidence estimates based on the substantial heterogeneity in the foot and ankle population in both conditions and procedures.

Despite the low incidence of VTED in foot and ankle surgery, and lack of consensus regarding chemical prophylaxis, the American Orthopedic Foot and Ankle Society (AOFAS) still recommends preoperative risk evaluation to determine if benefits may outweigh risks of chemical anticoagulation.[3]

RISK FACTORS

Classically, Virchow's triad of venous stasis, endothelial injury and hypercoagulability has been used to predict risk of thrombus formation. Stasis is particularly relevant to foot and ankle surgery given patients are often immobilized postoperatively for a prolonged period. These variables can be correlated with risk factors as listed in Table 3.

A risk assessment model can assist with determining which patients may be considered for VTED prophylaxis. The UK National Health Service (NHS) has used the Plymouth VTED trauma score for lower limb trauma in patients immobilized in a boot or cast to provide LMWH to patients scoring more than 3 points. In one study, the accuracy of the Plymouth assessment tool was estimated to be only approximately 55%, although better than other tools. Their risk assessment score is based on different patient

history elements with previous history of DVT/PE, pregnancy, Achilles tendon rupture, and coagulopathy each contributing 3 points (Table 4). Although the NHS internal auditing has shown that they have reduced their VTED events in orthopedics from 2.3 per month to fewer than 1 per month using the Plymouth tool, it has not been validated for the foot and ankle population.[9,14]

Variables with insufficient evidence supporting their role as risk factors include smoking, gender, race/ethnicity, pregnancy, and cardiovascular factors.[21] Tourniquet use and air travel (within 2 weeks of an operation) have had conflicting evidence regarding their extent as risk factors.[17,23]

DIAGNOSIS

The timely, accurate diagnosis of VTED can be challenging and requires a high index of suspicion given that the interval onset of VTED in the foot and ankle population is unclear. In one retrospective study of 115 patients who underwent Achilles tendon repair within an average 2.5-day interval, one-third of DVTs occurred preoperatively.[24] The investigators however, suggested that pharmacologic prophylaxis may not be necessary before surgery given the patients were not immobilized preoperatively. Arguably the more relevant clinical presentation is among those patients who present with symptomatic DVTs rather than those found on

Table 3 Purported risk factors for venous thromboembolism disease in foot and ankle surgery	
Primary Risk Factors per American Orthopedic Foot & Ankle Society (AOFAS)[3]	**Secondary Risk Factors per AOFAS**
Prior venous thromboembolism disease	Obesity
History of recent malignancy	Age >40 y
Prolonged lower extremity immobilization (ie, with plaster, at least 5 wk[22])	Oral contraceptive or hormone replacement therapy
	Family history of venous thromboembolism disease (most often overlooked)
	Venous stasis/varicose veins
	Higher injury severity score (correlated with more severe injuries of the foot and ankle)
	Diabetes
	Connective tissue disorders
	Non–weight-bearing status, hospitalization, bed rest >3 d
	Use of general anesthesia (as opposed to regional with monitored anesthesia care)
	Operative and nonoperative management of ankle fractures and Achilles tendon ruptures
	Hindfoot arthrodesis
	Total ankle replacement surgery

Data from Refs.[2,17,18,21]

Table 4
Summary of Plymouth guidelines for venous thromboembolism disease prophylaxis in orthopedics

Risk Factors	Score
Patient details	
Age ≥60	1
Body mass index ≥30	2
Inability to walk before accident/injury	2
Current medication	
Oral contraceptive pill	1
Hormone replacement therapy	1
Family history	
Known history of deep vein thrombosis (DVT) in immediate family member	2
Medical condition	
Varicose vein	1
Long-term medical condition requiring treatment	1
Abdominal surgery in last 6 wk	2
Active cancer	3
Previous history of DVT	3
Previous history of pulmonary embolism	3
Pregnant or within 6 wk of delivery	3
Achilles tendon rupture	3
Complex lower limb surgery	3
Known clotting disease	3

Score 0 to 2: mobilization as able.
Score 3 or more: enoxaparin 40 mg daily or equivalent.

screening studies. Patients who develop a DVT often present with some combination of pain, swelling, warmth, and/or erythema along the affected extremity. The challenging reality is that many of these signs and symptoms are also quite similar to those expected after injury as well as after surgical intervention. A positive Homan sign, specifically calf pain with the ankle dorsiflexed and the knee flexed, is neither particularly sensitive nor specific and can be positive in up to half of patients with or without a DVT.[25] Noninvasive duplex ultrasound has a reported sensitivity and specificity of more than 90% in diagnosing DVT.[10] Although ultrasound has been used to detect early peripheral DVT, the American Academy of Orthopedic Surgeons and Orthopedic Trauma Association both recommend against routine screening in asymptomatic orthopedic joint arthroplasty and trauma patients for DVT.[2,26] The ultimate goal of looking for a DVT is early detection of any potential signs, symptoms, and risk for PE. Computed tomography pulmonary angiography is used to definitely diagnose PE, but has no role as a screening tool given cost and the renal implications of contrast use, especially in elderly patients.

VENOUS THROMBOEMBOLISM DISEASE PROPHYLAXIS

A number of different prophylactic strategies exist to prevent VTED in the foot and ankle patient, ranging from mechanical prophylaxis to chemoprophylaxis. Full anticoagulation is generally reserved once the patient has developed a DVT or PE. The following section examines the evidence in efficacy of VTED prophylaxis for foot and ankle surgery and a summary is provided in Table 5.

The decision to use DVT prophylaxis or to treat a diagnosed DVT after foot and ankle surgery is further confounded by the fact that most DVTs affecting foot and ankle patients are distal to the popliteal fossa, which have a lower recurrence rate as well as a lower risk of progression to PE than more proximal DVTs.[27]

Table 5
Summary evidence of efficacy of different types of venous thromboembolism disease (VTED) prophylaxis in foot and ankle surgery

Modality of VTED Prophylaxis	Efficacy in VTED Prophylaxis
Mechanical	Unknown in foot and ankle, although routinely used
Aspirin	Insufficient evidence to support isolated use in high-risk patients
Low molecular weight heparin (LMWH)	Mixed evidence, but may be considered in higher risk patients who will be immobilized
Other agents: warfarin, factor Xa inhibitors, direct thrombin inhibitors	Can be used in place of LMWH if contraindicated

Furthermore, a shorter duration of treatment (6 as opposed to 12 weeks) seems sufficient to render a lower recurrence rate and fewer major hemorrhages.[28] The American College of Chest Physicians (ACCP) 2012 guidelines suggest for acute isolated distal DVT without severe symptoms or risk factors for extension such as multiple vein involvement, larger size thrombosis, active cancer, history of VTED, and inpatient status, serial imaging of the deep veins for 2 weeks should be performed. Only if patients have severe symptoms or risk factors, then anticoagulation should be initiated.[1]

Mechanical Prophylaxis

The concept of mechanical prophylaxis is predicated on the principle of graduated muscle contraction as a means of compressing veins to induce venous return. This type of treatment includes intrinsic isometric leg/calf/toe exercises, external elastic compression stockings, and sequential compression devices, such as calf or foot pumps. Intermittent compression pumps reduce venous stasis by facilitating increased venous flow velocity. Compressive stockings reduce the overall cross-sectional area of the limb, increase linear velocity of venous flow, and decrease venous distension. Its utility is often limited by the presence of a cast, splint, or other dressing on the operative extremity. Although regularly used, the efficacy and appropriate duration of these devices both intraoperatively and postoperatively are unknown in foot and ankle surgery.[25,29] The major advantage of mechanical compression, however, is their noninvasive nature and low associated morbidity.

One prospective trial randomized 372 patients to either LMWH or mechanical compression. These patients fell into one of the following categories: abbreviated injury scale ≥3, major head, spine, pelvic or lower extremity fractures.[30] Bilateral sequential compression devices (SCDs) were used in those without lower leg injury, and an arteriovenous impulse foot compression was placed over the foot when injury precluded SCD use. In this study, 2.4% of patients overall developed a DVT, with an incidence of 0.8% in those who received LMWH, 2.5% in the SCD group, and 5.7% in the arteriovenous impulse (AVI) group. Although this study suggests that mechanical prophylaxis can help reduce VTED rates, it is unclear whether the leg injury or the use of a foot rather than a leg compression device predicated a higher rate of DVT. Irrespectively, LMWH may be more effective superimposed on the fact that mechanical compression in foot and ankle surgery would be limited in its utility given the need for device application over the distal lower extremity as well as its use only during hospital admission.[30]

Aspirin

According to the AOFAS, and analogous to other forms of chemoprophylaxis, there is currently insufficient evidence to support the use of aspirin after foot and ankle surgery, although it should be noted that this form of chemical prophylaxis has recently been espoused as an effective prophylactic strategy after hip and knee arthroplasty.[31] Aspirin even at low doses has been consistently demonstrated to be effective against VTED and safe in reducing infection and other complications compared with other agents such as warfarin in the arthroplasty literature. Limited evidence exists specifically for the foot and ankle population. A retrospective study of 2654 patients undergoing foot and ankle surgery determined that of the 1078 who received aspirin 75 mg, it was ineffective in altering the rate of postoperative symptomatic VTED (0.47% in the aspirin group vs 0.39% in the no aspirin group, P = .985); however, the overall rates in both groups was very low.[31]

Based on the cardiology literature, there is no definitive dose of aspirin yet recommended and there may not be any clear benefit to higher doses of aspirin.[32] In fact, in a prospective, crossover study of 3192 patients receiving aspirin 325 mg twice daily and 1459 patients received 81 mg twice daily, there was a statistically insignificant difference of 0.1% VTED rate in the low dose compared with 0.3% in the higher dose group.[33] Indeed, the cardiology literature has begun to demonstrate an equivalent cardioprotective effect of lower dose (81 mg) and higher dose (325 mg) aspirin.[32,34] The ability to project this cardiology literature onto VTED, let alone VTED after foot and ankle surgery, remains unclear. The use of aspirin for VTED prophylaxis requires not only an understanding of its preventive potential, but also its implications for adverse events. Notably, as compared with other blood thinners, it may have a lower rate of adverse events, such as bleeding or wound ooze, postoperatively, which motivated much if its use after hip or knee arthroplasty.[35,36] Furthermore, limited evidence from rat and rabbit studies of radius and ulna fractures suggests that indomethacin and aspirin in a dose-dependent manner can potentially delay bone healing radiographically and mechanically, including at an equivalent level used in humans (325 mg).[37,38]

Low Molecular Weight Heparin

LMWH works on the coagulation cascade through its indirect inhibition of factor Xa. The evidence for the use of LMWH after lower leg injury or surgery is mixed. A Cochrane review of 6 randomized controlled trials with 1490 patients found that LMWH significantly reduced the incidence of VTED from 4.3% to 40% in surgical and nonsurgical patients requiring lower leg immobilization to a large range 0% to 37%.[10] However, in another meta-analysis of 22 studies of patients who underwent foot and ankle surgery, the incidence of VTED with or without LMWH was not significantly different whether assessed clinically (n = 43,381, 0.6% and 1.0%, respectively) or radiographically (n = 1666, 12.5% and 10.5%, respectively).[39] The AOFAS consensus panel recommends that if considering LMWH following a foot or ankle surgery, therapy should begin when immobilization is initiated and continued for the duration of immobilization, with non–weight-bearing status recognized as a modifiable risk factor, but without specific recommendation for starting chemoprophylaxis.[3,31] It is unclear whether this has explicit benefits preoperatively in addition to postoperatively, although the shorter blood-thinning effect of LMWH likely makes preoperative use more feasible as compared with aspirin, which has a longer effective half-life.

Other Chemical Prophylaxis

The AOFAS panel also agreed that when subcutaneous injections such as LMWH are not an option in the outpatient setting (eg, patient intolerance or nonadherence) and chemical prophylaxis is desired, warfarin with a targeted international normalized ratio (INR) 2.5 (acceptable range 2.0–3.0) or newer oral agents such as apixaban, dabigatran, or rivaroxaban that do not require INR monitoring are viable options.[3] One study of 200 patients found that oral rivaroxaban, a direct factor Xa inhibitor, was effective and potentially a safe alternative to LMWH in preventing VTED in patients with ankle fractures managed nonoperatively in a cast, with one instance of isolated distal DVT.[40] Fondaparinux is another option that exerts its effect by binding to antithrombin III to potentiate its inhibition of factor Xa. A controlled, multicenter study that analyzed 273 patients immobilized for a foot or ankle fracture randomized to either anti-Xa agent nadroparin (n = 92) versus fondaparinux (n = 92) versus control (n = 94) found via ultrasound that the incidence of DVT was 2.2%, 1.1%, and 11.7%, respectively.[41]

When there are contraindications to chemical prophylaxis, such as head injury or severe hemodynamic instability, but it is necessary or there is a recurrence of symptomatic DVT, an inferior vena cava (IVC) filter may be considered. There is no specific evidence in the use of IVC filters for foot and ankle surgery, and the ACCP cautioned that IVC filter efficacy for patients without a prior history of DVT is not well established.[21] IVC filters are thus not routinely used in foot and ankle patients.

It is of paramount importance to recognize that, as of today, there exist no large-scale, prospective, randomized controlled studies that assess the effect of thromboprophylaxis on the incidence of VTED in elective foot and ankle surgery. Additional studies are necessary to help providers and patients alike navigate this decision making.

Adverse Effects of Chemical Prophylaxis

Clearly, although it is imperative to determine which mechanical or chemical agents are truly effective against VTED in the foot and ankle population, one must keep in mind that it is equally critical to understand the tradeoffs that the use of these prophylactic modalities incur. In some cases, the risk or morbidity of adverse events as a side effect of these agents may outweigh any potential benefit. This balance is inherently complicated by the fact that, generally speaking, those chemical agents that have the highest efficacy against VTED also come with the greatest risk for side effects, such as bleeding events at the surgical site or elsewhere, including intracranial and gastrointestinal. Furthermore, one relatively rare but potentially devastating side effect associated with the use of heparin-based VTED chemoprophylactic agents is the risk of heparin-induced thrombocytopenia (HIT), a potentially fatal complication from an antibody immunologic process that can involve DVT, PE, leg ischemia, bleeding, stroke, myocardial infarction, and multisystem organ failure.[42] Presenting symptoms include hemodynamic instability with fevers, tachycardia, hypertension, diaphoresis, chills, dyspnea, and chest and abdominal pain. HIT has been reported to occur more frequently following orthopedic surgery compared with other types of surgery with absolute risk in orthopedic surgery of 0.2% for LMWH and 2.6% for unfractionated heparin.[43,44] These events are rare and it is unknown how often these adverse effects occur in foot and ankle surgery, although case reports exist of patient death after foot and ankle surgery due to 1 dose of a heparin product.[42] Notably, thrombocytopenia and major/minor bleeding events have been reported in patients undergoing total ankle replacement (TAR) surgery.[10,19] It is important to note that HIT specifically has not been reported with the use of aspirin or other unrelated, non–heparin-based agents.

EFFICACY OF VENOUS THROMBOEMBOLISM DISEASE PROPHYLAXIS IN DIFFERENT FOOT AND ANKLE SURGERY AND INJURY TYPES

Given the wide assortment of foot and ankle procedures, ranging from elective forefoot procedures to extensive traumatic reconstruction, it is intuitive that the rates of VTED would not be uniform across all surgeries. The following section strives to stratify rates of VTED and provide evidence, when available albeit limited for efficacy, in different foot and ankle injuries and surgeries with a summary of the data provided in Table 6.

Trauma

In one retrospective study of 1540 ambulatory patients with ankle fractures requiring open reduction and internal fixation, the incidence of VTED was 2.99%, with 2.66% involving a DVT, and 0.32% involving a nonfatal PE. In this study, 16.4% of the patients received either LMWH or warfarin, but the rate of VTED was not influenced by the use of either thromboprophylaxis, with incidences of 2.56% versus 2.37%, respectively.[45] Approximately 45% of the patients had at least 1 risk factor for VTED but the study did not find a significant difference in VTED events whether thromboprophylaxis was used or not. In a multicenter,

double-blind trial, 258 patients with isolated surgical lower leg fractures were randomized to subcutaneous dalteparin 5000 units or matching placebo once daily for 2 weeks with ultrasound at 2-week and 3-month follow-up. Incidence of either an asymptomatic or symptomatic VTED or proximal DVT in the dalteparin and placebo groups was 1.5% and 2.3%, respectively, without statistically significant difference.[46] In another double-blind, placebo-controlled study comparing with LMWH administered over 2 weeks, 2.3% of 814 patients who sustained a foot or ankle fracture experienced an imaging-confirmed, asymptomatic VTED event. The incidence of asymptomatic DVT was 0.98% in the LMWH group and 2.01% in the placebo group without significant difference.[47]

Total Ankle Replacement

A systematic review in patients who underwent TAR surgery found that the incidence of VTED ranged widely from 0.8% to 9.8%.[48] Barg and colleagues[19] found that in a large cohort of 655 patients status post TAR surgery, obese patients (defined in the study as BMI >35 kg/m^2), patients with a period of postoperative non–weight bearing, and those with prior history of VTED were at highest risk for VTED postoperatively. Another study retrospectively reviewed 637 patients who underwent a total of 664 TARs, with chemoprophylaxis used only in those patients who were on such medications preoperatively, or those with a known history of VTED or coagulopathy. Only 4 patients (0.6%) developed a symptomatic VTED event, including 3 DVTs and 1 PE.[49] It concluded that routine VTED prophylaxis was unnecessary

Table 6
Summary data using best available evidence for efficacy of VTED prophylaxis in different types of foot and ankle surgery and injury

Injury/Surgery Type	Evidence for VTED Prophylaxis
Trauma	No statistically significant reduction in DVT rate; DVT rate is higher, however, in fracture patients compared with other foot and ankle pathologies
Arthroplasty	Routine use of chemoprophylaxis not warranted except in case of known host risk factors; no specific evidence in terms of risk reduction from prophylaxis
Tendon injury namely Achilles rupture	Documented higher rate of DVT compared with other foot and ankle pathologies, but no statistically significant reduction in DVT rate; risk factors such as prolonged immobilization must be factored into decision for prophylaxis
Immobilization	Data remain unclear in decreased incidence of DVT with LMWH

Abbreviations: DVT, deep vein thrombosis; LMWH, low molecular weight heparin; VTED, venous thromboembolism disease.

except in the setting of prior VTED or known genetic predisposition.

Soft Tissue/Tendon Injury

The rate of VTED after acute Achilles tendon rupture may be uniquely elevated among foot and ankle injuries. Reported rates vary anywhere between 0.4% and 34% without the use of chemoprophylaxis, with much of this wide variability attributable to study design in which some studies use routine screening study among all subjects, and others report only those patients who develop symptomatic DVT.[12,50] A prospective case series of 100 patients with acute Achilles tendon rupture were screened with ultrasound and found to have a DVT rate of 34% whether operative or nonoperative management was pursued.[51] Furthermore, of the symptomatic DVT rate of 23.5% in a retrospective series, a third of the DVTs occurred preoperatively with age older than 40 a significant risk factor (P<.0026).[24] Chronic Achilles ruptures (>4 weeks from injury) also have a statistically significantly higher incidence of VTED compared with acute injury (P = .048) or elective repair.[52] Multiple studies suggest that early weight bearing confers lower VTED complications compared with longer duration of non–weight bearing.[53–55]

The literature appears inconclusive as to the ability of chemical prophylaxis to mitigate heightened rates of VTED after Achilles tendon rupture. Of 91 patients surgically treated for an Achilles rupture in a randomized, placebo-controlled, double-blind study, VTED rate was not significantly different at 34% in the dalteparin 5000 U daily for 6 weeks postoperatively group and 36% in the placebo group as diagnosed by ultrasound and confirmed with phlebography.[9] Another prospective, double-blind, placebo-controlled trial investigated the efficacy of subcutaneous reviparin (1750 anti-Xa units given once daily) in 183 patients with a below-knee fracture or rupture of the Achilles tendon requiring immobilization for at least 5 weeks. VTED incidence confirmed by venography within 1 week of removing immobilization or earlier if suggestive symptoms, was significantly lower at 9% in the reviparin group compared with 19% in the placebo group.[22] However, this study did not separately differentiate the benefits of reviparin for Achilles tendon ruptures relative to the fracture group. Nonetheless, due to retraction of the soleus muscle and its critical importance in maintaining venous return, one may consider VTED prophylaxis among patients with such injuries. Notably, some studies suggest that one-third of such VTED events after Achilles rupture may be preoperative,

suggesting that this is true even in patients managed nonoperatively.[24]

Below-Knee Immobilization

Significant controversy exists regarding the role of VTED prevention in those undergoing below-knee cast immobilization, with or without surgery. A recent Cochrane review of 1490 immobilized patients found rates of VTED ranging anywhere between 4.3% and 40.0%, with a decreased incidence in patients receiving LMWH with rates from 0% to 37%. However, 3 of the 6 prospective, randomized studies included in this meta-analysis study failed to show benefit afforded by pharmacologic prophylaxis.[10]

As stated previously, a prospective, randomized controlled trial that analyzed 273 nonsurgical patients immobilized for a foot or ankle fracture showed a significantly higher incidence of DVT (11.7%) in the placebo group compared with those who received either an LMWH or fondaparinux. Two clinically significant PEs occurred in the control group, with the remaining DVTs being asymptomatic, whereas no complications were reported in the prophylaxis groups. However, the clinical significance of the difference in DVT rate remains to be determined given that the DVTs were asymptomatic.[41] Another randomized, blinded study examined the efficacy of tinzaparin (LMWH) for DVT prophylaxis in 99 of 205 patients with at least 3 weeks of below-knee cast immobilization for fracture and tendon injuries. They noted a high incidence of DVT at 20% overall, diagnosed with venography on day of cast removal; however, there was no significant difference in the treatment (10%) versus control (17%) groups (P = .15). Nonetheless, the investigators cited that perhaps the tinzaparin at 3500 IU anti-Xa daily was underdosed to amount an effect.[11]

SUMMARY/DISCUSSION

The role of VTED prophylaxis after foot and ankle surgery remains unclear. In synthesizing the available literature, it appears that rates of VTED vary substantially given the diversity of foot and ankle surgery, injury, and host factors. It is most likely that, although the risk in aggregate of VTED in the foot and ankle population remains lower than the overall risk identified in the hip and knee population, it has yet to be properly defined. Additional large-scale, prospective studies are necessary to identify those that at risk. We suspect that there are subsets of the foot and ankle population that probably require absolutely no prophylactic measures and other subsets that should probably always have some form of prophylaxis, but the nature of these specific subpopulations as well as the type, duration, and dosing of an ideal agent for prophylaxis when indicated have yet to be defined. Currently, aggressive chemical prophylactic measures are probably not indicated in most cases of foot or ankle surgery, although when chemical prophylaxis is contemplated, the AOFAS consensus statement offers a reasonable multimodal approach to VTED prophylaxis. It particularly focuses on patients at high risk, which includes addressing any of the following risk factors[3,21]:

- Pregnancy or taking contraceptive medication preoperatively
- Increasing mobility
- Considering local rather than general anesthesia
- Using mechanical prophylaxis, early mobilization
- If considering the use of chemical prophylaxis, LMWH is effective at reducing the rate of clinically significant VTED and appears to be the most studied agent in current literature

Based on the limited evidence listed previously, one may consider the following recommendations for patients undergoing foot and ankle surgery:

- Patients with previous history of VTED should receive chemical prophylaxis for both reasons of surgery and period of immobilization
- Patients without previous history of VTED or risk factors and who can be mobilized likely do not need chemical prophylaxis
- Patients older than 50 with ankle fracture or older than 40 with Achilles tendon injury may benefit from VTED chemical prophylaxis

Clearly, future studies addressing VTED prophylaxis in foot and ankle surgery should differentiate incidence rates and conduct randomized controlled prospective trials to determine VTED efficacy and cost-effectiveness for different foot and ankle populations. Although the aggregate incidence and complication rate from VTED following foot and ankle injury or surgery are relatively low, it remains clinically paramount to also investigate the long-term potential morbidity after a VTED event. Further research also can examine more definitively whether smoking, gender, race/ethnicity, tourniquet use, and air travel, among others, may be risk factors for VTED. Although there is little doubt that high-risk patients would benefit from anticoagulation, it remains challenging to establish defined risk factors and their cumulative, interactive effect that constitute a high risk from the medium-risk patient. Specific evidence-based guidelines for therapeutic agents, dosages, and duration of treatment are desperately needed to provide better care to this population in the future.

REFERENCES

1. Falck-Ytter Y, Francis CW, Johanson NA, et al. Prevention of VTE in orthopedic surgery patients. Antithrombotic therapy and prevention of thrombosis, 9th ed: American College of Chest Physicians evidence-based clinical practice guidelines. Chest 2012;141(2 SUPPL). https://doi.org/10.1378/chest.11-2404.

2. Jacobs JJ, Mont MA, Bozic KJ, et al. American Academy of Orthopaedic Surgeons clinical practice guideline on: preventing venous thromboembolic disease in patients undergoing elective hip and knee arthroplasty. J Bone Joint Surg Am 2012;94(8):746–7.

3. AOFAS. Position statement: the use of VTED prophylaxis in foot and ankle surgery position statement. 2013. Available at: https://www.aofas.org/medical-community/health-policy/Documents/VTED-Position-Statement-approv-7-9-13-FINAL.pdf. Accessed July 5, 2017.

4. Chao J. Deep vein thrombosis in foot and ankle surgery. Orthop Clin North Am 2016;47(2):471–5.

5. Wolf J, Digiovanni CW. A survey of orthopedic surgeons regarding DVT prophylaxis in foot and ankle trauma surgery. Orthopedics 2004;27(5):504–8.

6. Mizel MS, Temple HT, Michelson JD, et al. Thromboembolism after foot and ankle surgery. A multicenter study. Clin Orthop Relat Res 1998;(348):180–5. papers://eb2db329-465b-4791-b47f-c3347d944097/Paper/p744.

7. SooHoo NF, Eagan M, Krenek L, et al. Incidence and factors predicting pulmonary embolism and deep venous thrombosis following surgical treatment of ankle fractures. Foot Ankle Surg 2011;17(4):259–62. Available at: http://www.embase.com/search/results?subaction=viewrecord&from=export&id=L51080477%5Cnhttps://doi.org/10.1016/j.fas.2010.08.009%5Cnhttp://hz9pj6fe4t.search.serialssolutions.com?sid=EMBASE&issn=12687731&id=doi:10.1016/j.fas.2010.08.009&atitle=Incidence+a. Accessed November 23, 2017.

8. Soohoo NF, Farng E, Zingmond DS. Incidence of pulmonary embolism following surgical treatment of metatarsal fractures. Foot Ankle Int 2010;31(7):600–3.

9. Lapidus LJ, Rosfors S, Ponzer S, et al. Prolonged thromboprophylaxis with dalteparin after surgical treatment of Achilles tendon rupture: a randomized, placebo-controlled study. J Orthop Trauma 2007;21(1):52–7.

10. Testroote M, Stigter W, de Visser DC, et al. Low molecular weight heparin for prevention of venous thromboembolism in patients with lower-leg immobilization. Cochrane Database Syst Rev 2008;(4):CD006681.

11. Jorgensen PS, Warming T, Hansen K, et al. Low molecular weight heparin (Innohep) as thromboprophylaxis in outpatients with a plaster cast: a venografic controlled study. Thromb Res 2002; 105(6):477–80.

12. Lapidus LJ, Ponzer S, Elvin A, et al. Prolonged thromboprophylaxis with Dalteparin during immobilization after ankle fracture surgery: a randomized placebo-controlled, double-blind study. Acta Orthop 2007;78(4):528–35.

13. Silverstein MD, Heit JA, Mohr DN, et al. Trends in the incidence of deep vein thrombosis and pulmonary embolism: a 25-year population-based study. Arch Intern Med 1998;158(6):585–93.

14. Mangwani J, Sheikh N, Cichero M, et al. What is the evidence for chemical thromboprophylaxis in foot and ankle surgery? Systematic review of the English literature. Foot (Edinb) 2015;25(3):173–8.

15. Felcher AH, Mularski RA, Mosen DM, et al. Incidence and risk factors for venous thromboembolic disease in podiatric surgery. Chest 2009;135(4):917–22.

16. Saragas NP, Ferrao PNF, Saragas E, et al. The impact of risk assessment on the implementation of venous thromboembolism prophylaxis in foot and ankle surgery. Foot Ankle Surg 2014;20(2):85–9. Available at: http://www.scopus.com/inward/record.url?eid=2-s2.0-84899981274&partnerID=40&md5=a3ad73ae7d7cbceb1b094589aedade88. Accessed November 23, 2017.

17. Hanslow SS, Grujic L, Slater HK, et al. Thromboembolic disease after foot and ankle surgery. Foot Ankle Int 2006;27(9):693–5.

18. Jameson SS, Augustine A, James P, et al. Venous thromboembolic events following foot and ankle surgery in the English National Health Service. J Bone Joint Surg Br 2011;93(4):490–7.

19. Barg A, Henninger HB, Hintermann B. Risk factors for symptomatic deep-vein thrombosis in patients after total ankle replacement who received routine chemical thromboprophylaxis. J Bone Joint Surg Br 2011;93(7):921–7.

20. SooHoo NF, Farng E, Krenek L, et al. Complication rates following operative treatment of calcaneus fractures. Foot Ankle Surg 2011;17(4):233–8.

21. Fleischer AE, Abicht BP, Baker JR, et al. American College of Foot and Ankle Surgeons' Clinical Consensus Statement: risk, prevention, and diagnosis of venous thromboembolism disease in foot and ankle surgery and injuries requiring immobilization. J Foot Ankle Surg 2015;54(3):497–507.

22. Lassen MR, Borris LC, Nakov RL. Use of the low-molecular-weight heparin reviparin to prevent deep-vein thrombosis after leg injury requiring immobilization. N Engl J Med 2002;347(10):726–30.

23. Simon MA, Mass DP, Zarins CK, et al. The effect of a thigh tourniquet on the incidence of deep venous thrombosis after operations on the fore part of the foot. J Bone Joint Surg Am 1982;64(2):188–91.

24. Makhdom AM, Cota A, Saran NCR. Incidence of symptomatic deep venous thrombosis after Achilles tendon rupture. J Foot Ankle Surg 2013;52(5): 584–7.

25. Urbankova J, Quiroz R, Kucher N, et al. Intermittent pneumatic compression and deep vein thrombosis prevention: a meta-analysis in postoperative patients. Thromb Haemost 2005;94(6):1181–5.

26. Sagi HC, Ahn J, Ciesla D, et al. Venous thromboembolism prophylaxis in orthopaedic trauma patients: a survey of OTA member practice patterns and OTA expert panel recommendations. J Orthop Trauma 2015;29(10):e355–62.

27. Riou B, Rothmann C, Lecoules N, et al. Incidence and risk factors for venous thromboembolism in patients with nonsurgical isolated lower limb injuries. Am J Emerg Med 2007;25(5):502–8.

28. Palareti G, Sartori M. Treatment of isolated below the knee deep vein thrombosis. Curr Atheroscler Rep 2016;18(7). https://doi.org/10.1007/s11883-016-0594-1.

29. Amaragiri SV, Lees TA. Elastic compression stockings for prevention of deep vein thrombosis. Cochrane Database Syst Rev 2010;(7). https://doi.org/10.1002/14651858.CD001484.pub3.

30. Knudson MM, Morabito D, Paiement GD, et al. Use of low molecular weight heparin in preventing thromboembolism in trauma patients. J Trauma 1996;41(3):446–59.

31. Griffiths JT, Matthews L, Pearce CJ, et al. Incidence of venous thromboembolism in elective foot and ankle surgery with and without aspirin prophylaxis. J Bone Joint Surg Br 2012;94(2):210–4.

32. Johnston A, Jones WS, Hernandez AF. The ADAPTABLE trial and aspirin dosing in secondary prevention for patients with coronary artery disease. Curr Cardiol Rep 2016;18(8):9.

33. Parvizi J, Huang R, Restrepo C, et al. Low-dose aspirin is effective chemoprophylaxis against clinically important venous thromboembolism following total joint arthroplasty: a preliminary analysis. J Bone Joint Surg Am 2017;99(2):91–8.

34. Raphael IJ, Tischler EH, Huang R, et al. Aspirin: an alternative for pulmonary embolism prophylaxis after arthroplasty? Clin Orthop Relat Res 2014;472: 482–8.

35. Patel V, Walsh M, Sehgal B, et al. Factors associated with prolonged wound drainage after primary total hip and knee arthroplasty. J Bone Joint Surg Am 2007;89(1):33–8.

36. An V, Phan K, Levy Y, et al. Aspirin as thromboprophylaxis in hip and knee arthroplasty: a systematic review and meta-analysis. J Arthroplasty 2016; 31(11):2608–16.

37. Lack WD, Fredericks D, Petersen E, et al. Effect of aspirin on bone healing in a rabbit ulnar osteotomy model. J Bone Joint Surg Am 2013;95(6):488.

38. Allen HL, Wase A, Bear WT. Indomethacin and aspirin: effect of nonsteroidal anti-inflammatory agents on the rate of fracture repair in the rat. Acta Orthop Scand 1980;51(1–6):595–600.

39. Calder JD, Freeman R, Domeij-Arverud E, et al. Meta-analysis and suggested guidelines for prevention of venous thromboembolism (VTE) in foot and ankle surgery. Knee Surg Sports Traumatol Arthrosc 2016;24(4):1409–20.

40. Haque S, Davies MB. Oral thromboprophylaxis in patients with ankle fractures immobilized in a below the knee cast. Foot Ankle Surg 2015;21(4): 266–8.

41. Bruntink MM, Groutars YME, Schipper IB, et al. Nadroparin or fondaparinux versus no thromboprophylaxis in patients immobilised in a below-knee plaster cast (PROTECT): a randomised controlled trial. Injury 2017;48(4):936–40.

42. Digiovanni CW. Current concepts review: heparin-induced thrombocytopenia. Foot Ankle Int 2008; 29(11):1158–67.

43. Girolami B, Girolami A. Heparin-induced thrombocytopenia: a review. Semin Thromb Hemost 2006; 32(8):803–9.

44. Martel N, Lee J, Wells PS. Risk for heparin-induced thrombocytopenia with unfractionated and low-molecular-weight heparin thromboprophylaxis: a meta-analysis. Blood 2005;106(8):2710–5.

45. Pelet S, Roger M-E, Belzile E, et al. The incidence of thromboembolic events in surgically treated ankle fracture. J Bone Joint Surg Am 2012;94(6):502.

46. Selby R, Geerts WH, Kreder HJ, et al, D-KAF (Dalteparin in Knee-to-Ankle Fracture) Investigators. A double-blind, randomized controlled trial of the prevention of clinically important venous thromboembolism after isolated lower leg fractures. J Orthop Trauma 2015;29(5):224–30.

47. Zheng X, Li DY, Wangyang Y, et al. Effect of chemical thromboprophylaxis on the rate of venous thromboembolism after treatment of foot and ankle fractures. Foot Ankle Int 2016;37(11): 1218–24.

48. Barg A, Barg K, Schneider SW, et al. Thromboembolic complications after total ankle replacement. Curr Rev Musculoskelet Med 2013;6(4):328–35.

49. Horne PH, Jennings JM, Deorio JK, et al. Low incidence of symptomatic thromboembolic events after total ankle arthroplasty without routine use of chemoprophylaxis. Foot Ankle Int 2015;36(6): 611–6.

50. Patel A, Ogawa B, Charlton T, et al. Incidence of deep vein thrombosis and pulmonary embolism after achilles tendon rupture. Clin Orthop Relat Res 2012;470(1):270–4.

51. Nilsson-Helander K, Thurin A, Karlsson JEB. High incidence of deep venous thrombosis after Achilles tendon rupture: a prospective study. Knee Surg Sports Traumatol Arthrosc 2009;17(10):1234–8.

52. Bullock MJ, DeCarbo WT, Hofbauer MH, et al. Repair of chronic Achilles ruptures has a high incidence of venous thromboembolism. Foot Ankle Spec 2017;10(5):415–20.

53. Persson A, Wredmark T. The treatment of total ruptures of the Achilles tendon by plaster immobilisation. Int Orthop 1979;3(2):149–52.

54. Speck M, Klaue K. Early full weightbearing and functional treatment after surgical repair of acute Achilles tendon rupture. Am J Sports Med 1998; 26(6):789–93.

55. Healy B, Beasley R, Weatherall M. Venous thromboembolism following prolonged cast immobilisation for injury to the tendo Achillis. J Bone Joint Surg Br 2010;92(5):646–50.

Patient-Reported Outcomes in Foot and Ankle Surgery

Kenneth J. Hunt, MD*, Eric Lakey, BS

KEYWORDS

- Patient-reported outcomes • PROMIS • AOFAS • SF-36 • VAS • OFAR • Foot and ankle
- Orthopedics

KEY POINTS

- The concept of tracking medical outcomes to provide better care has been around for more than 150 years, but most patient-reported outcome (PRO) tools in current use have been described in the past 25 years.
- Use of PROs to inform clinical practice and clinical research began increasing in popularity in the last decade of the twentieth century.
- There is currently an incredible quantity and variety of PRO measures available to the foot and ankle surgeon. These measures vary in length, degree of validation, and attributes measured. There is little consensus on which tools should be used for PRO collection in clinical practice.
- The emergence of Patient-Reported Outcomes Measurement Information System computer-adaptive tests and the proliferation of outcomes registries may encourage more widespread PRO collection as part of orthopedic practice and lead to consensus on which measures to collect.
- Participation in an existing registry can be a relatively easy means of incorporating PROs into practice and collecting valuable data for practice assessment and quality improvement.

INTRODUCTION

Health outcome measures are tools that capture the health status of a patient throughout an episode of care for treatment of an injury, condition, or health maintenance. These measures can generally be divided into clinical outcomes (as assessed by a clinician), laboratory outcomes (as seen with objective findings from laboratory tests, radiographs, and so forth), and PROs (or health status as perceived by patients). Interest in collection of PROs as part of standard clinical practice has increased substantially in recent years. This relates to several factors, including eligibility for full reimbursement from payors, fulfillment of American Board of Orthopaedic Surgery recertification criteria; an expanding market of secure, cloud-based survey tools;

and requirements of large hospital networks. Whatever the reasons, PROs are here to stay as a critical tool in assessing outcomes in foot and ankle surgery. The goal of this article is to describe common PROs in foot and ankle surgery, explore means of implementation into clinical practice, and assess the future of PROs in foot and ankle orthopedics.

HISTORY OF PATENT-REPORTED OUTCOMES

Florence Nightingale is generally considered a founder of modern evidence-based medicine.[1] As a field nurse during the Crimean War in the mid-1850s, she was distraught by the massive loss of life she observed during the war. As a dedicated statistician, she noticed that approximately 7

Disclosure Statement: No authors have financial interests related to the submitted work. Dr K.J. Hunt is Chair, Managerial Board of the Orthopedic Foot & Ankle Outcomes Research Network.
Department of Orthopaedic Surgery, University of Colorado School of Medicine, 12631 East 17th Avenue, Room 4508, Aurora, CO 80045, USA
* Corresponding author.
E-mail address: kenneth.j.hunt@ucdenver.edu

soldiers died from disease for every 1 soldier who died from combat wounds. Through simple interventions, such as improved hygiene nda better nutrition at the Scutari Hospital near modern-day Istanbul, she was able to reduce mortality among admitted soldiers from 42.7% in February 1855 to 2.2% by June 1855.[2] She returned to her native Britain in 1856 and lobbied for the formation of a royal commission that would track disease and mortality rates to aid in the identification of emergent public health concerns. Over the following decade, she lobbied for collection of data pertaining to hospital outcomes, trained versus untrained nurses, the relationship between housing and health status on the British census, and the incidence of maternal mortality for hospital and home births. By working to collect population-level health data and then acting to address the most prevalent and preventable forms of disease, Florence Nightingale paved the way as an early advocate for modern evidence-based medicine.

It was nearly 60 years later, in 1914, that Ernest Codman, MD, an early orthopedic specialist, cofounder of the American College of Surgeons, and creator of the first national tumor registry, published the "end results idea" wherein each patient received a note card that detailed presenting symptoms, treatments, and other relevant clinical details.[3] After at least a year, the success or failure of the treatment was also detailed on the note card. By encouraging the collection of outcomes data on an individual level, this concept pioneered the development of hospital standards by challenging physicians to assess their treatment outcomes and take appropriate measures to prevent new failures if previous outcomes were poor.

In more recent years, with the signing of the Patient Protection and Affordable Care Act in 2010, health care spending now accounts for 17.8% of the GDP,[4] and with the expansion of managed care, there have been renewed calls for a quality revolution in health care. In 1998, Arnold Relman, MD, charged, "We can no longer afford to provide health care without knowing more about its successes and failures."[5] In a 2010 editorial in *The New England Journal of Medicine*, Michael E. Porter, PhD, echoed these calls in stating, "Measuring, reporting, and comparing outcomes are perhaps the most important steps toward rapidly improving o2utcomes and making good choices about reducing costs."[6] Dr Porter's reminder is of the basic economic tenant that value = outcome ÷ cost and that the first step toward improving value in health care is to better track and understand outcomes.

In response to these calls for innovation, there has been a powerful push toward the widespread adoption PRO metrics to increase patient engagement, help move toward a model of value-based reimbursement, and aid in the practice of evidence-based medicine.[7] To better track and understand outcomes after treatment, there is a fundamental need for the following:

- Consistent, validated PRO metrics
- High-quality prospective comparative studies of treatments using validated PROs
- Efficient methods of data collection, storage, analysis, and dissemination

Toward this end, many professional societies and national organizations have taken the charge to establish and endorse guidelines for the collection and analysis of PROs. These include the International Society for Quality of Life Research,[8] the National Quality Forum,[9] the Patient-Reported Outcomes Measurement Information System (PROMIS) initiative at the National Institutes of Health (NIH),[10] and the American Orthopaedic Foot & Ankle Society (AOFAS) Orthopaedic Foot and Ankle Outcomes Research (OFAR) initiative.[11]

PATIENT-REPORTED OUTCOMES IN ORTHOPEDIC SURGERY

Early outcome measures in orthopedic surgery were somewhat limited. Prior to the advent of the more complex tools available today, patients were primarily assessed by objective and quantifiable measures like loss of life, loss of limb, return to work, and length of hospital stay. Toward the end of the twentieth century, the study of outcomes in medicine and in orthopedics began receiving more attention. Many of today's most popular PRO metrics originated in the 1990s (Fig. 1). One of the first modern outcome metrics was introduced in 1976 when Scott and Huskisson[12] described the visual analog scale (VAS). The VAS is a simple measure wherein the patient is instructed to mark their current level of pain on a 100-mm horizontal line representing the full spectrum of pain. The scale was validated for orthopedic conditions in 1980[13] and has been a mainstay of pain assessment in orthopedics for decades.

In 1989, Tarlov and colleagues[14] published the Medical Outcomes Study in *JAMA* wherein they developed a conceptual model of quality in health care that contains 3 tenets:

1. Structure
2. Process
3. Outcome

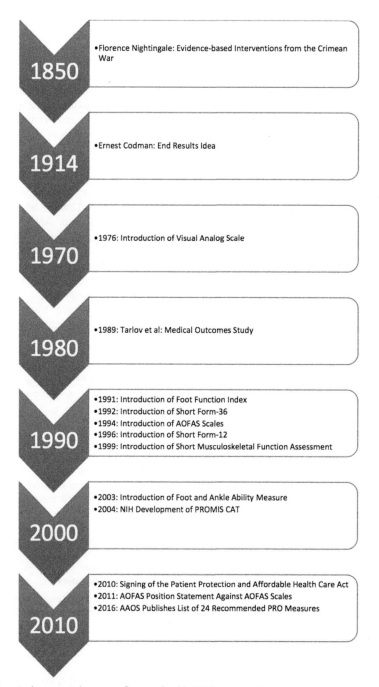

Fig. 1. Select historical events relevant to foot and ankle PROs research.

Tarlov and colleagues helped lay the conceptual groundwork for ensuing outcomes research by defining key elements of health care outcomes as clinical end points, functional status, general well-being, and satisfaction with care. In 1992, Ware and Sherbourne[15] designed and introduced a 36-Item Short Form Health Survey (SF-36) to measure overall patient-reported health status across 8 domains, including physical functioning, general mental health, and social functioning. In 1994, Douglas Bradham[16] adapted Tarlov and colleagues' conceptual model for orthopedics by emphasizing continuity of care over the long term with outcomes informing future care via feedback loops and by focusing primarily on functional outcome measures. Although much of the focus of practice guidelines and appropriate use criteria is on process metrics (eg, administration of perioperative antibiotics, deep vein thrombosis prophylaxis, and so forth), increasing attention is being paid to the importance of measuring outcomes.

Building on these early pioneers, today's orthopedic practice includes an expansive array of available PRO measures. Typically, PRO measures in orthopedics can be divided into 1 of 3 general classes: overall health, joint or anatomic region, and condition specific (Table 1). Recent reviews have found a wide variety of PROs used within any given field of orthopedics, including 206 unique metrics in spine surgery,[17] 73 in pediatric orthopedics,[18] and 89 in foot and ankle.[19] Even for discrete diagnoses, clinicians are reporting their outcomes data using 47 unique metrics in total knee arthroplasty,[20] 11 in total ankle arthroplasty,[21] 24 in adult spinal deformity,[22] and 21 in Achilles tendon rupture management.[23]

In 2016, the American Academy of Orthopedic Surgeons (AAOS) published a list of 24 recommended PRO measures for orthopedic surgeons that are open-access, brief, and clinically meaningful. Included in the recommendations are PROs focused on general quality of life, such as the Veterans RAND 12-Item Health Survey (SF-12) or the PROMIS computer-adaptive test (CAT), as well as a short list of metrics specific to a variety of joints and common orthopedic disease processes.[24] To date, there is no consensus among foot and ankle surgeons as to which metrics should be administered as a standard of patient care.

PATIENT-REPORTED OUTCOMES IN FOOT AND ANKLE SURGERY

There are a wide variety of PRO used in foot and ankle clinical research today. A recent review of the foot and ankle literature identified 89 unique metrics in use between 2012 and 2016.[19] Fig. 2 depicts the current distribution of PRO metrics in foot and ankle clinical research.[19] The top 3 metrics (AOFAS, VAS, and SF-36) altogether represented 48% of all PROs used in the literature. Custom questionnaires addressing patient satisfaction and functional status were prevalent and represented 13% of all PRO usage. The SF-12 and Foot and Ankle Outcome Score (FAOS) were the fourth and fifth most cited metrics overall and both represented 3% of PRO usage during that time. Other, less commonly used metrics were frequently cited and represented 33% of all PRO usage.

AOFAS scales have been commonly used since their introduction in 1994.[25] A meta-analysis of foot and ankle articles between 1990 and 2001 found that the AOFAS scales were the most commonly used metric across the study period.[26] A review of foot and ankle articles published from 2002 through 2011 found that AOFAS was by far the most commonly used outcome metric in each year of the study period.[27] AOFAS remained the most commonly used outcome metric in every year from 2012 through 2016.[19] Use of AOFAS scales, however, has declined relative to other outcome metrics since the release of a position

Table 1 Three major categories of foot and ankle patient-reported outcome measures		
Type of Measure	**Description**	**Examples**
Overall Health	These measures are used broadly and are not specific to orthopaedics. They may assess just one element such as the Visual Analog Score for pain or may be complex questionnaires	Visual Analog Scale for Pain, Short Form-36, EuroQol-5D
Joint or Anatomic Region	These measures are broadly applicable to specific joints or anatomic regions within the human body, such as the entire foot, just the forefoot, the hip, or back.	AOFAS Scales, Foot and Ankle Outcome Score, Foot Function Index, Harris Hip Score
Condition-Specific	These measures are designed to assess specific conditons, diagnoses, or treatments, such as Achilles tendon ruptures, ankle arthritis, or Achilles tendinopathy	Achilles Total Rupture Score, Ankle Osteoarthritis Score, Victorian Institute for Sports Assessment - Achilles

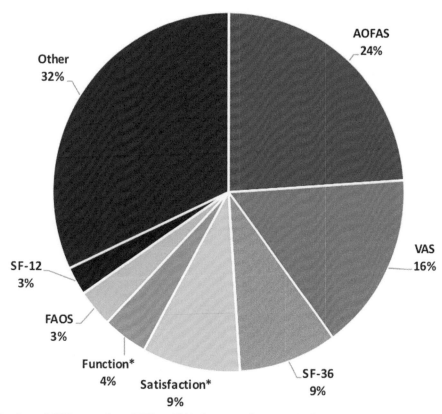

Fig. 2. Pie chart of PRO usage from 2012 to 2016. * unnamed, custom PRO measures.

statement by AOFAS recommending against its use as a sole outcome metric[28] (Fig. 3). In 2016, AOFAS was cited in just 47% of all outcomes articles.[19]

The second and third most frequently cited metrics are the VAS and the SF-36, respectively. The VAS has been the second most commonly used PRO in the foot and ankle orthopedics literature every year since at least 2001.[19,27] Furthermore, between 2012 and 2016, the VAS has been increasing in usage at an average rate of 4.5% per year and appeared in 44% of outcomes articles in 2016. If current trends continue, it is possible that the VAS may surpass the AOFAS scales in the next couple of years. Although the SF-36 is a general health measure, it has been among the top 5 most frequently cited PRO metrics in orthopedic foot and ankle surgery since its inception[19,26,27] (Table 2).

VALIDATION OF FOOT AND ANKLE PATIENT-REPORTED OUTCOMES
American Orthopaedic Foot & Ankle Society Scales
The AOFAS published a series of clinical rating scales in 1994 that were designed the cover

the gamut of foot and ankle conditions.[25] In all, there are 4 100-point rating scales, including ankle-hindfoot, midfoot, hallux, and lesser toes. AOFAS scales incorporate subjective and objective data to assess the patient in 3 primary domains: function, alignment, and pain. AOFAS scales are hybrid measures that take into account both PROs and physician-entered data, such as range of motion or gait assessments.

Although the AOFAS scales have been found responsive for specific conditions, such as ankle arthritis[29] as well as foot and ankle patients more broadly,[30] numerous studies have raised concerns about the AOFAS scales over the years. A survey of patients and clinicians found that up to half the measures in the AOFAS scales were considered not of primary importance by patients.[31] Furthermore, because the score uses absolute descriptors to describe health status, such as "no" and "none," that are rarely strictly true, patients must interpret these terms.[32] Similarly, the use of clinician-assessed scores increases the risk of interobserver variability due to variable examination techniques.[33] The AOFAS has been found to correlate poorly

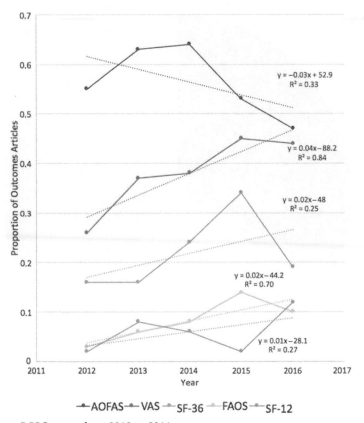

Fig. 3. Trends in top 5 PRO usage from 2012 to 2016.

with a host of generic PRO questionnaires, including the Musculoskeletal Function Assessment (MFA),[34] the SF-36,[35,36] and the QALY score (quality-adjusted life year).[37] There is also poor agreement between the AOFAS hallux

Author	Button & Pinney,[26] 2004	Hunt & Hurwit,[27] 2013	Hunt & LE[19]
Time period	1990–2001	2002–2011	2012–2016
First	AOFAS	AOFAS	AOFAS
Second	Mazur	VAS	VAS
Third	Maryland Foot Score	SF-36	SF-36
Fourth	SF-36	FFI	FAOS
Fifth	Good	AAOS	SF-12

Table 2
Most popular patient-reported outcome measures by time period

Data from Refs.[19,26,27]

subscale when evaluated prospectively and retrospectively.[38]

In September 2011, the AOFAS published a position paper echoing these concerns.[28] They recommended against continued use of the AOFAS scales and called for consolidation of the orthopedic community around a series of more validated and standardized outcome metrics. Although AOFAS scales remain the most popular scales in foot and ankle orthopedics, a recent review found that the popularity of AOFAS scales peaked in 2013 and 2014, appearing 0.64 times per outcomes article.[19]

Visual Analog Scale

The VAS for pain was introduced in 1976 as a metric that allows patients to graphically express their current level of pain on a 10-cm scale, ranging from no pain to the worst pain imaginable.[12] Although it has been highly validated for orthopedics,[13,39–41] it has low specificity, with a 3-cm decrease in the VAS score corresponding to the minimal clinically important difference for pain control.[42] It has also been suggested that changes in pain level may not be reflected linearly on the VAS.[40] A primary advantage of the VAS scale is that it is free and brief. It takes only moments for patients to complete and is an easy metric to compare treatment outcomes.

The 36-Item Short Form Health Survey and Veterans RAND 12-Item Health Survey

The SF-36 is a general health measure that was introduced in 1992 and includes 36 items addressing 8 domains of overall health status.[15] The SF-36 is widely validated for orthopedic conditions[43–45] and validation studies frequently compare instruments against the SF-36.[35,36,46] Although the SF-36 has been the third most popular outcome metric in foot and ankle orthopedics every year since 2003,[19,27] experts recommend pairing the SF-36 with an orthopedics-specific PRO: because it is a general health measure, it can be difficult to isolate orthopedic outcomes from changes in other health conditions that may be unrelated.[47]

The SF-12 is a shortened version of the SF-36 that was introduced in 1996 with the intention of reducing redundancies and decreasing the burden on the patient.[48,49] It shortens the survey to 12 items and reports a score in both physical and mental domains. It has been validated for orthopedic patients with minimal time burden on patients and minimal floor and ceiling effects.[50] It is also a general health measure and likely subject to the same concerns regarding interference as the SF-36. In 2016, the SF-12 was included as a recommended PRO measure for "General Quality of Life" by the AAOS[24] (Table 3). Both SF-36 and SF-12 are great tools for outcomes assessment in research. Including these as part of

Table 3 American Academy of Orthopaedic Surgeons recommended patient-reported outcome measures for foot and ankle surgeons	
Category	**Recommendations**
General quality of life	Veterans RAND 12 (SF-12), PROMIS (PROMIS 10 or CAT), EQ-5D
Treatment outcome	Single-assessment numeric evaluation
Foot and ankle	FAAM, FADI

This list is not comprehensive and is meant to steer data collection and reporting.

From American Academy of Orthopaedic Surgeons (AAOS). Patient reported outcome measures. Instruments for collection of orthopedic quality data. 2016. Available at: https://www.aaos.org/Quality/Performance_Measures/Patient_Reported_Outcome_Measures/?ssopc=1. Accessed July 11, 2017; with permission.

routine practice can be problematic, however, for a variety of reasons: a per use subscription fee, a scoring formula that is proprietary, and patient burden—most patients are not willing to repeatedly complete a 36-question survey.

Other Common and Validated Metrics

Although the AOFAS, VAS, and SF-36 scales are the most common outcomes scales in the foot and ankle literature,[19] there are a wide variety of commonly used, validated PROs available to foot and ankle surgeons.

The FAOS is a 42-item PRO metric for foot and ankle function[51] with good reliability and validity.[52] It has been validated for a wide variety of foot and ankle conditions, including adult-acquired flatfoot deformity,[51] hallux valgus,[53] hallux rigidus,[54] and ligament reconstruction.[55] It has been found a weak instrument for osteoarthritis of the ankle.[56] The length of this survey, however, can create significant patient burden.

The Foot Function Index (FFI) was developed in 1991 as a 23-item PRO that assesses foot function in 3 domains: pain, disability, and activity limitation.[57] Although it is a simple measure, it is reliable[58] and has been found to be a valid and response measure when compared with the SF-36.[29,59]

The Short Musculoskeletal Function Assessment (SMFA) was adapted in 1999 as a shorter version of the MFA.[60] At 46 items, the SMFA reports a dysfunction index that comments on pure function as well as a bother index, where patients are asked about how their function interferes with daily activities, such as sleep, sports, and family activities. Although it is not specific to foot and ankle orthopedics, it has been found to have validity similar to the SF-36.[58,60] A recent review found the SMFA to have high validity and reliability as well as moderate responsiveness.[61]

The Foot and Ankle Ability Measure (FAAM) was developed in 2003 as a 31-item scale that reports a score on both daily function and sports function.[62] It has been validated for foot and ankle orthopedics broadly[63] as well as for chronic ankle instability[64] and diabetes mellitus.[65] A recent study demonstrated that the FFI, SMFA, and FAAM are all highly correlated for foot and ankle trauma patients and that using more than 1 in clinical research may be unnecessary.[66]

Although the AAOS endorses the use of other measures, such as the EuroQol-5D (EQ-5D) for assessing general health status and the Foot and Ankle Disability Index (FADI) for foot and ankle function,[24] a recent review suggests these measures are infrequently used in foot and ankle orthopedics today.[19] Both the SF-12 and FAAM are also endorsed by the AAOS and commonly used in foot and ankle orthopedics today.[19]

NATIONAL INSTITUTES OF HEALTH PATIENT-REPORTED OUTCOMES MEASUREMENT INFORMATION SYSTEM INSTRUMENTS IN ORTHOPEDICS

Background on Patient-Reported Outcomes Measurement Information System

With PROs becoming increasingly popular, concerns have been raised about the time burden they may present to patients tasked with completing them.[67] CATs use item response theory to decide which questions to administer based on previous responses and may decrease testing times by more than 50%[11,67] with minimal losses in precision.[68]

The PROMIS is a system of PRO metrics that was developed by the NIH starting in late 2004.[69,70] It implements both short forms and CAT tools that consist of a series of item banks for key health domains, including physical function, depression, and fatigue.[10,71] Each item bank asks on average 4 to 6 questions and takes approximately 1 minute or less for a patient to complete,[72,73] allowing for the completion of numerous and select domains without creating undue burden on patients. Although there are currently 94 adult and 25 pediatric domains available on the PROMIS platform, most providers opt to administer approximately 3 to 5 PROMIS domains to maximize response rates and minimize the time commitment for the patient. PROMIS domains are responsive and compare favorably to legacy measures for a wide range of conditions, including substance abuse,[74] depression,[75] congestive heart failure,[76] back pain,[76] cancer,[77] chronic obstructive pulmonary disease,[78] and multiple sclerosis.[79] Use of PROMIS as a consensus metric may facilitate cross-provider communication and comparison of outcomes data across a variety of medical specialties.[80]

Patient-Reported Outcomes Measurement Information System in Orthopedics

PROMIS instruments have been validated for general orthopedic populations[81–86] as well as foot and ankle patients specifically.[87–89] PROMIS instruments are particularly noteworthy for decreasing administration time and minimizing floor and ceiling effects compared with legacy measurements. In foot and ankle, PROMIS instruments have been found superior to a variety of legacy measures, such as the SMFA, FAAM, and FFI.[81,90] A recent study found that the PROMIS physical function was more precise than an expensive gait-analysis system for evaluating improvement after knee ligament reconstruction; furthermore, administration times were decreased from 10 to 15 minutes to 1 minute and ceiling effects were not observed with PROMIS physical function.[72]

In addition to tracking outcomes data, PROMIS instruments may be used as a screening tool. In foot and ankle patients, PROMIS scores for both pain and physical function can predict with 95% specificity whether a patient will experience minimal clinically important difference from surgery.[88] When coupled with sound clinical judgment, CATs like PROMIS have the potential to help clinicians better understand prognoses, track outcomes data, and communicate with other providers. It is the many advantages of the PROMIS tools that led the AOFAS OFAR initiative to select these as the core outcome tools for the OFAR platform. The disadvantage of the PROMIS tools is that access to a CAT engine is needed to administer CAT tools to patients. Many electronic medical record (EMR) systems (including Epic [Epic Systems Corporation, Madison, Wisconsin]), however, now include CAT integration by using the NIH-funded CAT tool at AssessmentCenter.net.

THE FUTURE OF OUTCOMES ASSESSMENT

Implementing Patient-Reported Outcome Assessments in a Practice

Although frequently used in clinical outcomes research since the 1990s, there is an increasing emphasis on incorporating PROs into everyday orthopedic practice.[91] Any effort to integrate PROs into clinical practice should aim to collect meaningful data, use efficient collection and storage tools, and minimize patient burden. Care should be taken to avoid disrupting clinic work flow, overwhelming patients with long burdensome questionnaires, or collecting data that are redundant or of low value. Ideally, PRO data should be collected during an office visit and viewable in the EMR at the time of the visit. EMR integration will allow for PRO data to contribute to shared decision making during the visit as well as allow for health status tracking over time.[92] Although there is currently little guidance as to which specific tools should be used, the authors recommend use of at least,

1. A measurement of physical function
2. A measurement of average pain levels
3. A measurement of global health

In addition, an assessment of satisfaction with treatment can be a useful quality assurance tool.

Implementation studies in orthopedic clinical practices have stressed the importance of studying the flow of patients through the practice and identifying an optimal methodology to collect PROs that do not burden staff or otherwise disrupt the clinical practice.[93] For PROMIS scales, method of administration did not hinder score, validity, or reliability in a study comparing paper questionnaires, handheld devices, computers, and interactive voice response technology.[94] As such, the primary consideration in implementing PRO surveys is to maximize response rates and minimize disruptions. Recommendations have ranged from a pen-and-paper bubble questionnaire at intake that is then scanned into an EMR[95] to directing patients immediately after check-in to a dedicated survey room with computers.[92] Regardless of the route of administration, simple and inexpensive interventions can dramatically improve response rates. The addition of electronic tablet availability in the office and SMS completion reminders yielded PRO completion rates of 94% in an orthopedic population, up from 38% for patients who received only a letter encouraging completion.[96] The routine collection of 3 PROMIS domains throughout 30 departments at a large academic medical center demonstrated proof of concept: new patient registration times were unchanged, follow-up registration times increased by less than 30 seconds on average, and the average completion time was 3.5 minutes.[97]

Registries

As PROs are increasingly integrated into clinical practice, registries are poised to play a pivotal role in the collection and processing of PRO data. Registries are entities that help facilitate the collection, aggregation, and analysis of data from a wide network of peripheral sites. By collecting outcomes data throughout their network, registries can be the catalyst for interinstitutional research collaboration, postmarket surveillance of medical devices, and epidemiologic studies.

As PROs become increasingly important as a tool for measuring treatment efficacy, it is important for foot and ankle clinical researchers to administer a set of consensus PRO measures. Collection of a set of consensus PRO measures allows for outcomes data that are easily understood by clinicians, easily compared with other studies in the field, and easily tracked over time. Registries can collaborate with leading clinicians to select a series of validated measures

that should be collected for a given procedure, anatomic region, or medical specialty. By facilitating EMR integration and automatic collection of these select PRO measures, registries may be a vehicle for researchers to consolidate around a suite of consensus measures that are collected for every patient undergoing a certain procedure within a network. Registry networks also provide an experienced infrastructure that can ensure compliance with the evolving Health Insurance Portability and Accountability Act–related provisions that guide collection and sharing of patient data.

In 2012, the AOFAS established the OFAR Network[11] to serve as a national network for foot and ankle outcomes data aggregation and reporting. A pilot study was able to successfully enroll more than 300 patients across 10 institutions to complete 2 PROMIS domains and 2 legacy measures (FAAM and FFI) on the OFAR platform.[11] They reported 76% completion of preoperative PROs and 56% completion of 6-month postoperative PROs across all 10 sites. This pilot study demonstrates that a large and diverse nationwide network for the collection of PRO data is feasible. In just a few months, all 10 sites were successful in integrating PROs into their protocols and recruiting patients into the study. The OFAR Network is now scaling this consortium using a cloud-based platform, direct communication with EMRs, a patient portal, and automated patient alerts. Moving forward, outcomes registries like OFAR will be important players in the collection and aggregation of PROs data, development of national and regional benchmarks, and rapid dissemination of data that can help improve the quality of care for all providers.

SUMMARY

PROs have been an important element of foot and ankle clinical research for decades. PROs can be used to track patient outcomes, compare treatments, increase patient engagement, determine prognoses, and more. As a result of their utility, there has been a growing emphasis on incorporating PROs into routine clinical practice and collecting them for every patient. Newer PRO scales, like the PROMIS metrics, allow efficient collection of data using handheld and personal electronic devices, improving accuracy and reducing patient burden.

Through EMR integration, outcomes registries such as OFAR provide the framework for automatic data collection, aggregation, and analysis. In this manner, registries lower the barrier to entry for collecting PRO data and help standardize and streamline the process. Together, the union of outcomes registries, validated tools like PROMIS, and consensus legacy measures may represent an avenue for orthopedic providers to collect patient outcomes data in a way that is accurate, efficient, scalable, and consistent from one provider to another. The end goal is always to improve the quality of care provided, reduce the cost of that care, and improve the value of outcomes research on treatments and technologies in foot and ankle surgery.

REFERENCES

1. McDonald L. Florence Nightingale and the early origins of evidence-based nursing. Evid Based Nurs 2001;4(3):68–9.
2. Neuhauser D. Florence Nightingale gets no respect: as a statistician that is. Qual Saf Health Care 2003;12(4):317.
3. Dervishaj O, Wright KE, Saber AA, et al. Ernest Amory Codman and the end-result system. Am Surg 2015;81(1):12–5.
4. National health expenditures 2015 highlights. National Healthcare Expidenture Accounts: Centers for Medicare and Medicaid Services; 2015.
5. Relman AS. Assessment and accountability: the third revolution in medical care. N Engl J Med 1988;319(18):1220–2.
6. Porter ME. What is value in health care? N Engl J Med 2010;363(26):2477–81.
7. Lavallee DC, Chenok KE, Love RM, et al. Incorporating patient-reported outcomes into health care to engage patients and enhance care. Health Aff (Millwood) 2016;35(4):575–82.
8. User's guide to implementing patient-reported outcomes assessment in clinical practice. International Society for Quality of Life Research; 2015.
9. Patient reported outcomes (PROs) in performance measurement. National Quality Forum; 2013.
10. Intro to PROMIS®. Secondary intro to PROMIS®. Available at: http://www.healthmeasures. net/explore-measurement-systems/promis/intro-to-promis. Accessed June 29, 2017.
11. Hunt KJ, Alexander I, Baumhauer J, et al. The Orthopaedic Foot and Ankle Outcomes Research (OFAR) network: feasibility of a multicenter network for patient outcomes assessment in foot and ankle. Foot Ankle Int 2014;35(9):847–54.
12. Scott J, Huskisson EC. Graphic representation of pain. Pain 1976;2(2):175–84.
13. Reading AE. A comparison of pain rating scales. J Psychosom Res 1980;24(3–4):119–24.
14. Tarlov AR, Ware JE Jr, Greenfield S, et al. The Medical Outcomes Study. An application of methods for monitoring the results of medical care. JAMA 1989;262(7):925–30.
15. Ware JE Jr, Sherbourne CD. The MOS 36-item short-form health survey (SF-36). I. Conceptual framework and item selection. Med Care 1992;30(6):473–83.
16. Bradham DD. Outcomes research in orthopedics: history, perspectives, concepts, and future. Arthroscopy 1994;10(5):493–501.
17. Guzman JZ, Cutler HS, Connolly J, et al. Patient-reported outcome instruments in spine surgery. Spine (Phila Pa 1976) 2016;41(5):429–37.
18. Phillips L, Carsen S, Vasireddi A, et al. Use of patient-reported outcome measures in pediatric orthopaedic literature. J Pediatr Orthop 2016. https://doi.org/10.1097/bpo.0000000000000847.
19. Hunt KJ, Lakey E. Patient-reported outcome measures in foot and ankle research from 2012 to 2016. University of Colorado School of Medicine, in press.
20. Ramkumar PN, Harris JD, Noble PC. Patient-reported outcome measures after total knee arthroplasty: a systematic review. Bone Joint Res 2015; 4(7):120–7.
21. Naal FD, Impellizzeri FM, Rippstein PF. Which are the most frequently used outcome instruments in studies on total ankle arthroplasty? Clin Orthop Relat Res 2010;468(3):815–26.
22. Cutler HS, Guzman JZ, Al Maaieh M, et al. Patient-reported outcomes in adult spinal deformity surgery: a bibliometric analysis. Spine Deform 2015;3(4):312–7.
23. Kearney RS, Achten J, Lamb SE, et al. A systematic review of patient-reported outcome measures used to assess Achilles tendon rupture management: what's being used and should we be using it? Br J Sports Med 2012;46(16):1102–9.
24. Instruments for collection of orthopaedic quality data. American Academy of Orthopaedic Surgeons; 2016.
25. Kitaoka HB, Alexander IJ, Adelaar RS, et al. Clinical rating systems for the ankle-hindfoot, midfoot, hallux, and lesser toes. Foot Ankle Int 1994;15(7): 349–53.
26. Button G, Pinney S. A meta-analysis of outcome rating scales in foot and ankle surgery: is there a valid, reliable, and responsive system? Foot Ankle Int 2004;25(8):521–5.
27. Hunt KJ, Hurwit D. Use of patient-reported outcome measures in foot and ankle research. J Bone Joint Surg Am 2013;95(16):e118(1-9).
28. Pinsker E, Daniels TR. AOFAS position statement regarding the future of the AOFAS clinical rating systems. Foot Ankle Int 2011;32(9):841–2.
29. Madeley NJ, Wing KJ, Topliss C, et al. Responsiveness and validity of the SF-36, ankle osteoarthritis scale, AOFAS ankle hindfoot score, and foot

function index in end stage ankle arthritis. Foot Ankle Int 2012;33(1):57–63.

30. SooHoo NF, Vyas R, Samimi D. Responsiveness of the foot function index, AOFAS clinical rating systems, and SF-36 after foot and ankle surgery. Foot Ankle Int 2006;27(11):930–4.

31. Baumhauer JF, McIntosh S, Rechtine G. Age and sex differences between patient and physician-derived outcome measures in the foot and ankle. J Bone Joint Surg Am 2013;95(3):209–14.

32. Guyton GP. Theoretical limitations of the AOFAS scoring systems: an analysis using Monte Carlo modeling. Foot Ankle Int 2001;22(10):779–87.

33. Pynsent P, Fairbank J, Carr A. Outcome measures in orthopaedics and orthopaedic trauma. 2nd edition. CRC Press; 2004.

34. Pena F, Agel J, Coetzee JC. Comparison of the MFA to the AOFAS outcome tool in a population undergoing total ankle replacement. Foot Ankle Int 2007;28(7):788–93.

35. SooHoo NF, Shuler M, Fleming LL. Evaluation of the validity of the AOFAS clinical rating systems by correlation to the SF-36. Foot Ankle Int 2003; 24(1):50–5.

36. Ceccarelli F, Calderazzi F, Pedrazzi G. Is there a relation between AOFAS ankle-hindfoot score and SF-36 in evaluation of Achilles ruptures treated by percutaneous technique? J Foot Ankle Surg 2014;53(1):16–21.

37. Malviya A, Makwana N, Laing P. Correlation of the AOFAS scores with a generic health QUALY score in foot and ankle surgery. Foot Ankle Int 2007; 28(4):494–8.

38. Schneider W, Knahr K. Poor agreement between prospective and retrospective assessment of hallux surgery using the AOFAS Hallux Scale. Foot Ankle Int 2005;26(12):1062–6.

39. Ferreira-Valente MA, Pais-Ribeiro JL, Jensen MP. Validity of four pain intensity rating scales. Pain 2011;152(10):2399–404.

40. Kersten P, White PJ, Tennant A. Is the pain visual analogue scale linear and responsive to change? An exploration using Rasch analysis. PLoS One 2014;9(6):e99485.

41. Zampelis V, Ornstein E, Franzen H, et al. A simple visual analog scale for pain is as responsive as the WOMAC, the SF-36, and the EQ-5D in measuring outcomes of revision hip arthroplasty. Acta Orthop 2014;85(2):128–32.

42. Lee JS, Hobden E, Stiell IG, et al. Clinically important change in the visual analog scale after adequate pain control. Acad Emerg Med 2003; 10(10):1128–30.

43. Busija L, Osborne RH, Nilsdotter A, et al. Magnitude and meaningfulness of change in SF-36 scores in four types of orthopedic surgery. Health Qual Life Outcomes 2008;6:55.

44. Smith MV, Klein SE, Clohisy JC, et al. Lower extremity-specific measures of disability and outcomes in orthopaedic surgery. J Bone Joint Surg Am 2012;94(5):468–77.

45. Laucis NC, Hays RD, Bhattacharyya T. Scoring the SF-36 in orthopaedics: a brief guide. J Bone Joint Surg Am 2015;97(19):1628–34.

46. SooHoo NF, McDonald AP, Seiler JG 3rd, et al. Evaluation of the construct validity of the DASH questionnaire by correlation to the SF-36. J Hand Surg Am 2002;27(3):537–41.

47. Dawson J, Boller I, Doll H, et al. Minimally important change was estimated for the Manchester-Oxford Foot Questionnaire after foot/ankle surgery. J Clin Epidemiol 2014;67(6):697–705.

48. Ware J Jr, Kosinski M, Keller SD. A 12-item short-form health survey: construction of scales and preliminary tests of reliability and validity. Med Care 1996;34(3):220–33.

49. Jenkinson C, Layte R, Jenkinson D, et al. A shorter form health survey: can the SF-12 replicate results from the SF-36 in longitudinal studies? J Public Health Med 1997;19(2):179–86.

50. Gosling CM, Gabbe BJ, Williamson OD, et al. Validity of outcome measures used to assess one and six month outcomes in orthopaedic trauma patients. Injury 2011;42(12):1443–8.

51. Mani SB, Brown HC, Nair P, et al. Validation of the foot and ankle outcome score in adult acquired flatfoot deformity. Foot Ankle Int 2013;34(8): 1140–6.

52. Golightly YM, Devellis RF, Nelson AE, et al. Psychometric properties of the foot and ankle outcome score in a community-based study of adults with and without osteoarthritis. Arthritis Care Res (Hoboken) 2014;66(3):395–403.

53. Chen L, Lyman S, Do H, et al. Validation of foot and ankle outcome score for hallux valgus. Foot Ankle Int 2012;33(12):1145–55.

54. Hogan MV, Mani SB, Chan JY, et al. Validation of the foot and ankle outcome score for hallux rigidus. HSS J 2016;12(1):44–50.

55. Roos EM, Brandsson S, Karlsson J. Validation of the foot and ankle outcome score for ankle ligament reconstruction. Foot Ankle Int 2001;22(10): 788–94.

56. Mani SB, Do H, Vulcano E, et al. Evaluation of the foot and ankle outcome score in patients with osteoarthritis of the ankle. Bone Joint J 2015;97-b(5): 662–7.

57. Budiman-Mak E, Conrad KJ, Roach KE. The foot function index: a measure of foot pain and disability. J Clin Epidemiol 1991;44(6):561–70.

58. Pinsker E, Inrig T, Daniels TR, et al. Reliability and validity of 6 measures of pain, function, and disability for ankle arthroplasty and arthrodesis. Foot Ankle Int 2015;36(6):617–25.

59. SooHoo NF, Samimi DB, Vyas RM, et al. Evaluation of the validity of the Foot Function Index in measuring outcomes in patients with foot and ankle disorders. Foot Ankle Int 2006;27(1):38–42.

60. Swiontkowski MF, Engelberg R, Martin DP, et al. Short musculoskeletal function assessment questionnaire: validity, reliability, and responsiveness. J Bone Joint Surg Am 1999;81(9):1245–60.

61. Bouffard J, Bertrand-Charette M, Roy JS. Psychometric properties of the musculoskeletal function assessment and the short musculoskeletal function assessment: a systematic review. Clin Rehabil 2016;30(4):393–409.

62. Martin RL. The development of the foot and ankle ability measure [Doctoral Dissertation]. University of Pittsburgh; 2003.

63. Martin RL, Irrgang JJ, Burdett RG, et al. Evidence of validity for the foot and ankle ability measure (FAAM). Foot Ankle Int 2005;26(11):968–83.

64. Carcia CR, Martin RL, Drouin JM. Validity of the foot and ankle ability measure in athletes with chronic ankle instability. J Athl Train 2008;43(2):179–83.

65. Martin RL, Hutt DM, Wukich DK. Validity of the foot and ankle ability measure (FAAM) in diabetes mellitus. Foot Ankle Int 2009;30(4):297–302.

66. Goldstein CL, Schemitsch E, Bhandari M, et al. Comparison of different outcome instruments following foot and ankle trauma. Foot Ankle Int 2010;31(12):1075–80.

67. Bass M, Morris S, Neapolitan R. Utilizing multidimensional computer adaptive testing to mitigate burden with patient reported outcomes. AMIA Annu Symp Proc 2015;2015:320–8.

68. Jette AM, Haley SM. Contemporary measurement techniques for rehabilitation outcomes assessment. J Rehabil Med 2005;37(6):339–45.

69. Templin TN, Hays RD, Gershon RC, et al. Introduction to patient-reported outcome item banks: issues in minority aging research. Expert Rev Pharmacoecon Outcomes Res 2013;13(2):183–6.

70. Cella D, Riley W, Stone A, et al. The patient-reported outcomes measurement information system (PROMIS) developed and tested its first wave of adult self-reported health outcome item banks: 2005-2008. J Clin Epidemiol 2010;63(11):1179–94.

71. Cella D, Yount S, Rothrock N, et al. The patient-reported outcomes measurement information system (PROMIS): progress of an NIH Roadmap cooperative group during its first two years. Med Care 2007;45(5 Suppl 1):S3–11.

72. Papuga MO, Beck CA, Kates SL, et al. Validation of GAITRite and PROMIS as high-throughput physical function outcome measures following ACL reconstruction. J Orthop Res 2014;32(6):793–801.

73. Baumhauer JF. Patient-reported outcomes - are they living up to their potential? N Engl J Med 2017;377(1):6–9.

74. Pilkonis PA, Yu L, Dodds NE, et al. Validation of the alcohol use item banks from the patient-reported outcomes measurement information system (PROMIS). Drug Alcohol Depend 2016;161:316–22.

75. Pilkonis PA, Yu L, Dodds NE, et al. Validation of the depression item bank from the patient-reported outcomes measurement information system (PROMIS) in a three-month observational study. J Psychiatr Res 2014;56:112–9.

76. Schalet BD, Hays RD, Jensen SE, et al. Validity of PROMIS physical function measured in diverse clinical samples. J Clin Epidemiol 2016;73:112–8.

77. Jensen RE, Potosky AL, Reeve BB, et al. Validation of the PROMIS physical function measures in a diverse US population-based cohort of cancer patients. Qual Life Res 2015;24(10):2333–44.

78. Irwin DE, Atwood CA Jr, Hays RD, et al. Correlation of PROMIS scales and clinical measures among chronic obstructive pulmonary disease patients with and without exacerbations. Qual Life Res 2015;24(4):999–1009.

79. Amtmann D, Kim J, Chung H, et al. Comparing CESD-10, PHQ-9, and PROMIS depression instruments in individuals with multiple sclerosis. Rehabil Psychol 2014;59(2):220–9.

80. Bevans M, Ross A, Cella D. Patient-reported outcomes measurement information system (PROMIS): efficient, standardized tools to measure self-reported health and quality of life. Nurs Outlook 2014;62(5):339–45.

81. Hung M, Stuart AR, Higgins TF, et al. Computerized adaptive testing using the PROMIS physical function item bank reduces test burden with less ceiling effects compared with the short musculoskeletal function assessment in orthopaedic trauma patients. J Orthop Trauma 2014;28(8):439–43.

82. Brodke DJ, Saltzman CL, Brodke DS. PROMIS for orthopaedic outcomes measurement. J Am Acad Orthop Surg 2016;24(11):744–9.

83. Tyser AR, Beckmann J, Franklin JD, et al. Evaluation of the PROMIS physical function computer adaptive test in the upper extremity. J Hand Surg Am 2014;39(10):2047–51.e4.

84. Morgan JH, Kallen MA, Okike K, et al. PROMIS physical function computer adaptive test compared with other upper extremity outcome measures in the evaluation of proximal humerus fractures in patients older than 60 years. J Orthop Trauma 2015;29(6):257–63.

85. Hung M, Hon SD, Franklin JD, et al. Psychometric properties of the PROMIS physical function item bank in patients with spinal disorders. Spine (Phila Pa 1976) 2014;39(2):158–63.

86. Lyren PE, Atroshi I. Using item response theory improved responsiveness of patient-reported outcomes measures in carpal tunnel syndrome. J Clin Epidemiol 2012;65(3):325–34.

87. Hung M, Baumhauer JF, Latt LD, et al. Validation of PROMIS (R) Physical Function computerized adaptive tests for orthopaedic foot and ankle outcome research. Clin Orthop Relat Res 2013;471(11): 3466–74.

88. Ho B, Houck JR, Flemister AS, et al. Preoperative PROMIS scores predict postoperative success in foot and ankle patients. Foot Ankle Int 2016;37(9):911–8.

89. Hung M, Clegg DO, Greene T, et al. A lower extremity physical function computerized adaptive testing instrument for orthopaedic patients. Foot Ankle Int 2012;33(4):326–35.

90. Hung M, Baumhauer JF, Brodsky JW, et al. Psychometric comparison of the PROMIS physical function CAT with the FAAM and FFI for measuring patient-reported outcomes. Foot Ankle Int 2014;35(6):592–9.

91. Ayers DC, Bozic KJ. The importance of outcome measurement in orthopaedics. Clin Orthop Relat Res 2013;471(11):3409–11.

92. Ayers DC, Zheng H, Franklin PD. Integrating patient-reported outcomes into orthopaedic clinical practice: proof of concept from FORCE-TJR. Clin Orthop Relat Res 2013;471(11):3419–25.

93. Slover JD, Karia RJ, Hauer C, et al. Feasibility of integrating standardized patient-reported outcomes in orthopedic care. Am J Manag Care 2015;21(8):e494–500.

94. Bjorner JB, Rose M, Gandek B, et al. Method of administration of PROMIS scales did not significantly impact score level, reliability, or validity. J Clin Epidemiol 2014;67(1):108–13.

95. Beach WR. Collecting outcomes data in the private practice setting: why is it important and how to get the data without disrupting the workflow. Sports Med Arthrosc 2013;21(3):148–51.

96. Roberts N, Bradley B, Williams D. Use of SMS and tablet computer improves the electronic collection of elective orthopaedic patient reported outcome measures. Ann R Coll Surg Engl 2014;96(5):348–51.

97. Papuga MO, Dasilva C, McIntyre A, et al. Large-scale clinical implementation of PROMIS computer adaptive testing with direct incorporation into the electronic medical record. Health Systems 2017. https://doi.org/10.1057/s41306-016-0016-1.

Moving?

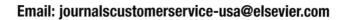

Make sure your subscription moves with you!

To notify us of your new address, find your **Clinics Account Number** (located on your mailing label above your name), and contact customer service at:

Email: journalscustomerservice-usa@elsevier.com

800-654-2452 (subscribers in the U.S. & Canada)
314-447-8871 (subscribers outside of the U.S. & Canada)

Fax number: 314-447-8029

Elsevier Health Sciences Division
Subscription Customer Service
3251 Riverport Lane
Maryland Heights, MO 63043

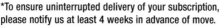

*To ensure uninterrupted delivery of your subscription, please notify us at least 4 weeks in advance of move.

Printed and bound by CPI Group (UK) Ltd, Croydon, CR0 4YY

08/05/2025

01864711-0010